Contemporary Medical Office Procedures

Third Edition

Doris D. Humphrey, Ph.D.
President
Career Solutions Training Group

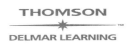

Contemporary Medical Office Procedures, Third Edition
by Doris D. Humphrey, PhD

Vice President, Health Care Business Unit:
William Brottmiller

Editorial Director:
Cathy L. Esperti

Acquisitions Editor:
Rhonda Dearborn

Editorial Assistant:
Natalie Wager

Developmental Editor:
Deb Flis

Marketing Director:
Jennifer McAvey

Marketing Coordinator:
Mona Caron

Technology Specialist:
Victoria Moore

Production Coordinator:
Jessica Peterson

Project Editor:
Bryan Viggiani

Art and Design Coordinator:
Connie Lundberg-Watkins

Library of Congress Cataloging-in-Publication Data

Humphrey, Doris.
  Contemporary medical office procedures / Doris D. Humphrey.—3rd ed.
     p. ; cm.
Includes bibliographical references and index.
  ISBN-13: 978-1-4018-6345-6
  ISBN-10: 1-4018-6345-0
  1. Medical assistants. 2. Medical offices—Automation.
  [DNLM: 1. Medical Secretaries. 2. Office Management. 3. Office Automation. W 80 H926c 2004] I. Title.

R728.8.H845 2003
651'.961— dc21
                                    2003055064

International Divisions List

Asia (Including India):
Thomson Learning
60 Albert Street, #15-01
Albert Complex
Singapore 189969
Tel 65 336-6411
Fax 65 336-7411

Australia/New Zealand:
Nelson
102 Dodds Street
South Melbourne
Victoria 3205
Australia
Tel 61 (0)3 9685-4111
Fax 61 (0)3 9685-4199

Latin America:
Thomson Learning
Seneca 53
Colonia Polanco
11560 Mexico, D.F. Mexico
Tel (525) 281-2906
Fax (525) 281-2656

Canada:
Nelson
1120 Birchmount Road
Toronto, Ontario
Canada M1K 5G4
Tel (416) 752-9100
Fax (416) 752-8102

UK/Europe/Middle East/Africa:
Thomson Learning
Berkshire House
1680-173 High Holborn
London WC1V 7AA
United Kingdom
Tel 44 (0)20 497-1422
Fax 44 (0)20 497-1426

Spain (includes Portugal):
Paraninfo
Calle Magallanes 25
28015 Madrid
España
Tel 34 (0)91 446-3350
Fax 34 (0)91 445-6218

Contents

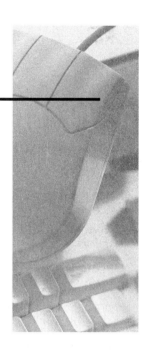

PREFACE   vii

HOW TO USE THIS BOOK   xi

HOW TO USE THE MEDICAL ASSISTING
ADMINISTRATIVE SKILLS CD-ROM   xiii

PART I   Today's Medical Environment   1

CHAPTER 1   THE MEDICAL ENVIRONMENT   3

Medical Offices   4
The Language of Medicine   9
Medical Specialties, Subspecialties, and
  Dental Specialties   12
Computers in Contemporary Medicine   14

CHAPTER 2   THE MEDICAL STAFF   19

The Medical Assistant   20
The Roles of Medical Professionals   24
Working with the Medical Professionals   25

CHAPTER 3   MEDICAL ETHICS   35

Medical Ethics and the Law   36
Ethics Statements of the Medical Associations   37
Social Policy Issues   42
Computers and Ethics   49
The Medical Assistant's Role in Ethical Issues   51

CHAPTER 4	MEDICAL LAW	57
	State Medical Practice Acts	58
	The Physician and the Law	60
	Confidentiality	69
	Telecommunications and Confidentiality	72
	Confidentiality Agreements	73
	The Physician in Court	73
	Fax Transmittal Cover Sheet	73
	Good Samaritan Laws	78
	The Physician and Controlled Substances	78
	Drug Schedules	79

PART II Patient Relations 83

CHAPTER 5	INTERACTING WITH PATIENTS	84
	Interpersonal Communication	85
	Importance of Verbal and Nonverbal Communication	89
	Computers and Relationships with Patients	92
	Managing Patient Activities	93
	Discussing Finances and Billing	95
	Handling Emergencies	96

CHAPTER 6	TELECOMMUNICATIONS	103
	Answering the Telephone	105
	Screening Calls	106
	Placing Local and Long-Distance Calls	113
	Using the Telephone Directory	118
	Using Answering Services and Telephone Answering Devices	119
	Telecommunications for Diagnosis and Treatment	120

CHAPTER 7	SCHEDULING APPOINTMENTS	125
	Scheduling According to a System	127
	Maintaining the Appointment Schedule	128
	Preparing a Daily List of Appointments	135
	Scheduling Patients for Other Medical Units	136
	Follow-Up Appointments	137

PART III Computers and Information Processing in the Medical Office 143

CHAPTER 8	COMPUTERIZING THE MEDICAL OFFICE	144
	High Tech Medical Offices	145
	Medical Software Applications	147

Developing Practice Lists and Reports 150
Inventories 152
Miscellaneous Computer Tips 155

CHAPTER 9   MEDICAL DOCUMENTS AND WORD PROCESSING   161

Letter Writing 162
Developing Your Communications 167
Writing for the Physician's Signature 167
Composing at the Computer 167
Sources of Input 169
Word Processing Software 173
Output 173

CHAPTER 10   PROFESSIONAL ACTIVITIES, TRAVEL
ARRANGEMENTS, AND POSTAL AND
DELIVERY SERVICES   193

The Medical Assistant's Professional Activities 194
Managing Travel 198
Postal and Delivery Services 204

CHAPTER 11   MANAGING MEDICAL RECORDS   213

Methods for Keeping Records 215
Trends and Issues in Medical Record Keeping 216
Creating a Medical Record 216
Problem-Oriented and Source-Oriented
   Medical Records 223
File Management 230
Rules for Filing 231
The Medical Assistant's Role in Record Keeping 235

PART IV   Automating Medical Office Financial Management   239

CHAPTER 12   PEGBOARD ACCOUNTING AND COMPUTERIZED
ACCOUNT MANAGEMENT   240

Pegboard Accounting 241
Banking 245
Payroll Accounting Procedures 250
Computerized Account Management 252

CHAPTER 13   BILLING AND COLLECTION   261

Billing Patients 262
The Collection Process 268
Truth-in-Lending 277

CHAPTER 14   HEALTH INSURANCE AND CODING   285

                    Types of Health Insurance Coverage   287
                    Prospective Payment System   296
                    Filing an Insurance Claim   297
                    Completing a Universal Health Insurance Claim Form   302

PART V   **Becoming a Career Medical Assistant**   311

CHAPTER 15   SEEKING EMPLOYMENT   312

                    Finding and Keeping a Job   313
                    Researching Employment Opportunities   315
                    The Job Application Process   317
                    Interviewing for a Position   323
                    Continuing the Education Process   327
                    Office Management   328

Appendices   339

APPENDIX A   MEDICAL ASSISTANT ROLE DELINEATION CHART   340

APPENDIX B   CAAHEP STANDARDS   342

APPENDIX C   ABHES COURSE CONTENT REQUIREMENTS
                    FOR MEDICAL ASSISTANTS   343

APPENDIX D   REGISTERED MEDICAL ASSISTANT
                    (RMA [AMT]) CERTIFICATION
                    COMPETENCY SUMMARY   346

                    GLOSSARY   349

                    INDEX   355

Preface

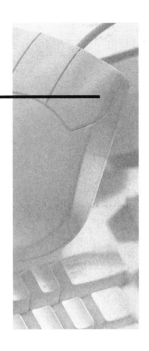

Health care professionals spend countless hours attending to patients and their families. They provide specialized services that patients need to lead healthy lives. The work of a medical office is unique. It combines a high level of caring about people and attention to the day-to-day details of running a practice. During an era when managed care is evolving and affecting almost every facet of medical care, the well-informed and well-trained medical assistant can be a central force in keeping a practice running smoothly.

Contemporary Medical Office Procedures, Third Edition, provides what you need to know to be a successful medical assistant—from how to communicate so patients can understand, to how to keep cash flowing into the practice, to how to grow in your career. You will not find a better resource to help you begin your medical assisting career.

WHY DO I NEED THIS BOOK?

Contemporary Medical Office Procedures, Third Edition, is practical. It highlights what you need to know and eliminates what is not needed. The subjects are broad enough to inform you in all the administrative medical assisting areas, and the content is presented in enough detail to teach you how to do what you will be required to do.

WHAT TYPES OF SUBJECTS ARE COVERED?

You will start by learning about the environment of medicine today. You will learn why physicians have mixed feelings about managed care and how this method of financing health care will affect your career from your first day on the job to the last.

Materials to help you communicate better with patients and their families and with the staff and physician are included. One place you will put these communication skills to work is in scheduling appointments, trying to find the one right spot for a professional man or woman who thinks there is no time to get sick or have a checkup.

You will learn the "nuts and bolts" of making travel arrangements, managing medical records, coordinating insurance payments, doing the daily bookkeeping required in a busy practice, and billing patients. Some of these tasks require understanding medical coding and knowing how to complete insurance claim forms. You will learn how to do each of these and more.

HOW WILL I REMEMBER EVERYTHING?

You do not have to remember everything. Just take *Contemporary Medical Office Procedures*,

Third Edition, along as a desk reference to your first job. The book and workbook are full of forms, examples, and illustrations to show you how to complete many administrative tasks. For example, lay the book illustration beside a blank health insurance claim form (CMS-1500), and you can fill in the blank form item for item by the directions provided in the book. It could not be easier.

SHOULD I BE PREPARED FOR A COMPUTERIZED OFFICE OR A TRADITIONAL OFFICE?

Do not worry. You are covered. *Contemporary Medical Office Procedures*, Third Edition, gives you training in both types of administrative work. Because many computer functions in a medical office are based on traditional pen and paper methods, you need to know both anyway.

WHAT ABOUT THE INTERNET?

You will get plenty of Internet practice. Every chapter has at least one section devoted to an interesting Internet activity.

HOW IS *CONTEMPORARY MEDICAL OFFICE PROCEDURES* ORGANIZED?

It is practical. The way this book is arranged will make sense to you. It has five broad topical areas that break down into more specific areas. Here is a preview:

- Today's Medical Environment
- Patient Relations
- Computers and Information Processing in the Medical Office
- Automating Medical Office Financial Management
- Becoming a Career Medical Assistant

WHO SHOULD USE THIS BOOK?

Contemporary Medical Office Procedures, Third Edition, should be used by anyone planning a career in medical assisting, medical office management, medical financing and insurance, and other aspects of administrative medical work. The book can be viewed both as introductory, for people who need a broad overview of medical office procedures, and specialized, for those who must learn specific information regarding office functions.

SHOULD I GET STARTED?

Yes. It is time to be on your way to a demanding and rewarding career. Good luck as you train to become an administrative medical assistant. You have a bright future ahead.

FOR THE INSTRUCTOR: A LEARNING PLAN

Contemporary Medical Office Procedures, Third Edition, is easy to use. In every chapter, you will find the following features, arranged in the same sequence each time.

- Performance-based competencies
- A story relating to the topic of each chapter, told by a medical assistant
- Vocabulary of important terminology from the chapter
- Practical, simple, thorough information on the topic of the chapter
- *In Your Opinion* questions that allow each student to think critically
- Many examples, forms, and illustrations that show how to do what is discussed
- Internet activities that relate to the chapter content
- A Student Checklist that directs the learner to additional activities in the workbook and on the CD-ROM in the back of the book.
- Performance-based activities that allow readers to practice what they learned
- *Expanding Your Thinking* activities that allow learners to be creative and solve problems

What's New in the Third Edition?

Special, new or expanded discussions develop topics that every medical assisting learner should understand before taking the first job. Major changes include:

- New stories at the beginning of each chapter
- Content updated throughout based on the AAMA Medical Assistant Role Delineation Chart that replaced DACUM
- Expanded discussion of AAMSA
- Expanded discussion of professional and work ethics
- Expanded discussion of payroll and banking
- Addition of the Health Insurance Portability and Accountability Act
- Addition of information about office management topics
- Expanded vocabulary sections
- Expanded discussion of scheduling concepts
- New photos and forms
- Internet activities

COMPREHENSIVE TEACHING/LEARNING CORRELATED MATERIALS

Although the textbook for *Contemporary Medical Office Procedures*, Third Edition, offers an abundance of materials, there is more. You will want to take advantage of everything the full package has to offer.

Delmar's Medical Assisting Administrative Skills CD-ROM

A free CD-ROM, included with each book, contains interactive activities to help reinforce concepts learned in the book. See How to Use the Medical Assisting Administrative Skills CD-ROM on page xiii.

Student Workbook to Accompany Contemporary Medical Office Procedures, Third Edition

The workbook provides a wealth of additional material for learners to gain more hands-on, practical experience. Activities include review questions, vocabulary review, case studies, medical forms to complete, and simulated "day-in-the-life" activities that provide learners with practice completing administrative tasks that would be performed in an actual medical office.

(Order No. 1-4018-7068-6)

Instructor's Guide

Making your job easier and less time consuming while helping you provide the training your students need is the primary goal of the Instructor's Guide. With that in mind, the following items are included for your use.

- Answers to Performance-Based Activities and Expanding Your Thinking Activities in the text
- Answers to activities in the workbook
- Instructional suggestions
- Evaluation recommendations

(Order No. 1-4018-4023-X)

Delmar's Medical Assisting CD-ROM

This CD-ROM is a multimedia interactive program developed specifically for the field of medical assisting. The CD-ROM's menu structure is based on AAMA's role delineation study plus an add-on Managed Care Segment. The CD-ROM can be used as a stand-alone program or as an integrated enhancement to any medical assisting textbook.

(Order No. 0-8273-8404-1)

Delmar's Medical Assisting Exam Review by J. P. Cody

This exam review book is a comprehensive guide that prepares certification candidates to successfully pass either the CMA exam sponsored by the American Association of Medical Assistants or the RMA exam sponsored by the American Medical Technologists.

(Order No. 0-8273-7183-7)

REVIEWERS

The author and Delmar Learning would like to thank the reviewers for their insights, comments, and suggestions for the third edition of the book. They include:

Kay E. Biggs, BS, CMA
Medical Assisting Program Coordinator
Columbus State Community College
Columbus, Ohio

Adrienne Lynne Carter, Med, NRMA, CMA
Vocational Education Instructor
University of California at San Bernardino
San Bernardino, California

Lisa D. Ezzell, BA
Medical Assisting Adjunct Instructor
Polk Community College
Kodak, Tennessee

Mimi Goulet, RN, CCN, CERN
Instructor
Oswego County BOCES
Mexico, New York

Marsha Hemby, BA, RN, CMA
Department Chair, Medical Assisting
Pitt Community College
Greenville, North Carolina

How to Use This Book

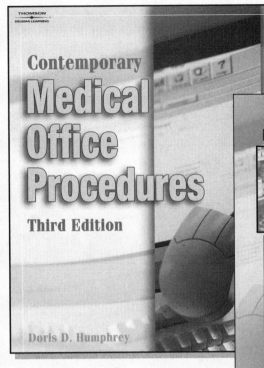

CHAPTER 3

Medical Ethics

RTLAND, MAINE

I moved here from Boston about three months ago to begin my career as a medical assistant. Last Friday, Liz, the other medical assistant in our office, invited me to get together for pizza with several MAs from other practices. We had a great time. It was nice to meet some new people and hear about their work.

One of their stories surprised me. Bill had noticed in his pediatric office that some of the patients were scheduling, then canceling and rescheduling their appointments. He thought this seemed strange, but the always a backlog of patients, so he had no trouble filling their sp he discovered something unusual — the one thing the canceling had in common was lack of health insurance.

He and Annie, another MA in the practice, went to the office and asked what was going on. She told them she had decided to the practice by calling the uninsured patients and telling them t had to reschedule. All the uninsured patients kept getting shuffle bottom of the deck.

We all agreed that this was unethical. I pointed out that t Principles of Medical Ethics says doctors should support access to care for all people. Annie said she had mentioned the same thi office manager, who pointed out that another one of the principl physician is free to choose whom to serve.

For the rest of the evening, we talked about this office behavior. I think the doctors should be informed that their office is discriminating against the uninsured. But what if the office m covering for the doctors who already know about the practice! was their idea! Bill and Annie have to decide what to do.

Erin McClintock
Medical Assistant

PERFORMANCE-BASED COMPETENCIES

After completing this chapter, you should be able to:

1. Identify five important social policy issues related to medicine and discuss the ethical implications of each.
2. Outline procedures for maintaining the confidentiality of computerized records.
3. Create examples of ethical dilemmas that might involve a medical assistant and discuss different ways of resolving them.
4. Compare the value of improved medical technology with the ethical problems that may result.

Contemporary Medical Office Procedures, Third Edition, is designed to provide learners with the knowledge and skills necessary for career success in administrative medical assisting. Several features are designed to enhance the reader's learning experience, including:

1. Scenarios — Stories related to the chapter content, told by a medical assistant, provide personal and specific examples of experience in the medical office. The stories help the reader relate to the material discussed in the chapter and provide a glimpse of the rewards and challenges encountered in the practice setting.
2. Performance-Based Competencies — The performance-based competencies are based on actual skills that are "doable" and "measurable."

3. Vocabulary — Important terms readers should be aware of as they study the content in each chapter are listed in the vocabulary sections.
4. In Your Opinion — Questions throughout each chapter encourage critical thinking by challenging learners to form opinions on thought-provoking issues.

VOCABULARY

Association Organization that advocates special interests through information or lobbying.
Business class Flight class that offers more amenities than coach, but fewer than first.
Direct flight Flight that connects two cities without a plane change.
Domestic mail services Mail service the United States Postal Service.
Internet search Locating informatic Internet.
Itinerary Schedule of travel, includi and arrival times, flight numbers, lo telephone numbers.
Keywords Words that identify the you want to locate through the Inte
Literature search Review of publish the library or by computer to find articles on a specified topic.
Non-stop Flight that connects two cities without making intermediate stops.
Objective The intent of the process.
Orient To provide an informational overview.

IN YOUR OPINION

1. Who makes the ultimate decision about the type of care a patient receives? For example, when do you think that a daughter or son has a right to decide what level of care is appropriate for an elderly parent?
2. What are some of the risks of establishing policy statements about patient treatments?
3. How do you feel about physician-assisted suicides?

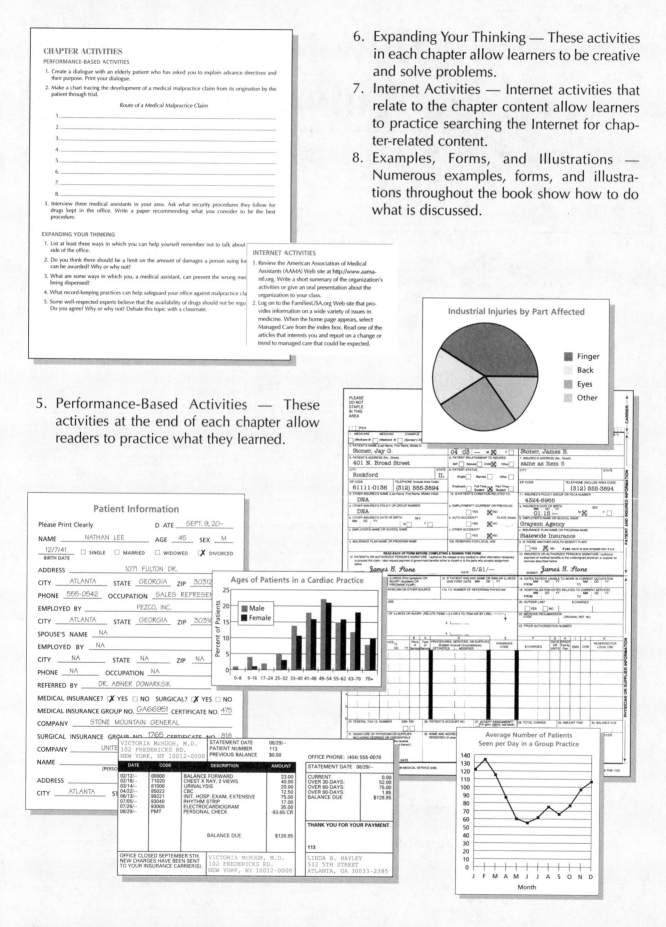

CHAPTER ACTIVITIES

PERFORMANCE-BASED ACTIVITIES

1. Create a dialogue with an elderly patient who has asked you to explain advance directives and their purpose. Print your dialogue.
2. Make a chart tracing the development of a medical malpractice claim from its origination by the patient through trial.

Route of a Medical Malpractice Claim

1. _____
2. _____
3. _____
4. _____
5. _____
6. _____
7. _____
8. _____

3. Interview three medical assistants in your area. Ask what security procedures they follow for drugs kept in the office. Write a paper recommending what you consider to be the best procedure.

EXPANDING YOUR THINKING

1. List at least three ways in which you can help yourself remember not to talk about [...] side of the office.
2. Do you think there should be a limit on the amount of damages a person suing for [...] can be awarded? Why or why not?
3. What are some ways in which you, a medical assistant, can prevent the wrong me[...] being dispensed?
4. What record-keeping practices can help safeguard your office against malpractice cla[...]
5. Some well-respected experts believe that the availability of drugs should not be regu[...] Do you agree? Why or why not? Debate this topic with a classmate.

INTERNET ACTIVITIES

1. Review the American Association of Medical Assistants (AAMA) Web site at http://www.aama-ntl.org. Write a short summary of the organization's activities or give an oral presentation about the organization to your class.
2. Log on to the FamiliesUSA.org Web site that provides information on a wide variety of issues in medicine. When the home page appears, select Managed Care from the index box. Read one of the articles that interests you and report on a change or trend to managed care that could be expected.

6. **Expanding Your Thinking** — These activities in each chapter allow learners to be creative and solve problems.
7. **Internet Activities** — Internet activities that relate to the chapter content allow learners to practice searching the Internet for chapter-related content.
8. **Examples, Forms, and Illustrations** — Numerous examples, forms, and illustrations throughout the book show how to do what is discussed.

5. **Performance-Based Activities** — These activities at the end of each chapter allow readers to practice what they learned.

How to Use the Medical Assisting Administrative Skills CD-ROM

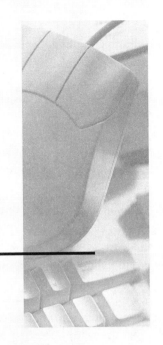

The *Medical Assisting Administrative Skills CD-ROM* is designed to accompany *Contemporary Medical Office Procedures*, Third Edition, so you can review and reinforce important concepts you are learning in the textbook. By using the CD-ROM, you will challenge yourself and make your study of medical assisting concepts more effective and fun.

ADMINISTRATIVE SKILLS CD-ROM

The Administrative Skills CD-ROM is designed with you, the user, in mind. Several medical assistants lead you on a verbal guided tour through the medical office.

An introductory tour gives you an overview of the entire office. To navigate through the office, click on the area you wish to visit.

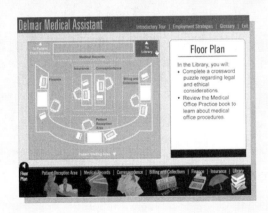

The medical assistant will give you an overview of the tasks and responsibilities associated with each area, and guide you through your many choices. In the patient reception area, for example, you may click on the active areas such as the computer, the phone, the answering machine, or the patient to branch into different content areas.

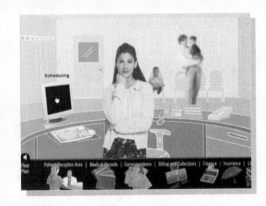

The medical assistant will give you instruction so that you understand the various aspects of each area. Activities include multiple choice questions with correct and incorrect responses noted, scheduling appointments by dragging and dropping the information into the appointment book, filling out a message pad, and maintaining a telephone log.

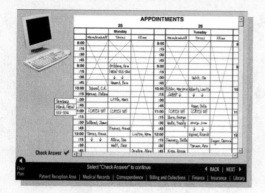

In the library, you can test your knowledge of legal and ethical principles by completing a crossword puzzle, and play interactive games related to administrative medical assisting.

A comprehensive glossary allows you to check your understanding of important key words and phrases.

In other areas, such as billing and collections, you will be asked to complete a patient receipt by entering information into the correct area, fill out a daily log sheet, use the pegboard system, complete a super bill and ledger card by entering and highlighting information, complete a patient charge slip, write a check, and complete a deposit slip.

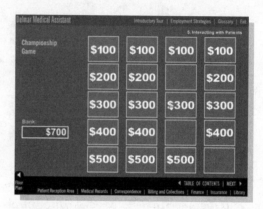

PART I

Today's Medical Environment

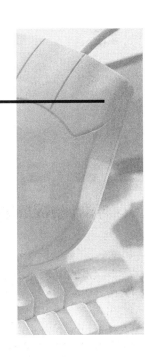

Both the quality and the costs of health care in the United States have spiraled upward in recent years. To a degree, the spirals are intertwined: quality care costs more. There are other reasons for health care cost increases. Diseases that have surfaced in the last generation, such as acquired immunodeficiency syndrome (AIDS), and a return of diseases once thought to have been eradicated, such as tuberculosis, have contributed to the increase. Another factor leading to the rise in expenditures is the extended life span of U.S. citizens, because an older population consumes more medical services. Overall costs are also increasing in response to the threat of biological terrorism.

Medical costs have skyrocketed so much in recent years that many families, especially those in which workers have lost employer-paid health benefits, receive below-standard care or no care at all. Entire segments of the U.S. population have life expectancies, infant mortality rates, and diseases comparable to some third-world countries. In addition, many patients wait too long to seek treatment for routine illnesses and must eventually be rushed to a hospital emergency room or trauma center. This is a very expensive practice, and all too often is too little, too late.

The delivery and financing of quality health care are issues currently being debated among physicians, economists, commentators, politicians, and patients. The discussions are often emotionally charged, because they directly involve questions such as: "Will Medicare still exist when I retire?", "Why are some medications available abroad but we cannot purchase them here?", "Why should my health care become more expensive just to subsidize the costs for drug addicts who do not take responsibility for their own health?", "Why are all of us affected because of the costs of malpractice insurance?" We are all affected by malpractice insurance costs in two ways: by doctors who increase their fees to help pay their insurance premiums, and by the increasing numbers of doctors leaving their practices because of insurance costs.

Since the 1930s, the United States has followed a worldwide trend of greater government financing of health services. Many countries, such as the United Kingdom, Canada, and Germany, provide comprehensive government health services for all citizens at limited or no cost to the individual. In the United States, our traditions of individual payment responsibility and abundant choice have meant less government involvement than in many other countries.

However, in the years between World War II and the introduction of Medicare and Medicaid in 1965, the federal government paid about 20% of each health care service. By 1975, this figure had grown to 40%; today between 60% and 65% of every health care dollar is paid by public funds. This is a 300% increase in forty years.

Our high cost of health care is attributable to several factors, including (1) an aging population that requires treatment for a longer time, (2) a culture that places its elderly in public nursing homes instead of caring for them privately, (3) earlier diagnosis and treatment of diseases, (4) technology that keeps people alive longer, (5) fear of malpractice suits that may lead physicians to use unnecessary or duplicate tests, (6) the attitude that life should be prolonged, even in the case of terminal illness, and (7) duplication among hospitals of expensive equipment and facilities, such as magnetic resonance imaging (MRI) scanners, trauma centers, and intensive care units.

As a medical assistant, your opportunities for employment are outstanding. Projections indicate that more than five of ten jobs in the future will be related in some way to health care. These positions may be clinical or administrative. They will be varied and there will be a lot of them. By 2010, the entire health services sector will increase by 2.8 million jobs. That increase will be driven in large part by advances in medical technology that prolongs life and also by a rapidly increasing population of older people. The need for medical assistants will grow faster than the average for all jobs. Between 2000 and 2010, the need for medical assistants is projected to grow by 57%, zooming from 329,000 to 516,000. The opportunities are limitless; in fact, many of the jobs you may perform are not yet in existence. Much of the medical equipment you will use has not yet been invented.

Although you may be most familiar with private physician practices and general hospitals, other delivery systems will play a prominent role in the future. Of particular importance are health maintenance organizations (HMOs).

Ambulatory centers, regional and national research organizations, extended care centers, therapy and rehabilitation centers, testing and research laboratories, and specialized clinics for the treatment of specific diseases are examples of other facilities and organizations that support health care. In each of these settings, the need exists for well-trained clinical and administrative support staff.

Helping to shape the health care landscape is the Centers for Medicare & Medicaid Services (CMS), formerly known as the Federal Health Care Financing Administration (HCFA, pronounced hickfa), the powerful agency that runs the Medicare and Medicaid programs. One of CMS's requirements—the standardized coding system used to describe medical procedures—affects almost all medical assistants. The code adopted by CMS for the first level of its three-level system is the same as that developed by the American Medical Association. It is called the Physician's Current Procedural Terminology and is referred to as CPT. Additionally, CMS requires doctors to submit, along with each Medicare claim, an ICD-coded report of the diagnosis or diagnoses made regarding the patient/claimant. ICD stands for International Statistical Classification of Diseases and Related Health Problems. It is typically the responsibility of the medical assistant to process Medicare claims and to be familiar with the appropriate codes.

The Health Insurance Portability and Accountability Act (HIPAA) of 1996 limits the ability of insurance companies to deny coverage to applicants because of preexisting conditions. For instance, it prohibits insurers from using genetic testing results to deny coverage. Additionally, it broadened the standardization of diagnostic and procedure coding and required insurance companies to comply with the standards.

The medical environment is filled with ethical dilemmas, and as you pursue your career you may have strong opinions about these issues. For example, recent ethical debates involve the use of fetal brain tissue for some treatments. Advances in genetic engineering allow physicians to bypass disease cycles in some patients.

This is a momentous time to be enrolled in a health services course of study. During the next several years, you will be involved personally in many of the radical changes occurring in the health care delivery and financing systems. As you read the chapters in this part, follow the news for the latest developments involving genetic research, technological advances, the effects of personal habits on health, and the political and economic implications of our health care systems. The debate will make you a better health care employee and enhance your ability to make informed decisions about your future.

REFERENCES

U.S. Department of Labor, Bureau of Labor Statistics. *Occupational Outlook Handbook,* 2002–2003.

U.S. Department of Labor, Bureau of Labor Statistics. Occupational employment projections to 2010, *Monthly Labor Review,* November, 2001. Table 4, Occupations with the largest job growth, 2000–2010.

CHAPTER 1

The Medical Environment

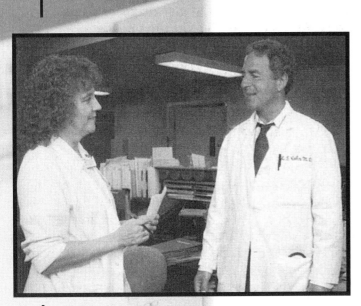

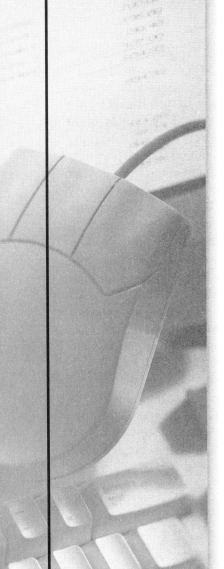

ST. LOUIS, MISSOURI

Each morning over breakfast I keep one eye on the television news and one on the paper. I like to stay informed, but mostly I want to keep on top of what's going to be next in health care services. That's the field I've been working in for about ten years, and the future is always changing. I took this job back when the national debate on health care reform started. Since then the debate has stopped and then started again. It's like a roller coaster ride. What happens can affect my job.

The doctors I work for have a successful group practice specializing in pediatrics. But with the influence of managed competition, they're thinking about other ways to structure their practice. It's difficult to continue offering high-quality medical care, pay increasingly huge malpractice insurance fees, keep patient fees affordable, and allow a reasonable income for the doctors. I know some doctors who have had to leave their specialties because insurance costs are so steep. In fact, I saw on television that one hospital emergency room is open only half-time because so many of its doctors have quit practicing because of high malpractice insurance premiums.

My doctors attend health reform meetings often. I know that whatever happens they'll research all the new ways to set up a medical practice before they make any decision about our office. I'm not worried for myself. They'll need me no matter what they do. But it would be nice to be able to reduce my anxieties.

Mary Alvarez
Medical Assistant

After completing this chapter, you should be able to:

1. Analyze the projected reforms in health care and support and debate two of the most important issues.
2. Detail the advantages of a managed care system and supplement your points with examples.
3. Compare and contrast the responsibilities a specialist and a subspecialist may have in treating the same patient.
4. Correlate each of the body systems to the appropriate specialties.

VOCABULARY

Centers for Disease Control and Prevention Federal medical research center located in Atlanta, Georgia.

Fee-for-service Payment system in which the full bill is paid each time a patient visits the physician.

Managed competition Medical care in which physicians and hospitals compete for patients.

Medical specialties Branches of medicine that concentrate on specific body systems.

On call Medical care in which physicians are available on an as-needed basis, no matter the time of day. Doctors in a single practice are always on call. Doctors in a group practice can rotate the responsibility.

Residency Three years of specialty training that occurs after a physician finishes medical school.

Root medical word Basic medical word used in combination with other words or prefixes and suffixes.

Third-party reimbursement A form of payment for medical services where someone other than the patient — a third party — pays the doctor or hospital. Third parties include insurance companies, health maintenance organizations, and Medicare and Medicaid. Under the *fee-for-service* payment system, fees can be paid directly by the patient, or by a third party; either way, it is considered a fee paid for a service received.

The high cost of quality health care is bringing change in the U.S. health care arena. Knowledge about how reimbursement systems operate helps to drive for improvements in those systems. At the same time, knowledge about new medical procedures — almost always expensive — helps to drive up costs. And these days, more of us recognize early when we are ill. That is because state-of-the-art technology can diagnose every conceivable type of illness, from strokes to acquired immunodeficiency syndrome (AIDS), and new treatments and medications are continually becoming available.

Concerns about rising health care costs and increased regulations have led many solo practitioners to merge with other physicians into large group practices, or to leave medicine. Some hospitals and physicians are establishing large networks capable of meeting every possible patient need from the cradle to the grave. Other hospitals are electing to develop one segment of their business in a certain specialty or procedure. For example, one hospital in a large city may become the principal treatment center for heart disease. Concentrating on the care of one body system can reduce costs while providing quality service.

MEDICAL OFFICES

Medical offices take many forms. They may be privately owned and operated by one or more physicians or by a for-profit private company employing its own physicians. Some medical offices and facilities are operated, directly or indirectly, by a local or state government, or by the federal government. Veterans' Administration hospitals, for example, are federally operated. Usually, government-controlled medical offices are larger than private practices and employ many physicians. Often, they serve "uncompensated care" patients who are unable to pay. They are located in metropolitan areas or in a wing of a city-owned or state-owned hospital.

The number of medical assistants employed in solo practices is deceasing yearly, as physicians merge practices. A 1998 survey by the American Association of Medical Assistants (AAMA) shows that most medical assistants are employed in partnership or group physician practices. Figure 1–1 shows the employment work settings for medical assistants.

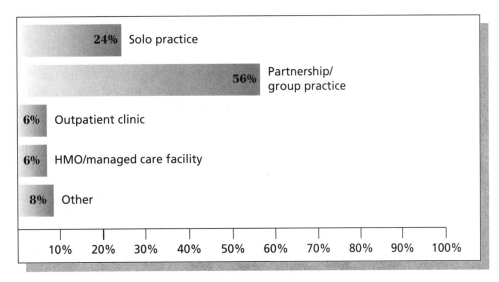

FIGURE 1–1   Percent of medical assistants employed by type of practice (Courtesy of the American Association of Medical Assistants)

Medical Practices

A medical doctor is a physician with years of training in the diagnosis, treatment, and prevention of disease. After four years of college or university education, four years of medical school, and at least three years of specialty training under supervision, called **residency**, a physician is ready to begin their career. Physicians who prefer to practice alone open solo- or single-physician practices. Physicians who prefer to practice with associates join a group.

Solo-Physician Practice

When a physician maintains a solo practice, arrangements must be made with another physician to treat patients when the primary care physician is unavailable. The practice is limited in the number of patients it can effectively serve. Solo-physician practices usually charge based on a **fee-for-service**. In this form of payment, the patient or insurance company pays the full bill for each visit.

Many patients prefer the warm, close relationship they enjoy with the physician and staff of a single-physician practice. Patients like to know they will see the same physician each time they visit, and they develop a loyalty to the practice (Figure 1–2). Some experts consider a close relationship with the physician an important factor in patient health.

Group Practice

Several physicians may associate as partners to share the expenses of operating a practice. The high costs of medical technology, paperwork, premiums for malpractice insurance, and expenditures for office space are more affordable when shared. For this reason, physicians who combine offices and staffs recognize an immediate savings.

The importance of accurate medical records and other documentation cannot be overstated. The documentation is important, of course, in

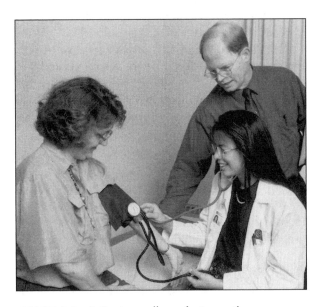

FIGURE 1–2   Patients usually prefer to see the same physicians each time.

tracking a patient's history. Beyond that, however, records are important in defending the thousands of malpractice lawsuits that are filed against physicians each year. As a result, case histories, laboratory test results, doctors' notes, and other medical reports must be transcribed and stored with the patient's records.

When a group of physicians pool their resources and form a practice, one of the advantages is saved money in shared overhead and staff. There are advantages beyond cost savings that draw physicians to group practices. By forming a group, physicians assure their patients that a doctor will always be available, even when the primary care physician is away. In addition, large group practices often are able to provide some laboratory tests on-site. For example, blood or urine may be tested and analyzed while the patient waits, avoiding a return trip to the doctor's office or a trip to another facility. When saving time is important to the patient, a group practice offering on-site laboratory services is a strong incentive.

Physicians in a group practice usually have more flexible schedules because they alternate times when they are "**on call.**" One of the greatest disadvantages of a medical career is the lack of time flexibility; a physician in a single practice is always **on call**, frequently receiving calls in the middle of the night. In a group practice where the physicians practice the same specialty, the time required to be on call is reduced.

A group practice also offers a new physician the advantage of associating with experienced doctors and building a practice more quickly. When established physicians in a group have all the patients they can treat effectively, they commonly assign new patients to the most recent member of the group.

The new physician in a group practice also saves part of the expense of opening a new office by joining an established group. These days, many doctors enter practice owing large amounts of money from student loans.

Ambulatory Centers

Ambulatory centers, also known as "urgent care centers," are usually private, for-profit centers that offer routine medical services for extended hours, some for twenty-four hours a day. They are in direct competition with private physician practices. This idea has sometimes been called "franchised" medicine because centers with the same name owned by one company have sprung up in cities all around the country. Ambulatory centers are often staffed by salaried physicians who do not participate in the profits of the company. Some experts predict an increase in the number of ambulatory centers; furthermore, they see competition for less expensive services drawing patients away from traditional practices.

Clinics

Clinics usually are set up to serve a specific medical need or a specific geographic area. Large group practices are often considered clinics. When a clinic serves a specialty, such as cardiology or pediatrics, all physicians who work in the clinic practice the same specialty or offer related services. By combining the knowledge and skill of several physicians, the clinic can provide advanced levels of patient care. Wellness centers, sports-injury clinics, rehabilitation facilities, and women's clinics are examples of specialty practices.

Clinics that serve geographic areas may offer their patients a broad range of specialties. Often located in the center of large cities or in isolated locations, these clinics provide medical assistance to patients of all ages for most illnesses and diseases. When a medical problem is beyond the scope of the physicians staffing the clinic, the patient is referred to another medical facility.

Clinics may be private, as with large group practices, or they may be operated by a government entity. Public health clinics historically have provided low-cost inoculations for school-age children. Clinics for patients unable to pay are operated by some city governments.

Medical Centers

Medical centers offer many of the same services as clinics because they treat a variety of illnesses; however, they are usually much larger. Except for their names, it is sometimes difficult to distinguish between a large medical center and a hospital. Medical centers may be private or public, but because of their size and operating costs, most large medical centers are supported by public funds.

Managed Competition Organizations

Controlling health care costs and making services more affordable is the goal of **managed competition**. Under this type of plan, insurance buyers band together in large "alliances" to bargain with competing networks of physicians, hospitals, and other health care providers for the best care at the best price. Theoretically, managed competition bargaining will encourage lower costs and greater efficiency by establishing a schedule of fees and reducing unnecessary tests. Critics of managed competition complain that insurance company auditors, instead of doctors, may make the decisions about when patients should or would be allowed more care.

Six types of managed competition attract the most attention. Figure 1–3 contrasts these six types of managed competition organizations.

Medical Institutions

Medical institutions differ in the services they offer. Whereas some medical institutions exist solely to diagnose and treat disease, others do research or offer rehabilitation.

Research Centers

Research centers seek to broaden medical knowledge and to find answers to major health questions. Equipped with the latest medical technology, research centers are staffed by physicians, scientists, laboratory technicians, teachers, and others in related occupations. Research centers may have direct contact with patients, as in research hospitals, or they may do laboratory research with body tissue, cells, organs, and fluids to provide answers to health questions.

Frequently, the work of research centers is experimental, and many decades may pass before an answer is found that remedies a public health problem. For example, after decades of scientific study, physicians and scientists in major research centers have told us that cigarette smoking contributes to lung cancer. Laws have been enacted forcing tobacco companies to add a warning to cigarette advertising, and, increasingly, public and private buildings and spaces have become smoke free. Lawsuits by states have cost tobacco companies hundreds of millions of dollars in reparation for tobacco-related deaths.

The **Centers for Disease Control and Prevention** (CDC) in Atlanta, Georgia is a government agency that employs 8,500 people and provides research in a wide range of programs. Its primary responsibility is to safeguard health by preventing and controlling disease. For example, each year, scientists at the CDC announce the results of the previous year's study of influenza outbreaks internationally and predict how influence will affect U.S. citizens during the next flu season. The CDC identifies the group (e.g., the aged) that will be most affected by future outbreaks and recommends proper preventives. Among its publications are research findings concerning AIDS, genetic mapping, and the development of a blood test to detect breast cancer.

Laboratories

A medical laboratory is a room or building equipped for scientific experimentation, research, testing, or clinical study of materials, fluids, or tissues obtained from patients. An experimental laboratory is a component of almost all research facilities, except for those that study only medical records. In addition to doing research, independent laboratories provide the routine analysis of patient materials, fluids, and tissues. When a patient has a routine blood test, the analysis is conducted by a physician's office laboratory or by an independent laboratory. Using the modern laboratory's sophisticated technology, a technician or physician can determine the cause of a patient's medical problem and follow through with the proper treatment.

Laboratories provide a valuable service in treating disease by focusing years of experimentation on a specific problem. A laboratory researcher is like a detective seeking a clue in a baffling case. Answers to some of our most challenging medical questions have been found through laboratory experimentation. The National Institutes of Health (NIH) conducts research across many fields, from aging and cancer to mental health and incontinence. For example, take the field of anxiety disorders, sometimes appearing as panic attacks. What was untreatable a short time ago is now treatable, thanks in good part to the research efforts of the National Institute of Mental Health, part of NIH. Treatments are extremely effective, typically combining

Exclusive Provider Organizations (EPOs)

In this approach to managed care, subscribers receive benefits for obtaining services from a network of providers who contract with the managed care plan. These are "exclusive" providers and agree not to take work for any other managed care organization. A network provider can be a sole practitioner or a hospital, or anything in between.

Typically, subscribers must have their health needs coordinated by their primary care physician. That means that visits to specialists are covered only if recommended by a primary care physician.

Health Maintenance Organizations (HMOs)

Health maintenance organizations are formed with an eye to controlling costs. HMOs sell health care at a fixed, prenegotiated price, usually to insurance carriers, large companies, or other groups who band together to purchase health care for everyone in the group. HMOs offer all types of care, often under one roof. The emphasis is on preventive care or wellness, because the HMO receives the same monthly payment whether the subscriber or member has been sick or well during the month.

Most of the physicians providing care in the HMOs are hired employees who receive a standard salary, no matter how many patients are seen, treatments performed, or tests ordered. If the cost of providing health services for all patients in a group during a month is greater than the fee paid for services, the HMO loses money. Conversely, if the HMO contains costs, it is profitable. HMOs compete with one another for large contracts.

Integrated Delivery System (IDS)

This approach to managed care features providers such as physicians' groups, hospitals, and ambulatory service centers that affiliate to provide joint health care services to subscribers. By subscribing to the plan, patients can choose their provider depending on the circumstance at the time.

Point-of-Service Plan (POS)

HMOs and PPOs can offer greater flexibility in managed care by using a point-of-service plan. Under the plan subscribers have not only the option of going to a physician or facility that is part of the plan, they also are free to "self-refer" to a non-HMO provider. When subscribers self-refer, however, they usually have to pay a significant deductible fee and coinsurance charges as high as 25%.

Preferred Provider Organizations (PPOs)

A preferred provider organization could be called a health care price club, where individuals receive discounts because they are members of an organization that buys in volume. PPOs discount their health care services to large employers, union members, or major insurance companies when they refer all their members to a single PPO.

High volume is the key to profitability for PPOs. Physicians are not employees of the PPO as they are of the HMO; therefore, they can continue to provide service under the traditional fee-for-service arrangement.

Triple Option Plan

This approach to managed care is often called a cafeteria plan because of the flexibility of options open to subscribers — HMO, PPO, or traditional health insurance. Triple option plans protect insurers from covering subscribers who are sicker than the general population. Insurers determine the cost of coverage by assessing the age, sex, health, and occupation of each employee. Creating such a pool of subscribers and assessing their status allows insurers to spread their risks of paying out large sums of money. For that reason, such pools of subscribers are called risk pools.

FIGURE 1–3 Six types of managed competition

medication and specific types of psychotherapy. Meanwhile, new medications to treat anxiety disorders are being tested and others are under development.

Nursing Homes

Contemporary nursing homes offer many services to all age groups. Some nursing homes act as rehabilitation units for the physically disabled and for accident victims, whereas others offer services for the aged. The care may be short-term, with the nursing home acting as a temporary therapy facility after a patient's hospitalization, or it may involve long-term assisted living.

Specialized Care Centers

Specialized care centers have received attention in recent years, primarily from the publicity surrounding several drug treatment centers. For example, the Betty Ford Drug Treatment Center in California has become widely known because of famous people who seek treatment there; however, this type of medical institution is not a new phenomenon. Specialized care centers for the treatment of polio, tuberculosis, malaria, and similar diseases affecting large numbers of people have been available since the beginning of modern medicine. Today, in addition to the traditional specialized care centers, newer centers specialize in psychiatric care, rehabilitation care, head trauma care, and outpatient surgical care.

Hospitals

Hospitals provide medical care and surgery for the sick and injured. Private physicians serve on the staff of one or more hospitals and refer their patients to the hospitals they serve. Physicians may also have "visiting physician" privileges at other hospitals, though they may not routinely admit their patients to them.

A hospital's size is measured by the number of rooms and beds it provides. Some hospitals are small; others may have hundreds of rooms. Hospitals may be categorized as general hospitals, teaching hospitals, or research hospitals. General hospitals may be found in almost every town, and several general hospitals may serve the population in large cities. They provide the community with both routine and special health care services. A teaching hospital is usually affil-iated with a medical school, and medical students participate in treating patients under the supervision of staff physicians. A research hospital, as the name implies, is an institution with twin goals of treating patients and performing research. A research hospital may also be a teaching hospital.

Hospitals are licensed by state or local licensing groups. Each state may license hospitals as it chooses. One cannot assume that a hospital licensed in one state meets the same health care standards as a similar hospital in another state. Federal hospitals, such as Veterans' Administration hospitals, are regulated by the federal government.

IN YOUR OPINION

1. What are the advantages and disadvantages, economic and otherwise, of practicing alone or in a group?
2. As a medical assistant, how will "managed care" affect your work in a solo practice, a group practice, an ambulatory center, a hospital, or one of the other facilities named? Why?
3. How does working in a laboratory compare with working in a well-baby clinic?

THE LANGUAGE OF MEDICINE

Case histories, consulting reports, doctors' notes, and other medical documents contain many words that, if spelled or used incorrectly, could result in improper diagnosis and treatment of a patient. Therefore, you as a medical assistant must thoroughly understand medical terminology in order to produce accurate reports. A brief explanation of medical terminology is given in this section. However, a complete understanding requires one or more courses in anatomy and physiology, medical terminology, the language of medicine, or similar courses.

Root Words, Prefixes, and Suffixes

Many medical words are formed by combining a root, or basic word, and a prefix or suffix. For example, the root **neur-** refers to the nervous system, and the root **orth-** means "straight" or "in proper order." When these roots are used with a prefix or suffix, they form medical words. Therefore, **neurology** means the branch of medicine that deals with the nervous system, and **orthopedics** means the branch of medicine that deals with disorders that require restructure, such as setting a broken leg. A combining form, usually the vowel "o," is added to root words to aid in pronunciation. A sample of root words with prefixes or suffixes is shown in this chart:

Prefix	Root Word	Suffix	Meaning
	cardi- (heart)	-ology (study of)	study of the heart
	cardi- (heart)	-ologist (specialist)	a specialist who studies the heart
contra- (against)	indicated (point out)		points out inappropriate form of treatment
	derma- (skin)	-(t)ology (study of)	study of the skin
ex- (out)	-cise (cut)		cut out
	gastro- (stomach)	-scopy (look)	look in the stomach (with a medical (instrument)
peri- (around)	cardium (heart)		fibrous sac enclosing the heart

Abbreviations

Abbreviations for laboratory tests, chemical elements, measurements, medications, dosages, and names of organizations often replace medical words in reports. A sample of common abbreviations is given in the following chart. Refer to a medical dictionary for a complete list of abbreviations.

Abbreviation	Complete Word or Name
b.i.d.	twice a day
CBC	complete blood count
CPE	complete physical exam
CT	computed tomography
EEG	electroencephalogram
EENT	eye, ear, nose, throat
EKG/ECG	electrocardiogram

continues

continued

Abbreviation	Complete Word or Name
EMG	electromyogram
h.s.	at bedtime
IV	intravenous
mg	milligram
mm	millimeter
MRI	magnetic resonance imaging
p.r.n.	as needed
q.h.	every hour
q.2h.	every two hours
q.i.d.	four times a day
RBC	red blood count
segs	segmented neutrophiles (white blood cells)
T3, T4, R7	thyroid profile
t.i.d.	three times a day
UA	urinalysis
VA	visual acuity
WBC	white blood count

Body Systems

An understanding of human anatomy helps the medical assistant determine whether words are correct in a medical report, especially if the dictation is garbled or the handwriting difficult to decipher. Body systems are discussed briefly in this section.

Circulatory System

The circulatory system consists primarily of the heart, the blood vessels, the blood, and the lymphatic system. The heart pumps blood that travels through blood vessels to organs of the body. It cleanses the organs of waste and provides them with oxygen and food. Cardiologists, vascular surgeons, and hematologists study and treat the circulatory system.

Digestive System

All the organs and glands associated with ingestion and digestion of food make up the digestive system, including the mouth, pharynx, esophagus, stomach, small intestine, appendix, and large intestine. The digestive system breaks down food into simple substances that the cells can use, absorbs food as needed, and eliminates leftovers in the forms of wastes. Gastroenterology is the study of the digestive system.

Endocrine System

The glands that regulate body functions are a part of the endocrine system, and specialists who diagnose and treat these glands are called endocrinologists. The endocrine system plays a major role in regulating growth, in the reproductive process, and in the way the body uses food. The primary endocrine glands include the adrenal glands, pituitary gland, parathyroid glands, thyroid gland, and sex glands.

Integumentary System

The organ system that refers to the skin and related appendages, including nails and hair, is called the integumentary system. The skin is the largest organ of the body and measures about 20 square feet on a 150-pound person. The outer layer of the skin is made up of dead cells and is called the epidermis. The middle layer of skin, the dermis, maintains an even temperature. The innermost layer of skin, the subcutaneous layer, helps retain body heat, cushions the tissues against blows, and provides extra fuel for the body. The study of the skin is called dermatology.

Muscular System

The body has more than 600 muscles that contract and pull tissue to create body movement. Skeletal muscles move the bones that allow us to walk, throw a ball, or make other voluntary movements. Smooth muscles, which are found in the internal organs, move food through the digestive system. They also control the width of the blood vessels and the size of the breathing passages. Physicians who study the muscular system are called rheumatologists.

Nervous System

The nervous system regulates and coordinates the activities of all the other systems of the body. It enables the body to adjust to changes that occur within itself and its surroundings. The central nervous system, which is made up of the brain and spinal cord, receives messages from the senses and sends instructions. A neurologist is the specialist in the study of the nervous system. A neurosurgeon specializes in the surgical treatment of the nervous system.

Respiratory System

The organs that allow breathing make up the respiratory system. They include the nose, mouth, pharynx, larynx, trachea, bronchi, and lungs. The primary jobs of the respiratory organs are to provide the body with oxygen and to rid it of carbon dioxide. Breathing allows humans to inhale air as the lungs expand and to exhale as the lungs push air out. Physicians who treat respiratory diseases are called pulmonary specialists.

Reproductive System

The organs of the reproductive system enable men and women to have children. The male reproductive organs are the testicles, scrotum, and penis. Physicians who diagnose and treat problems with these organs are called urologists. The female reproductive organs are the ovaries, fallopian tubes, uterus, and vagina. Physicians who specialize in the treatment of female reproductive problems are called gynecologists. Physicians who treat women during pregnancy and childbirth are called obstetricians.

Skeletal System

The skeleton of an adult consists of about 200 bones that support and protect the body. The skull protects the brain, the ribs protect the heart and lungs, and the spinal column protects the spinal cord. The skeletal system and muscles together allow the body to move. The study of the skeletal system is called orthopedics.

Urinary System

The urinary system, made up primarily of the two kidneys, filters various wastes from the blood and flushes them from the body in a fluid called urine. About 1,700 quarts of blood flow through the kidneys each day. Physicians who treat the urinary system are called urologists. Physicians who treat only diseases of the kidneys are called nephrologists.

MEDICAL SPECIALTIES, SUBSPECIALTIES, AND DENTAL SPECIALTIES

The complexity of the body's structure and the way it functions calls for a thorough understanding of the body systems and a knowledge of the effect that each system has on the healthy or diseased body. That is the reason most physicians today choose to specialize or subspecialize.

Medical Specialties

Specialists are physicians who concentrate on certain body systems, specific age groups, or complex scientific techniques developed to diagnose or treat certain disorders. **Medical specialties** developed originally because of the rapidly expanding body of knowledge about health and illness and the constantly evolving new treatments for disease. Today, no one physician can hope to master the total field of medical knowledge or to maintain the skills necessary for all diagnostic tests, treatments, and procedures.

A specialist's training begins after the physician receives an M.D. degree from a medical school. The first year of residency is called an internship. Resident physicians dedicate themselves to a period of three to seven years of full-time experience in a hospital or ambulatory center, caring for patients under the supervision of experienced teaching specialists. Educational conferences and research experience are also part of the training.

Specialty boards certify that physicians have met published standards, including testing. Twenty-four specialty boards are recognized by the American Board of Medical Specialties (ABMS). To be certified as a medical specialist by one of these boards, a physician must complete its requirements. Not all physicians choose to become certified.

Medical Subspecialties

A subspecialist is a physician who, after completing training in a general medical specialty, takes additional training in a more specific sub-area of that specialty. This training increases the specialist's depth of knowledge in the specialty field. For example, cardiology is a subspecialty of internal medicine; pediatric surgery is a subspecialty of surgery; and child psychiatry is a subspecialty of psychiatry. The training of a subspecialist requires an additional one or more years of full-time education in a program called a fellowship.

A brief description of the specialties and subspecialties recognized by the ABMS is given in Figure 1–4.

Dental Specialties

The practice of dentistry has changed in the last ten years. This can be attributed to differing dental care needs of the population, greater use of support personnel, and technological advances that affect the materials and techniques dentists employ. Because nine of ten dentists practice privately, they handle the business aspects of running an office as well as the diagnosis and treatment of dental disease. Dental assistants help the dentists with a variety of administrative tasks, from keeping the books to ordering supplies.

About 21% of all dentists practice in one of nine specialty areas listed below. Each is recognized by the American Dental Association.

- Orthodontist — Straightens and aligns teeth. This is the largest group of dental specialists.
- Oral and maxillofacial surgeon — Operates on the mouth and jaws. This is the second largest group of dentists.
- Oral and maxillofacial radiologist — Produces and then interprets radiant energy images and data for the diagnosis of diseases and disorders
- Pediatric dentist — Specializes in children's dentistry
- Periodontist — Treats gum diseases
- Prosthodontist — Develops artificial teeth or dentures
- Endodontist — Provides root canal therapy
- Public health dentist — Provides community dental health
- Oral pathologist — Treats diseases of the mouth

Specialties and Subspecialties

Allergy and immunology   Evaluates, diagnoses, and manages disorders involving the immune system, such as asthma, eczema, and adverse reactions to drugs, foods, and insect bites.

Anesthesiology   Provides pain relief and maintenance of a stable condition during a surgical, obstetric, or diagnostic procedure.

Colon and rectal surgery   Diagnoses and treats diseases of the intestinal tract, rectum, and anus, including such conditions as hemorrhoids, polyps, cancer, colitis, and diverticulosis.

Dermatology   Prevents, diagnoses, and treats benign and malignant disorders of the skin and related mouth tissues, external genitalia, hair, and nails.

Emergency medicine   Manages immediate intervention to prevent death or further disability, usually based in an emergency department or trauma center.

Family practice   Treats the general health of the individual and the family.

Internal medicine   Provides care for nonsurgical illnesses of adolescents and adults.

  Cardiovascular medicine   Manages complex diseases of the heart, lungs, and blood vessels.

  Critical care medicine   Manages acute, life-threatening disorders such as shock, coma, heart failure, and drug overdoses in intensive care and other settings.

  Diagnostic laboratory immunology   Uses laboratory tests to diagnose and treat disorders of the body's immune system.

  Endocrinology   Concentrates on disorders of the endocrine glands, such as the thyroid and adrenal glands.

  Gastroenterology   Treats the digestive organs, including the stomach, bowels, liver, and gallbladder.

  Geriatrics   Study of aging patients.

  Hematology   Diagnoses and treats diseases of the blood, spleen, and lymph glands, such as anemia, clotting disorders, sickle cell disease, and leukemia.

  Infectious diseases   Deals with infectious diseases of all types and in all organs.

  Medical oncology   Diagnoses and treats benign and malignant tumors.

  Nephrology   Treats disorders of the kidneys.

  Pulmonary diseases   Manages diseases of the lungs and other chest tissues, including conditions such as bronchitis and emphysema.

  Rheumatology   Focuses on diseases of the joints, muscles, bones, and tendons.

Medical genetics   Study of inherited diseases/conditions and search for the genetic defect causing them.

Neurological surgery   Evaluates and treats diseases of the brain, spinal cord, and nerves.

Neurology   Treats all categories of disease involving the central, peripheral, and autonomous nervous system.

Nuclear medicine   Uses the nuclear properties of radioactive and stable nuclides to evaluate conditions of the body.

Obstetrics and gynecology   Cares for disorders of the female reproductive system, the fetus, or the newborn.

  Gynecologic oncology   Treats cancer of the female reproductive system.

  Maternal-fetal medicine   Cares for patients during high-risk pregnancies.

Ophthalmology   Provides comprehensive care of the eyes.

Orthopedic surgery   Preserves and restores the extremities, spine, and associated body structures.

Otolaryngology   Treats disorders of the ears, respiratory, and upper alimentary systems, medically and surgically.

FIGURE 1–4   Specialties and subspecialties *(continues)*

Pathology   Diagnoses the causes of disease and predicts the course of disease.

    Blood banking   Maintains an adequate, safe blood supply.

    Chemical pathology   Uses understanding of the chemical systems of the body in diagnosing and monitoring diseases.

    Dermatopathology   Diagnoses and monitors diseases of the skin.

    Forensic pathology   Investigates and establishes the cause of death.

    Immunopathology   Monitors the course of disease by applying immunological principles to the analysis of tissues, cells, and body fluids.

    Medical microbiology   Isolates and identifies microbes that cause disease.

    Neuropathology   Diagnoses diseases of the nervous system and skeletal muscles.

Pediatrics   Treats the health of children from birth to young adulthood.

Physical medicine and rehabilitation   Evaluates and restores patients with many types of disabilities.

Plastic surgery   Repairs, replaces, and reconstructs defects of form and function of the skin and its underlying systems.

Preventive medicine   Focuses on maintenance of healthful lifestyle habits that prevent disease.

Psychiatry   Diagnoses and treats mental, emotional, and behavioral disorders.

Radiology   Uses x-rays to picture, diagnose, and treat diseases.

    Therapeutic radiology   Uses radiant energy to treat cancer.

    Diagnostic radiology   Uses x-rays as a diagnostic tool.

    Nuclear radiology   Uses other imaging techniques in diagnosis.

    Radiological physics   Regulates safe radiological practices.

    Therapeutic radiological physics   Treats diseases using x-rays and related sources in diagnosis.

    Medical nuclear physics   Uses radionuclides to diagnose and treat disease.

General surgery   Provides surgical procedures.

    General vascular surgery   Surgically treats disorders of the blood vessels, excluding those of the heart, lungs, and brain.

    Pediatric surgery   Surgically treats infants, children, and adolescents.

    Surgical critical care   Cares for critically ill patients and postoperative patients.

Thoracic surgery   Evaluates and surgically treats conditions within the chest, such as congenital defects and heart diseases.

Urology   Treats disorders of the adrenal glands and of the genitourinary system.

FIGURE 1–4   *(continued)*

COMPUTERS IN CONTEMPORARY MEDICINE

Computers are used for diagnosing and treating disease and for managing medical facilities. They tell a physician whether a patient's vital signs are normal, track the course of the patient's health after surgery, and record the costs of the patient's treatment. The pattern of an illness can be traced by computer, and the appropriate test or procedure can be identified from the pattern.

Computers in Private Practice

In the past few years, the number of computers in private practice has soared. Physicians are taking advantage of computerized patient accounting, billing, scheduling, payroll completion, word processing, and database management. Medical record management, tracking, diagnosis, and data referral are other important applications. Another reason for the increased use of computers by physicians is access by modem to online databases such as Medline that helps the physician provide better treatment. The physician or medical assistant can retrieve the most recent and technical medical journals quickly and easily, including journals published abroad.

As a medical assistant preparing to enter the medical job market, you can expect to work with computers daily. You can also expect to continue your education by taking additional courses in your field. As technology develops, new applications will be added to your responsibilities, and you must continue learning.

Computers in the Hospital

Computers are used in hospitals to maintain a record of each patient's health, handle administrative responsibilities, cross-check drugs, and develop illness patterns. Nurses read physicians' instructions from a computerized database before giving medications. They enter notes about the patient's condition for the physician to read during hospital rounds.

Computers are involved in many aspects of high technology diagnoses. Magnetic resonance imaging (MRI) scans, for example, are used to produce a cross-sectional image of the head, back, knee, or other body area. The patient rests inside a tube while a magnetic force rotates around the patient "taking pictures" from every angle. Computers can analyze and refine data from the image making machine.

IN YOUR OPINION

1. Why do physicians spend the additional time required to become a specialist?
2. What additional training and experience do you think is necessary for a medical assistant working in a subspecialty?
3. Why are health maintenance organizations (HMOs) so controversial?

INTERNET ACTIVITIES

1. Review the American Association of Medical Assistants (AAMA) Web site at http://www.aama-ntl.org. Write a short summary of the organization's activities or give an oral presentation about the organization to your class.
2. Log on to the FamiliesUSA.org Web site that provides information on a wide variety of issues in medicine. When the home page appears, select Managed Care from the index box. Read one of the articles that interests you and report on a change or trend to managed care that could be expected.

STUDENT STUDY CHECKLIST

Workbook

1. Complete Chapter 1 exercises in the workbook.
2. Complete Chapter 1 simulations in the workbook that access the CD-ROM in the back of your book.

Administrative Skills CD-ROM

1. Go to the Library on the CD-ROM and play the interactive games for Chapter 1.
2. Take the Introductory Tour of the CD-ROM and study the many types of work found in a medical office. After the tour, identify the features of medical office work that appeal to you most.

REFERENCES

American Board of Medical Specialties. *Approved Specialty Boards and Certificate Categories.* Evanstan, IL.

Eisenbert, R. S. Human body. In *The World Book Encyclopedia* (Vol. 9), 2002.

Healthcare business issues. (Vol. 9) Report by Arthur Andersen LLP, 2000.

Humphrey, Doris D. *Pediatric Associates, P.C. — The Medical Secretary.* Cincinnati, OH: South-Western, 1997.

Sormunen, Carolee. *Terminology for Allied Health Professionals,* 5th ed. Clifton Park, NY: Delmar Learning, 2003.

Venes, Donald and Clayton L. Thomas, eds. *Taber's Cyclopedic Medical Dictionary*, 19th ed. Philadelphia: F.A. Davis Company, 2001.

U.S. Health and Human Services Commission, testimony before the Senate Finance Committee, October 24, 2001 (testimony of Don Gilbert).

U.S. Department of Labor, Bureau of Labor Statistics. *Occupational Outlook Handbook*, 2002–2003.

CHAPTER ACTIVITIES

PERFORMANCE-BASED ACTIVITIES

1. Read two articles from the Internet written on health care reform issues within the last three months. Select two important issues and create a short paper that supports the need for change. Use facts and examples. Debate these issues with another student in the class. Use the chart below to prepare short paper notes for your debate.

   Most important issues   *Facts*   *Examples*

   1. _____

   2. _____

2. Complete the following chart to communicate clearly the advantages and disadvantages of a managed care system for a medical practice.

   Advantages and Disadvantages of Managed Care

   Advantages   *Disadvantages*

   1. _____

   2. _____

   3. _____

   4. _____

   5. _____

3. Using the chart below, compare and contrast the responsibilities of an internal medical specialist and a cardiovascular subspecialist in treating the same patient.

   Responsibilities of a Specialist and Subspecialist

   Internist   *Cardiovascular Specialist*
   Responsibilities   *Responsibilities*

   1. _____

   2. _____

   3. _____

   4. _____

4. What are the areas of overlapping responsibility between an internal medicine specialist and a cardiologist? What is the value to the patient of having each specialist involved in treatment?

   Overlapping Responsibilities   *Value of a Specialist Plus a Subspecialist*

   1. _____

   2. _____

   3. _____

   4. _____

Overlapping Responsibilities   *Value of a Specialist Plus a Subspecialist*

5. _____

6. _____

5. Using Figure 1–4 and the body systems identified in this chapter, associate each of the body systems to the appropriate medical specialty(s).

Body System Relationship to Specialty

Body System   *Specialty/Subspecialty*

1. _____

2. _____

3. _____

4. _____

5. _____

6. _____

7. _____

8. _____

9. _____

10. _____

EXPANDING YOUR THINKING

1. A friend who wishes to work in the medical field asks you for advice about different types of medical facilities where jobs might be available. What will you tell your friend?

2. Your employer has agreed to talk to a group of college students about medical specialties and subspecialties and asks you to develop a brief outline for the talk. Create an outline that includes the following points:

   a. The difference between a medical specialty and a medical subspecialty

   b. The difference in training for a specialist and subspecialist

   c. Examples of specialties and their subspecialties

3. Describe the types of changes required when two practices merge into one. What do you think are the advantages and disadvantages of merging with another group?

CHAPTER 2

The Medical Staff

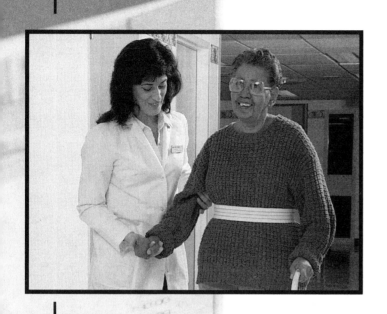

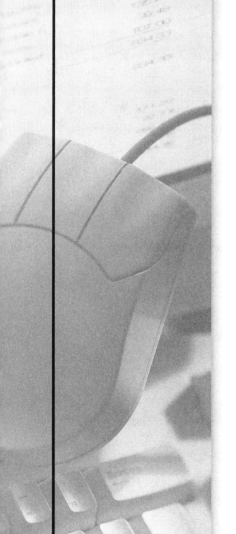

DENVER, COLORADO

I just completed my first week of working for Femcare Associates, a small clinical practice focusing on OB/GYN issues but also offering services in internal and general practice medicine for women who prefer working with female physicians. Nothing in my experience as a student prepared me for the range and pace of this work.

At Femcare, three MAs work with two doctors. One of us is a CMA, which means Certified Medical Assistant. This practice believes in cross-training, which has always made sense to me. We are all expected to perform a variety of duties, everything from greeting the patients to administering selected tests ordered by the doctors. We rotate, so that one day I handle administrative duties and the next I assist one of the doctors. Let me give you an idea of what last week was like.

On Monday, Wednesday, and Friday, Glenda and I worked the back of the office. Both of the doctors had office hours, so we saw about forty patients each day. We prepared the treatment rooms and interviewed the patients to find out about changes they had experienced since their last visit. We took vital signs and performed a urinalysis for each patient. Then we stayed in the treatment rooms with the patient to help the doctor during the exam.

Although most patients were there for routine prenatal or annual checkups, some things aren't so routine. That's when I'm glad I received good training. One patient, a young mother-to-be, was recently diagnosed with breast cancer. She is facing several tough decisions because some treatment options could hurt her unborn baby. Another patient, an elderly woman brought in by her daughter, simply refused to cooperate. It took all of my interpersonal skills to resolve her concerns.

Tuesday and Thursday were my days to handle the front office. I greeted patients and helped new ones fill out the introductory medical history questionnaire. I entered that information into the computer. When patients left, I scheduled their next visit. And in between all that I also helped answer the phone and made calls to insurance companies regarding outstanding claims. It was a whirlwind start, and I'm still learning. Does it sound like a good first week to you?

Akila Powers
Medical Assistant

PERFORMANCE-BASED COMPETENCIES

After completing this chapter you should be able to:

1. Compare and contrast the clinical and administrative responsibilities of a medical assistant.
2. Analyze and project the demand for medical assistants in view of a changing health care environment.
3. Identify and discuss interpersonal skills that nurture a team concept among the medical staff.
4. Make recommendations for education and credentialing that will enhance a medical office assistant's career.

VOCABULARY

AAMA The American Association of Medical Assistants, a professional organization for all practicing medical assistants, certified and noncertified.
Ambulatory care centers Twenty-four-hour medical centers that treat patients with minor illnesses or injuries.
CAAHEP Commission on Accreditation of Allied Health Education Programs, a group that accredits a school's medical assisting program. Medical assistants who wish to sit for the CMA examination should select a CAAHEP-approved school for their education.
CMA Certified Medical Assistant, a credential earned by passing the comprehensive examination offered by the American Association of Medical Assistants.
CPT Current Procedural Terminology
Credentialing Examination that certifies the medical assistant in administrative and clinical procedures.

Multiskilled medical assistant Medical assistant who is trained in both administrative and clinical duties.
OMA Ophthalmic Medical Assistant, a credential earned through the Joint Commission on Allied Health Personnel in Ophthalmology.
Physician extenders Paramedical staff trained to support the physician by performing some tasks previously performed only by the physician.
RDC The Role Delineation Chart, developed by the Endowment of the American Association of Medical Assistants to define the basic competencies for an entry-level medical assistant professional.
RMA Registered Medical Assistant, a credential earned by passing the comprehensive examination offered by the American Medical Technologists.

The size of a medical practice determines the number of employees and the scope of their duties. A solo practice may require only a nurse and a multiskilled medical assistant, whereas a group practice may require several physicians, nurses, laboratory technicians, and medical assistants.

The role of the medical assistant is changing from a loosely defined support function to a professional, highly visible career. The demand for well-trained medical assistants possessing a wide range of human relations and technology skills grows each year.

THE MEDICAL ASSISTANT

In 1954, a group of medical assistants met to establish a professional organization. With support, guidance, and encouragement from the American Medical Association (AMA), the American Association of Medical Assistants (AAMA) was founded in 1955. It is the only association in the world devoted exclusively to the medical assisting profession.

The AAMA has forty-three state societies nationwide and more than fifty local chapters. AAMA members include practicing medical assistants (administrative, clinical, office managers), medical assisting educators, students, and others interested in the profession. Its three primary responsibilities are accreditation, certification, and continuing education. The profession of medical assisting was formally recognized by the U.S. Department of Education in 1978.

In 1991, the AAMA Board of Trustees approved the present definition of medical assisting:

> Medical assisting is an allied health profession whose practitioners function as members of the health care delivery team and perform administrative and clinical procedures.

The term **medical assistant** refers to a broad category of medical office professionals. Receptionists, medical transcriptionists, appointment schedulers, billing clerks, and phlebotomists are all medical assistants. Sometimes several medical assistants are responsible for different tasks, or a multiskilled medical assistant may assume all of these responsibilities. Medical assistants work in a wide variety of specialties and subspecialties. Figure 2–1 illustrates the distribution of medical assistants across specialty fields.

The medical assistant's job can be separated into two distinct categories: (1) administrative responsibilities, which include both routine and special office tasks, and (2) clinical responsibilities, which involve helping the physician examine and treat patients. In larger offices, medical assistants usually specialize in either the administrative or the clinical aspect of the job, whereas the multiskilled medical assistant frequently works in an ambulatory center or in a solo practice where fewer medical assistants are on duty at one time.

Medical assistants receive their education in community colleges, universities, and vocational schools, or through on-the-job training. Although there are no general licensing requirements for medical assistants, some states require the successful completion of a test or a short course as a prerequisite for performing procedures such as taking x-rays, drawing blood, or giving injections. Some employers prefer to hire either experienced workers or certified applicants.

Certification

Voluntary certification is offered through several professional organizations. The American Association of Medical Assistants sponsors the certification examination for a large number of practicing medical assistants throughout the United States. Individuals who pass the exam receive the Certified Medical Assistant credential. Figure 2–2 shows the **CMA** pin awarded by the AAMA. The American Medical Technologists awards the Registered Medical Assistant (RMA) credential and the Joint Commission on Allied Health Personnel in Ophthalmology awards the Ophthalmic Medical Assistant (**OMA**) credential.

The AAMA adopted a policy in 1998 that requires any candidate for the AAMA Certification Examination to be a graduate of a medical assisting program accredited by the Commission on Accreditation of Allied Health Education Programs (**CAAHEP**). The policy addressed the problem of medical assistants whose right to practice clinical procedures was being challenged by some states. These states had begun to require

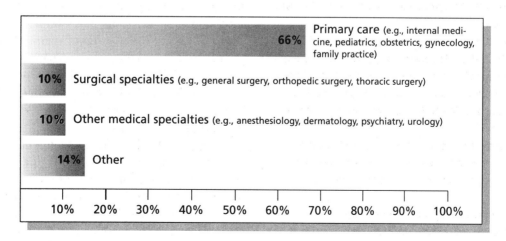

66% Primary care (e.g., internal medicine, pediatrics, obstetrics, gynecology, family practice)

10% Surgical specialties (e.g., general surgery, orthopedic surgery, thoracic surgery)

10% Other medical specialties (e.g., anesthesiology, dermatology, psychiatry, urology)

14% Other

10% 20% 30% 40% 50% 60% 70% 80% 90% 100%

FIGURE 2-1 Medical assistant employment by type of specialty (Courtesy of the American Association of Medical Assistants)

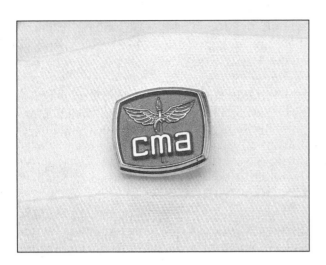

FIGURE 2-2 Pin awarded to medical assistants on successful completion of the certification examination (Courtesy of the Association of Medical Assistants)

licensure or certification before certain clinical tasks could be performed.

Anticipated benefits of the AAMA's certification policy are:

1. Safeguard the quality of care to the consumer
2. Ensure the CMA's role in the rapidly evolving health care delivery system
3. Continue to promote the identity and stature of the profession

Eligibility for taking the AAMA certification examination is clearly defined. Graduates of medical assisting programs accredited by the Accrediting Bureau of Health Education Schools (ABHES) with twelve months of full-time health work experience are eligible to take the AAMA certification examination. The status of a medical assistant's credentials (whether current or lapsed) is a public record available through the AAMA. Effective January 2003, all certified medical assistants who are employed or seeking employment must have current status as a CMA to use the credential.

You should seriously consider sitting for a **credentialing** examination and continuing education seminars or workshops after you begin work. A credentialed medical assistant is viewed as the "cream of the crop" and often can move into administrative and office management positions.

Career Opportunities

Employment of medical assistants is expected to grow faster than the average for all occupations through the year 2010 due to expansion of the health services industry. According to the 2002–2003 *Occupational Outlook Handbook*, employment growth will be spurred by the increasing number of group and health care practices that use support personnel. These outpatient settings are where medical assistants primarily work. Job openings will also be created because experienced medical assistants will leave the occupation by moving to other health service careers or through retirement. In light of this high turnover and the preference for trained personnel, job prospects should be excellent for medical assistants with formal training or experience, particularly those with certification.

The current era of cost containment in health service has provided an increased demand for generalist health care workers possessing basic skills in multiple areas. Medical assistants in the future will be expected to be broadly trained, both in administrative and clinical tasks and in the use of computers and other technology. The medical assistant's responsibilities are varied, interesting, and rewarding. Anyone who likes to work with people, who has a desire to help others, and who is willing to learn will enjoy this challenging profession.

The Multiskilled Medical Assistant

Competitive pressures on medical practices, hospitals, and other health care facilities have resulted in an emphasis on efficiency and reduction of idle time. Today's health care professionals handle a variety of administrative and clinical tasks. This trend is especially evident in the medical assisting profession where, in 1985, the broad CMA credential replaced the pediatric, administrative, and clinical specialties once available beyond the initial CMA credential. Medical assistants who were awarded the specialty credentials before 1985 may re-certify through continuing education units (CEUs).

Ambulatory care centers, often staffed twenty-four hours a day, seven days a week, are projected to grow at a rapid pace, and an increased need for **multiskilled medical assistants** will parallel this growth. Because it is not economical to staff a center with several different employees possessing specialized skills, the medical assistant with both administrative and clinical training will be in high demand.

Responsibilities of the Position

Medical assistants perform a variety of administrative and clinical duties. Administrative duties include answering the telephone, greeting patients and other callers, recording and filing patient data and medical records, completing medical reports and insurance forms, handling correspondence, scheduling appointments, arranging for hospital admission and laboratory services, completing record keeping and billing, and transcribing dictation. Clinical duties include recording patient height, weight, temperature, and blood pressure; obtaining medical histories; performing basic laboratory tests; preparing patients for and assisting in examinations; sterilizing instruments; drawing blood, preparing patients for x-rays and EKGs; and applying dressings.

Computer use is an important part of both the administrative and clinical duties of a medical assistant's job. Any machine that shows a digital readout is computer based, and the number and kind of these machines are increasing. Patient temperature can be taken with a thermometer attached to a small hand-held device that shows a digital readout. Computers analyze blood and urine and do many other laboratory tests in the medical office.

Computers have revitalized many boring, time-consuming administrative tasks traditionally completed by hand. If you had gone to work as a medical assistant twenty years ago, you would probably have spent several days preparing the monthly billing manually and by typewriter. Now, patient billing is completed in a few hours by a computer programmed for the task.

The Role Delineation Study Analysis

In 1979, the AAMA conducted an analysis of the medical assisting career to determine the responsibilities of people employed in the profession.

Using a process called DACUM, which stands for Developing A CUrriculuM, the analysts developed a chart listing the skills performed daily by medical assistants. The analysis has undergone several revisions as major changes in medical science and in the health care delivery system have affected the medical assistant's responsibilities. In 1997, the DACUM was replaced with the Role Delineation Chart, which resulted from the Medical Assistant Role Delineation Study.

For the Role Delineation Study, the AAMA invited a sample of currently practicing CMAs to discussion groups at the headquarters of the national Board of Medical Examiners in Philadelphia. A random sample of CMAs were also mailed a survey. Those participating included CMAs in current practice who were not educators and who represented a variety of geographic locations and work settings, with various work experience and different practice focuses.

The oversight committee concluded from the information obtained that the scope of practice for medical assistants did not expand as much as anticipated. The findings indicated medical assistants were spending more time and needed more depth of knowledge performing the same or similar tasks identified in previous DACUM studies. The Committee evaluated, combined, and categorized the content of the information from the Role Delineation Study into areas of competency for entry-level medical assistants.

The medical assistant role delineation chart lists the responsibilities the analysts developed. It identifies ten general areas of competence and seventy-four individual skills required of medical assistants. In reading each statement, you should precede it with the words, "The medical assistant should be able to . . . ."

Review the medical assistant role delineation chart carefully. The range of responsibilities is broad, from Listen and Observe, which is considered an entry-level skill, to Manage Personnel and Benefits, an advanced skill.

Job Titles and Job Sites

Medical assistant job titles often describe specific responsibilities. Typical titles include medical secretary, office manager, receptionist, word processing specialist, computer operator, billing clerk, bookkeeper, records manager, transcriptionist, and laboratory technician. According to the AAMA, medical assistants held about 252,000 jobs across the United States in 1998.

IN YOUR OPINION

1. Which medical assisting responsibilities do you think you will like best?
2. How can a medical assistant show interest in assuming extra responsibilities?
3. Why did you decide to pursue a career as a medical assistant?

THE ROLES OF MEDICAL PROFESSIONALS

As a medical assistant, you will work with a variety of health care professionals who diagnose and treat diseases, help those with disabilities, provide laboratory services, advise patients on ways to maintain and improve their health, and attempt to prevent disease. The following section will help you understand how the methods, procedures, and technology differ among health care deliverers.

Physicians

Physicians perform medical examinations, diagnose illnesses, treat injuries and diseases, and advise patients. In the past, almost all medical practices were owned by a physician or a group of physicians; however, practice patterns have changed. Today, many younger physicians work in salaried positions in health maintenance organizations, ambulatory centers, government institutions, and other health care facilities.

Physician Extenders

During the 1960s, physicians investigated other resources to extend their practices. The idea of **physician extenders**, identified as Physician Assistants (PAs), Certified Registered Nurse Practitioners (CRNPs), and Certified Midwives, was created to relieve doctors of some time-consuming tasks. Vietnam veteran medical personnel, nurses, and others with patient care experience took advantage of additional training at medical teaching centers and hospitals.

Today, these medical providers perform a wide range of duties. Based on the licensure requirements of their states, they may interview patients, take medical histories, perform physical examinations, order laboratory tests, make tentative diagnoses, prepare patients for treatment, and, in some states, write prescriptions. They always work with a supervising physician. Physician extenders frequently work in long-term care institutions and rural settings where they fill a vacuum caused by a shortage of local physicians. Employment of physician extenders is expected to grow faster than the average for other medical occupations through the year 2010.

Nurses

Nurses are licensed professionals who observe, assess, and record symptoms, dispense medications, and aid in patients' convalescence and rehabilitation. They also provide instruction in proper care to patients and their families and help people understand the importance of diet, exercise, and daily habits to health improvement. Sometimes they perform routine laboratory and office work, especially in solo and small practices.

After completing years of education and training, including some of the same courses required for physicians, nurses are licensed to practiced as registered nurses (RNs) or licensed practical nurses (LPNs or LVNs in some states). Registered nurses train from two to five years after high school, and they supervise licensed practical nurses, who usually train for one year after high school. An LPN/LVN may continue their education and eventually become licensed as a registered nurse.

In general, nurses see patients more often and spend more time with them than physicians. Physicians often pass directions for care and instructions for medication along to a nurse for administration.

Medical Technologists and Technicians

As advanced diagnostic techniques, laboratory procedures, and treatment methods develop through medical technology, new jobs are created for people who operate the highly specialized equipment. Known as medical technologists and technicians, these people often carry titles associated with the equipment they use, for example, radiologic technologist, electrocardiograph technician, and dialysis technician. Others who test body fluids and tissues are called laboratory technologists or technicians. Projections indicate that 50% of the technology that will be used by today's eighth graders when they begin their careers has not yet been invented.

Medical Records Personnel

Medical records employees manage an information system of patient records that meet medical, administrative, ethical, and legal requirements. **Medical records administrators** direct the activities of large departments, handling thousands of patient records yearly. Their job is to develop systems for efficient documentation, storage, and retrieval of records. **Medical records technicians** compile, organize, and evaluate patients' records for completeness and accuracy (Figure 2–3). They use standard coding and classification systems such as ICD-9 (*International Statistical Classification of Diseases and Related Health Problems*, Ninth Edition, renamed from *International Classification of Diseases*, Ninth Edition) and CPT-5 (*Current Procedural Terminology*,

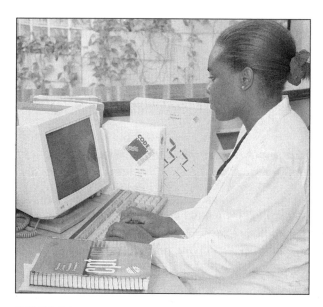

FIGURE 2-3 Medical records technicians evaluate patients' records.

Fifth Edition) to list symptoms, diseases, operations, procedures, therapies, and diagnoses on each patient's record. Physicians are primary users of patient records; however, nonconfidential information may also be supplied to insurance companies, government agencies, public health agencies, and other institutions.

The size of a medical facility determines the degree of responsibility of its medical records personnel. In private practices and small facilities, one person may be responsible for managing all aspects of record keeping, whereas in larger facilities an administrator and several technicians and clerks may be required. Credentialing for medical records personnel is available through the American Health Information Management Association, which awards professional credentialing for the following: Registered Health Information Administrator (RHIA), Registered Health Information Technician (RHIT), Certified Coding Specialist (CCS), Certified Coding Specialist-Physician based (CCS-P), and Certified Coding Associate (CCA).

IN YOUR OPINION

1. Compare the medical assistant's duties to those of the physician's extenders. Which position do you think is most important to the future growth of a physician practice?
2. How do you think national health insurance will change the role of medical professionals?
3. What is the importance of a medical record employee's job?

WORKING WITH THE MEDICAL PROFESSIONALS

In your role as medical assistant, you will work with all the health care professionals. Most of your work will be of a support nature, including registering the patient on arrival, organizing patient records for the physician and nurse to review, maintaining an even flow of patient traffic for the physician, and preparing the bill before the patient leaves. If you have additional clinical responsibilities, you may prepare the treatment room, locate and retrieved supplies needed by the physician or nurse, apply bandages, and give injections.

As a member of the health care team, you must respect and support all your coworkers. This means you must understand the professional responsibilities of each person and provide the help they need, recognizing that every task is important if the physician, nurse, or laboratory employee requires assistance in patient care.

Medical assistants often increase their value to a medical practice simply by being willing to assume extra responsibilities. With motivation, enthusiasm, the desire to work hard, good judgment, and good training, you can become very important to the success of a practice. You will determine whether you have a job or a career, and you can ensure your own success by becoming a valuable support employee for the physician and other professionals.

Working with the Physician and the Health Care Team

Physicians spend many years in training to treat the physical and mental ills of individuals in our society. Their study is intense, encouraging a fast-paced and demanding life style that can carry over to the physician's private practice after formal education is completed. The nurses, laboratory technologists, and medical assistants

work under intense pressure at times. For this diverse team of professionals to best use their efforts, each must work at top efficiency and use good interpersonal skills. Several characteristics that add to a medical assistant's success are discussed in the next section.

Honesty

A medical assistant's honesty must be beyond reproach. Because the physician is responsible for an employee's actions, a dishonest employee can unknowingly involve a physician in a crime or malpractice lawsuit. A medical assistant who dishonestly alters a patient's record because of a mistake reflects on the physician and may cause a malpractice lawsuit, in the same way, a bookkeeper or accountant who reports dishonest tax information involves the physician in a crime.

Dishonesty does not always involve a crime. The person who lies about a minor infraction of office policy and the person who does not tell the whole truth are dishonest. Consider the situations in Figure 2–4; some may seem unimportant, but all are dishonest and can destroy a medical assistant's career.

Cooperation

"No man is an island unto himself" is a famous quotation that characterizes the necessity of cooperation among members of the medical

Honesty	Dishonesty
Correctly reporting daily work hours	Failing to report late arrival; "stretching" breaks and lunch hours; conducting personal business, such as phone calls and chores, during scheduled work hours
Taking responsibility for errors and omissions, correcting errors and planning ways to prevent errors in the future	Blaming others for errors, complaining, and being defensive
Properly accounting for money, office supplies, medical supplies, and drugs	"Borrowing" from petty cash, taking drug samples or supplies without permission, making personal telephone calls without logging them
Accepting responsibility for mistakes	Blaming others

FIGURE 2–4 Comparison of honesty and dishonesty

office staff. Although each person has special responsibilities, all the responsibilities combine into one major effort to treat patients. When several people work toward a common goal, each must support all the others involved in the effort. One person who does not cooperate can spoil the success formula.

A cooperative person suppresses personal goals if those goals do not agree with the group goal. For example, as a medical assistant you will not be able to eat lunch each day at 11:30 AM if routine lunch hours are scheduled for 12:30 PM. Your desire to answer the telephone and greet patients may not be met if the day's agenda calls for you to mail monthly statements.

Cooperation is pleasurable, and the rewards are both personal and financial. Personal reward comes through ego support and good will from colleagues, whereas monetary recognition results in salary increases. Cooperative people are well liked and their services are in demand. A list of ways a medical assistant can show cooperation is given in Figure 2–5.

Assertiveness

Assertiveness refers to making a point positively or putting your views forward. Assertiveness is sometimes confused with aggressiveness; however, the two terms are not the same. Aggressiveness means pushiness or the desire to attack; it is considered a negative term when applied to relationships with others. On the other hand, assertiveness is a positive characteristic that means standing up for yourself or speaking when a comment is needed.

As a medical assistant, you should be assertive and offer new ideas when they improve office procedures or activities. If you have a personal concern or a complaint, such as a promised pay increase that you have not received, or if you feel resentment because other employees seem not to be sharing the work, you should discuss the problem with the physician or office manager. However, if you are a new employee, you should understand fully why a chore or responsibility is handled in its particular way before offering a suggestion. You should allow plenty of time to pass before bringing up a personal concern. You may be embarrassed if you are assertive without having all the facts.

The best approach is to delay making a move until you are absolutely satisfied that your question or remark is justified. It is a good idea to ask advice from someone you trust or a person who has been employed in a similar job before you approach the physician or office manager. Then, when you are confident you have waited long enough, use your most professional manner. State the problem or suggestion clearly, objectively, and without emotion. You

Problem	Cooperation Shown by
Fellow employee must leave fifteen minutes early to pick up a child at daycare	Offer to cover for employee during absence
You dislike a coworker	Be polite to all coworkers
You disagree with a decision	Explain why you disagree, then support the final decision
A hostile patient verbally attacks a new employee who made a mistake	You step in to mediate
The day after the cleaning crew has cleaned the office, a child spills grape juice on the carpet	Quickly and quietly mop it up
Emergency situations	Do whatever is necessary to assist in the situation

FIGURE 2–5 Suggestions for cooperation

may be slightly nervous; that is a natural feeling when you are discussing an important matter with a superior. However, once you have communicated your point, you will probably feel more confident. Be sure to use good oral skills to make your point and to read the feedback. If nonverbal feedback indicates that your point is not being well received, tactfully drop the subject and reconsider your position before speaking up again. You may want to consider submitting your idea or concern in writing. Be sure to sign and date your letter or memorandum. To clarify the differences between assertiveness and aggressiveness, several examples are given in Figure 2–6.

Dependability

In a busy medical office, employees must be able to depend on one another. As a medical assistant, you should know what needs to be done, when it needs to be done, and how to do it. The physician depends on the medical assistant to make the right decision or to ask questions as necessary with little direct supervision.

When you are dependable, you arrive at work on time each day and you finish your work without being reminded, even though you may have to stay after hours (Figure 2–7). You take sick leave only when you are sick, and you use

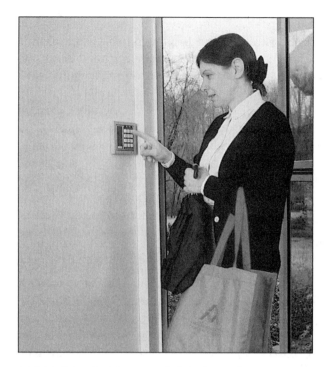

FIGURE 2–7 Arriving on or before time reflects a responsible attitude.

only the allotted time for lunch. You tackle unpleasant tasks without complaint and without being asked or reminded. People who are undependable usually lose their jobs because they cannot be counted on when needed.

Assertive	Aggressive
Thursday will be my six-month anniversary of employment. I would like to schedule a review with you at your convenience.	I work twice as hard as everyone else around here for less money. I thought I would get a raise by now.
I think it would be possible to shorten our billing cycle by combining steps.	Your billing cycle here is really Stone Age. I can't believe how much time you waste doing all those steps.
I will need to leave early tomorrow afternoon. Would you prefer that I stay late tonight, come in early tomorrow, or make up the time some other way?	I'm leaving early today. I'll make it up.
I must complete this report for Dr. Joyce, but I'll be happy to help you when I'm finished.	How come I get stuck with all the work? I'm not supposed to do filing; you are.

FIGURE 2–6 Comparison of assertive and aggressive behaviors

8:30 AM:	I'm sorry, Dr. Richter, I won't be in today. My daughter has the day off from school.
Day preceding monthly billing:	We can't do the billing tomorrow, Dr. Richter, because I forgot to order return envelopes.
After lunch:	Gee, I'm sorry I'm late, Dr. Richter. The mall was having a great sale.
In conversation with another medical assistant:	Janie, I know I said I would work late for you tonight, but Rob just called to take me out.
In conversation with a patient:	Mrs. Cristini, I'm sorry I didn't mail the insurance forms. I just forgot.

Loyalty

The employees of a medical office must be loyal to the physician and to other staff members. Loyalty carries a responsibility to defend the physician and colleagues tactfully from unworthy remarks from patients, outsiders, and other employees.

When a person works with the public, many opportunities exist for disloyal words and acts. A medical assistant who is in close contact with many different people during the day learns that some people like to gossip, complain, or ask "nosy" questions. A loyal medical assistant remains silent or defends the practice when patients or other employees engage in negative conversation.

Compare the loyal and disloyal medical assistants quoted here:

Loyal Medical Assistant

Situation One

(Listens to patient's question about the physician's recent divorce): "Dr. Levine doesn't tell us about his personal life, so I don't know where his children are living."

Situation Two

(Listens to a fellow employee complain about delay of the lunch hour): "I'm hungry, too, but I don't think it's Dr. Levine's fault that we're behind. Two patients were very late for their appointments."

Disloyal Medical Assistant

Situation One

(Listens to fellow employee complain about the physician's irritability): "I agree. Dr. Levine has been a real pain lately, and I don't like it at all."

Situation Two

(Listens to a sales representative's insult about the office furniture): "Yes, we do have old-fashioned furniture, but between you and me, we'll probably have it another five years. Dr. Levine is a real penny pincher."

Coordinating with the Hospital Staff

Hospital employees you will work with most often include billing personnel regarding fees and codes, scheduling personnel who admit patients, and laboratory technicians who process samples. When working with hospital staff, your communication, cooperation, and assertiveness skills are important. As a representative of the physician, you must make sure the interests of your patients are carefully considered; however, the degree of urgency and the availability of hospital personnel to perform services may at times appear to be at odds with the patient's needs.

Patients being admitted to a hospital present a challenge in terms of coordination, and it is the medical assistant who is primarily responsible for making the arrangements. Because hospitals sometimes have a limited number of beds and can admit only a specified number of patients, the admittance scheduler may have to determine which patients are admitted first. You must learn to discriminate between the patient's need for hospitalization and the hospital's limited access to beds. If you find yourself pushing for a faster hospitalization than the scheduler wishes to provide, review the patient's needs with the physician to determine if you have any flexibility in scheduling. You should possess the human relations skills to reach a solution that satisfies everyone.

When you work with a hospital's billing department, you may be asked to contribute information that helps in coding procedures, treatments, and services. This is an important responsibility that requires diligence, attention to detail, and the desire to provide the best information. The hospital and the doctor's remuneration depends on the responsible handling of billing matters between the medical assistant and the hospital billing assistant.

Coordinating with the hospital staff should be viewed as an opportunity to create and build a good working relationship. An adversarial relationship can develop when the medical assistant and the hospital personnel do not understand the limitations imposed by the systems within which they work. You should guard your relationship carefully because you and the hospital staff are mutually dependent.

Interacting with Other Outside Professionals

As a representative of the practice, the medical assistant has a responsibility to offer a positive image. Rescue teams, independent laboratories, and other allied health units call the medical office for instructions, information, and questions. Often, their first and last contact is the medical assistant, and any opinion they form will be based on this encounter. By using interpersonal skills and good communication, you can make a good first and last impression.

Be courteous, helpful, and cooperative with outside professionals, and they will respond in a like manner. Because you will request the services of these deliverers often and regularly, you should treat them as allies. Although they do not work in a salaried position for the physician, personnel from outside agencies play an important role in the day-to-day activities of the practice. The practice can be adversely affected if related units do not experience cooperation with the medical office assistant.

IN YOUR OPINION

1. What personal characteristics do you think are most important in a medical assistant?
2. Do you think an undependable medical assistant may injure or harm a patient?
3. How would you handle working with a person who is aggressive?

INTERNET ACTIVITY

1. Go to the Web site http://www.aama-ntl.org. Click on "Education and Certification," "Student Information," and "AAMA Role Delineation Study." Read about the Role Delineation Study and identify ways that the chart can be useful to the medical assisting profession.

STUDENT STUDY CHECKLIST

Workbook

1. Complete Chapter 2 exercises in the workbook.
2. Complete Chapter 2 simulations in the workbook that access the CD-ROM in the back of your book.

Administrative Skills CD-ROM

1. Go to the Library on the CD-ROM and play the interactive games for Chapter 2.

REFERENCES

American Association of Medical Assistants. *Medical Assistant Role Delineation Chart*, 2003.

American Association of Medical Assistants. 1998 Medical Assisting Employment Issues Survey.

Fordney, Marilyn T. and Joan J. Follis. *Administrative Medical Assisting*, 4th ed. Clifton Park, NY: Delmar Learning, 1998.

Lindh, Wilburta Q., Marilyn S. Pooler, Carol D. Tamparo. *Administrative Medical Assisting*, 2nd ed. Clifton Park, NY: Delmar Learning, 2002.

CHAPTER ACTIVITIES

PERFORMANCE-BASED ACTIVITIES

1. Summarize the differences between a multiskilled medical assistant and a medical assistant who handles only clinical or administrative medical responsibilities. Using correct grammar and format, compose a short paper expressing your opinion of which type of career is best for you. Give reasons for making this choice.

2. On the following chart, contrast the duties of a medical assistant who works in a solo physician practice to one who works in a large group clinic. What are the advantages and disadvantages of each?

    Solo Practice　　　　　　　　　　　　　*Clinic*

    Advantages

    1. _____
    2. _____
    3. _____

    Disadvantages

    1. _____
    2. _____
    3. _____

3. Evaluate the advantages of credentialing in terms of securing and maintaining a position as a medical assistant.

    Advantages of Credentials

    Getting a job

    1. _____
    2. _____
    3. _____

    Advancing in a career

    1. _____
    2. _____
    3. _____

    Advancing on the career ladder

    1. _____
    2. _____
    3. _____

4. On the following lines, list the personal characteristics of a medical assistant that improve relationships with patients and other staff members. Compare the list with your own traits and develop a plan for improving your relationship characteristics.

Improving Relations

Personal Characteristics Needed   *Do I possess These Traits? (Yes or No)*

1. _____

2. _____

3. _____

4. _____

5. _____

6. _____

My Personal Plan for Improvement

Goal

When

How will I achieve my goal?

1. _____

2. _____

3. _____

4. _____

5. Log on to an Internet search engine and read a recent article on health care reform. Project changes in health care that might influence the number or types of jobs available to medical assistants between now and the year 2010.

Characteristics of Health Care Reform That Might Influence the
Number and Type of Medical Assisting Jobs Available in the Future

Fee-for-Service System   *Managed Care*

EXPANDING YOUR THINKING

1. Describe how you would handle a fellow employee who is showing negative personal characteristics. How would such behavior adversely affect the general morale and productivity of the medical office?

2. What would you do if:

   a. a patient complains because she has been waiting for fifteen minutes to see the doctor.

   b. a patient tells you he heard that the physician and his wife are getting a divorce.

   c. a young mother whose six-week-old baby is ill brings her two-year-old child with her to the medical office. The two-year-old causes problems in the reception area.

   d. an elderly patient tells you that the medicine the physician gave her at her last visit made her sicker.

   e. another medical assistant, the receptionist, complains to you that the physician took too long with a patient, thus delaying the schedule and causing patients to be impatient with the receptionist.

   f. one of the nurses confides in you that she is pregnant and unmarried.

   g. you overhear two physician partners talking about a staff member they plan to replace because the person is tardy too often.

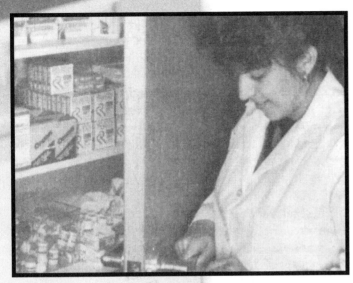

CHAPTER 3

Medical Ethics

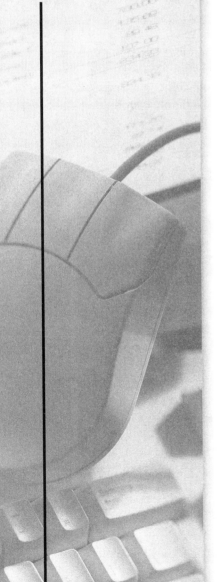

PORTLAND, MAINE

I moved here from Boston about three months ago to begin my career as a medical assistant. Last Friday, Liz, the other medical assistant in our office, invited me to get together for pizza with several MAs from other practices. We had a great time. It was nice to meet some new people and hear about their work.

One of their stories surprised me. Bill had noticed in his pediatric office that some of the patients were scheduling, then canceling and rescheduling their appointments. He thought this seemed strange, but there was always a backlog of patients, so he had no trouble filling their spots. Then he discovered something unusual — the one thing the canceling patients had in common was lack of health insurance.

He and Annie, another MA in the practice, went to the office manager and asked what was going on. She told them she had decided to improve the practice by calling the uninsured patients and telling them the doctor had to reschedule. All the uninsured patients kept getting shuffled to the bottom of the deck.

We all agreed that this was unethical. I pointed out that the AMA Principles of Medical Ethics says doctors should support access to medical care for all people. Annie said she had mentioned the same thing to the office manager, who pointed out that another one of the principles says a physician is free to choose whom to serve.

For the rest of the evening, we talked about this office manager's behavior. I think the doctors should be informed that their office manager is discriminating against the uninsured. But what if the office manager is covering for the doctors who already know about the practice? What if it was their idea? Bill and Annie have to decide what to do.

Erin McClintock
Medical Assistant

PERFORMANCE-BASED COMPETENCIES

After completing this chapter, you should be able to:

1. Identify five important social policy issues related to medicine and discuss the ethical implications of each.
2. Outline procedures for maintaining the confidentiality of computerized records.
3. Create examples of ethical dilemmas that might involve a medical assistant and discuss different ways of resolving them.
4. Compare the value of improved medical technology with the ethical problems that may result.

VOCABULARY

Bioethics Branch of medical ethics concerned with moral issues resulting from high technology and sophisticated medical research. Social issues such as abortion, fetal research, artificial insemination, and euthanasia are important bioethical questions.

Confidentiality Maintaining secrecy about all information regarding patients, including placing the fax machine in a secure location, storing patient files out of the view of everyone except the medical staff, and securing computer records so they are visible only to individuals with a pass code.

DNR Do Not Resuscitate order permits the patient to die without cardiopulmonary resuscitation. This order is commonly used in treating terminally ill or elderly patients.

Durable power of attorney Document that provides broad powers of medical authority to an individual often either a family member or an attorney, who is given legal power to decide what extraordinary measures should be taken with a patient when the patient is too sick to decide. A durable power of attorney usually accompanies a DNR in the patient's hospital record.

Genetic counseling Counseling related to gene disorders. Prospective parents often receive genetic counseling regarding the likelihood of bearing a child with genetic disorders.

Genetic engineering Advanced, complex, and often controversial means of isolating and replacing part or all of a "mutant" gene to reduce or eliminate the chances that a person will develop a particular disease.

Genetics Study of genes and their role in illness and disease. Gene therapy is an exciting, emerging field of medical study because it promises a cure for some illnesses now considered terminal.

Living will Legal document, signed by an individual, that provides precise instructions about the amount of extraordinary care to be delivered in the event of a life-threatening medical situation.

Medical ethics Term applied to the principles governing medical conduct. Medical ethics deals with the relationship of the physician to the patient, the patient's family, fellow physicians, and society.

Medical law Standards set by elected officials in the state and nation. An illegal act is always unethical according to the American Medical Association's Principles of Medical Ethics, but an unethical act may not be illegal.

Patient's Bill of Rights Established by the American Hospital Association in 1972, the Patient's Bill of Rights provides basic guidelines for the care of hospitalized patients.

Patient Self-Determination Act Federal law requiring all hospitals and nursing homes to explain in detail the extraordinary care their state permits. These facilities must alert patients of their right to execute living wills or appoint a health care proxy through a durable power of attorney.

MEDICAL ETHICS AND THE LAW

Medical ethics refers to moral conduct or to what is right or wrong based on religious teachings from the Judeo-Christian, Buddhist, Islamic, and other religious traditions, and the Hippocratic Oath (Figure 3–1). Medical ethics are often stricter than standards set by law, but they are never less strict. Ethical dilemmas in medicine occur when (1) legal enforcement does not appear to provide justice, (2) there is no obvious right or wrong behavior, (3) right behavior appears to have the wrong outcome, and (4) personal sacrifice is the consequence of following one's ideals.

One of the most pressing issues in modern medicine is the question, "What is ethical con-

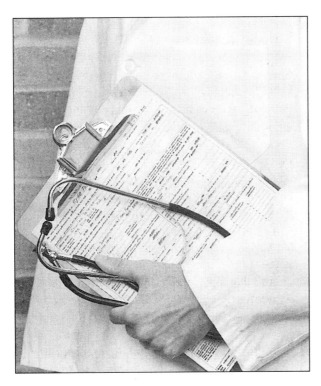

FIGURE 3–1 Medical ethics refers to moral conduct. Codes of ethics remind medical professionals of proper conduct and of their duty to patients.

duct?" Abortions are legal, but are they ethical? Should extraordinary measures be used to prolong life in a newborn with mental and physical deficiencies who is likely to survive only a short time? Will the current experimentation in **genetic engineering** lead to other experimentation that may be unethical? Should extraordinary measures be used for a patient in the last stages of a terminal illness? The greatest minds in the legal and medical profession today are struggling with these and other complex ethical questions.

IN YOUR OPINION

1. Who makes the ultimate decision about the type of care a patient receives? For example, when do you think that a daughter or son has a right to decide what level of care is appropriate for an elderly parent?
2. What are some of the risks of establishing policy statements about patient treatments?
3. How do you feel about physician-assisted suicides?

ETHICS STATEMENTS OF THE MEDICAL ASSOCIATIONS

The system by which a profession sets standards of right and wrong behavior for its members is called its code of ethics. Through these codes, the professions attempt to maintain high standards of competence, to strengthen the relationship among members, and to promote the welfare of the whole community.

Medical professionals, including physicians, nurses, medical assistants, laboratory employees, and others may join an organization in their career field that establishes a statement of ethics or a professional code for its members. Although an organization cannot guarantee that its members will abide by the code, it serves as a reminder of proper conduct. Members who ignore the code and who are reported may be expelled from the organization. Membership does not exempt a member from being charged with a crime if the conduct is both unethical and illegal.

The earliest written code of medical ethics, called the **Code of Hammurabi**, was conceived by the Babylonians around 2000 BC. It was so specific and detailed that it probably would not be applicable today. The Oath of Hippocrates, written by a Greek physician around 400 BC, is a better-known statement of ethical principles that has been accepted throughout history as a standard of behavior for physicians.

The **Oath of Hippocrates** does not impose authority over or prescribe punishment for a physician, but it does give the medical profession a sense of duty to humankind. The oath (1) protects the rights of the patient, (2) appeals to the inner and finer instincts of the physician, and (3) includes rules for the relationship between a doctor and a patient. Many medical students still take the Oath of Hippocrates before graduation and display it in their offices once they begin to practice medicine.

AMA Principles of Medical Ethics

The American Medical Association (AMA) assumes leadership in the United States for setting standards of ethical medical behavior for physicians. In 1847, the AMA adopted its first ethical guidelines, based on a **Code of Medical Ethics** written by Thomas Percival, an English physician, philosopher, and writer.

Ethical behavior, according to the AMA Judicial Council, refers to (1) moral principles and practices, (2) the customs and usage of the medical profession, and (3) matters of medical policy. The word **unethical** is used to describe behavior that fails to conform to ethical standards. When a physician is accused of unethical conduct, the AMA Judicial Council has the authority to dismiss the accusation, issue a warning or criticism, or expel the physician from membership in the Association. However, the AMA does not have the authority to bring legal action against a member for unethical behavior.

The **2003** revision of the **Principles of Medical Ethics** is given in Figure 3–2. These principles speak of human dignity, honesty, responsibility to society, confidentiality, continued study, freedom of choice, and responsibility to an improved community.

American Hospital Association

In recent years, patients have become better informed about medical services. Startling medical breakthroughs are publicized by the media, including daily reports on the progress and prognosis of patients undergoing experimental procedures. Media attention to medicine advises us of many previously unknown options in health care, and an important patients' rights movement has grown out of this newfound knowledge. In the past, the patient rarely questioned a physician's diagnosis, procedure, or treatment, but today's educated patient is not as accepting. By joining together, private citizens have brought significant pressure on the medical community to protect patients' rights. As a result, patients and their families are more actively involved in treatment and in decisions involving surgery than in the past.

This change in patients' attitudes is apparent in the 1993 case of the Lakeberg twins. The twins, conjoined at the chest and sharing a single six-chamber heart, were born in Chicago. Their doctors decided against surgery. However, the parents, Kenny and Reitha Lakeberg, persisted

Principles of Medical Ethics, June 2001

Preamble

The medical profession has long subscribed to a body of ethical statements developed primarily for the benefit of the patient. As a member of this profession, a physician must recognize responsibility to patients first and foremost, as well as to society, to other health professionals, and to self. The following Principles adopted by the American Medical Association are not laws, but standards of conduct which define the essentials of honorable behavior for the physician.

Principles of Medical Ethics

I. A physician shall be dedicated to providing competent medical care, with compassion and respect for human dignity and rights.

II. A physician shall uphold the standards of professionalism, be honest in all professional interactions, and strive to report physicians deficient in character or competence, or engaging in fraud or deception, to appropriate entities.

III. A physician shall respect the law and also recognize a responsibility to seek changes in those requirements which are contrary to the best interests of the patient.

IV. A physician shall respect the rights of patients, colleagues, and other health professionals, and shall safeguard patient confidences and privacy within the constraints of the law.

V. A physician shall continue to study, apply, and advance scientific knowledge, maintain a commitment to medical education, make relevant information available to patients, colleagues, and the public, obtain consultation, and use the talents of other health professionals when indicated.

FIGURE 3–2 Principles of Medical Ethics. (Reprinted with permission from the American Medical Association, copyright 2001) *(continues)*

VI. A physician shall, in the provision of appropriate patient care, except in emergencies, be free to choose whom to serve, with whom to associate, and the environment in which to provide medical care.

VII. A physician shall recognize a responsibility to participate in activities contributing to the improvement of the community and the betterment of public health.

VIII. A physician shall, while caring for a patient, regard responsibility to the patient as paramount.

IX. A physician shall support access to medical care for all people.

Adopted by the AMA's House of Delegates
June 17, 2001

FIGURE 3–2 *(continued)*

in seeking medical intervention and transferred their daughters to Children's Hospital in Philadelphia. One twin died in surgery, as the medical team knew she would. Doctors estimated a survival of only a few months or years for the second twin. Great public controversy erupted over this case. Should the one million dollars spent for an almost hopeless operation have been used on medical care for other sick babies, or for preventive prenatal care for other patients?

Treatment decisions about a parent, spouse, child, or other family member are often difficult to make, considering the technological advances available to prolong life. Medical ethicists are now trying to come to grips with how to help patients better control their own destinies. **Living wills** and durable powers of attorney are other means for patients to make their wishes known.

A living will gives patients the opportunity to state in advance, while they are capable of doing so, what type of medical treatment they would consent to or refuse in the future. Also, known as "advance directives," a living will generally follows a set format of "if/then" statements. The "if" refers to the patient's condition; for example, "if I am terminally ill." The "then" statement involves the treatments the patient would want

withheld or withdrawn, for example, "then I direct my attending physician to withhold or withdraw life-sustaining treatment that serves only to prolong the process of dying." A **durable power of attorney** allows patients to designate a responsible person to make decisions on their behalf. Often a family member or trusted friend is designated. Living wills and durable powers of attorney are discussed further in Chapter 4.

In 1972 the American Hospital Association established a Statement on a **Patient's Bill of Rights**, which has become the standard for the medical community. In 2003 the American Hospital Association revised the Patient's Bill of Rights and renamed it **The Patient Care Partnership**, shown in Figure 3–3. The focus of the Partnership is on:

- high quality medical care
- a clean and safe environment
- patient involvement in his or her personal care
- discussion of the treatment plan with the patient
- gaining complete information from the patient
- protection of the patient's privacy
- help for preparing the patient to leave the hospital
- help with the bill and filing insurance claims

A federal law, the **Patient Self-Determination Act**, requires all hospitals, nursing homes, and health maintenance organizations to ask on admission whether a patient has a living will or a proxy and, if so, to note its provisions in the patient's chart.

American Association of Medical Assistants

Although medical assistants usually are not involved in life-and-death ethical decisions, you will probably confront ethical dilemmas that will cause frustration, anxiety, guilt, and a great deal of soul searching. Should you, for example, allow the mayor or school principal to see the physician ahead of other patients who have been waiting longer? Should you keep silent about foul language another employee uses in front of patients? Should you break a promise to work late when a more appealing option becomes available?

The Patient Care Partnership: Understanding Expectations, Rights, and Responsibilities

When you need hospital care, your doctor and the nurses and other professionals at our hospital are committed to working with you and your family to meet your health care needs. Our dedicated doctors and staff serve the community in all its ethnic, religious, and economic diversity. Our goal is for you and your family to have the same care and attention we would want for our families and ourselves.

The sections below explain some of the basics about how you can expect to be treated during your hospital stay. They also cover what we will need from you to care for you better. If you have questions at any time, please ask them. Unasked or unanswered questions can add to the stress of being in the hospital. Your comfort and confidence in your care are very important to us.

What to Expect During Your Hospital Stay

- **High quality hospital care.** Our first priority is to provide you the care you need, when you need it, with skill, compassion, and respect. Tell your caregivers if you have concerns about your care or if you have pain. You have the right to know the identity of doctors, nurses, and others involved in your care, as well as when they are students, residents, or other trainees.

- **A clean and safe environment.** Our hospital works hard to keep you safe. We use special policies and procedures to avoid mistakes in your care and keep you free from abuse or neglect. If anything unexpected and significant happens during your hospital stay, you will be told what happened and any resulting changes in your care will be discussed with you.

- **Involvement in your care.** You and your doctor often make decisions about your care before you go to the hospital. Other times, especially in emergencies, those decisions are made during your hospital stay. When they take place, making decisions should include:

  ▶ *Discussing your medical condition and information about medically appropriate treatment choices.* To make informed decisions with your doctor, you need to understand several things:
     - The benefits and risks of each treatment.
     - Whether it is experimental or part of a research study.
     - What you can reasonably expect from your treatment and any long-term effects it might have on your quality of life.
     - What you and your family will need to do after you leave the hospital.
     - The financial consequences of using uncovered services or out-of-network providers.
     Please tell your caregivers if you need more information about treatment choices.

  ▶ *Discussing your treatment plan.* When you enter the hospital, you sign a general consent to treatment. In some cases, such as surgery or experimental treatment, you may be asked to confirm in writing that you understand what is planned and agree to it. This process protects your right to consent to or refuse a treatment. Your doctor will explain the medical consequences of refusing recommended treatment. It also protects your right to decide if you want to participate in a research study.

  ▶ *Getting information from you.* Your caregivers need complete and correct information about your health and coverage so that they can make good decisions about your care. That includes:
     - Past illnesses, surgeries, or hospital stays.
     - Past allergic reactions.
     - Any medicines or diet supplements (such as vitamins and herbs) that you are taking.
     - Any network or admission requirements under your health plan.

FIGURE 3–3 The Patient Care Partnership: Understanding Expectations, Rights, and Responsibilities (Reprinted with permission of the American Hospital Association, copyright 2003.) (continues)

▶ *Understanding your health care goals and values.* You may have health care goals and values or spiritual beliefs that are important to your well-being. They will be taken into account as much as possible throughout your hospital stay. Make sure your doctor, your family, and your care team know your wishes.

▶ *Understanding who should make decisions when you cannot.* If you have signed a health care power of attorney stating who should speak for you if you become unable to make health care decisions for yourself, or a "living will" or "advance directive" that states your wishes about end-of-life care, give copies to your doctor, your family and your care team. If you or your family need help making difficult decisions, counselors, chaplains, and others are available to help.

- **Protection of your privacy.** We respect the confidentiality of your relationship with your doctor and other caregivers, and the sensitive information about your health and health care that are part of that relationship. State and federal laws and hospital operating policies protect the privacy of your medical information. You will receive a Notice of Privacy Practices that describes the ways that we use, disclose, and safeguard patient information and that explains how you can obtain a copy of information from our records about your care.

- **Help preparing you and your family for when you leave the hospital.** Your doctor works with hospital staff and professionals in your community. You and your family also play an important role. The success of your treatment often depends on your efforts to follow medication, diet, and therapy plans. Your family may need to help care for you at home.

  You can expect us to help you identify sources of follow-up care and to let you know if our hospital has a financial interest in any referrals. As long as you agree we can share information about your care with them, we will coordinate our activities with your caregivers outside the hospital. You can also expect to receive information and, where possible, training about the self-care you will need when you go home.

- **Help with your bill and filing insurance claims.** Our staff will file claims for you with health care insurers or other programs such as Medicare and Medicaid. They will also help your doctor with needed documentation. Hospital bills and insurance coverage are often confusing. If you have questions about your bill, contact our business office. If you need help understanding your insurance coverage or health plan, start with your insurance company or health benefits manager. If you do not have health coverage, we will try to help you and your family find financial help or make other arrangements. We need your help with collecting needed information and other requirements to obtain coverage or assistance.

While you are here, you will receive more detailed notices about some of the rights you have as a hospital patient and how to exercise them. We are always interested in improving. If you have questions, comments, or concerns, please contact _____.

FIGURE 3–3 *(continued)*

The American Association of Medical Assistants (AAMA) is an association of medical secretaries, receptionists, medical office managers, and back office medical assistants who work with physicians. Recognizing that its members face ethical dilemmas every day, the Association has established a standard of ethics to guide them through their daily activities. The AAMA **Code of Ethics**, a part of the organization's bylaws, enumerates responsibilities of service, confidentiality, honor, improving knowledge, and improving the community. The AAMA Code of Ethics is shown in Figure 3–4.

American Association of Medical Assistants Code of Ethics

The Code of Ethics of AAMA shall set forth principles of ethical and moral conduct as they relate to the medical profession and the particular practice of medical assisting.

Members of AAMA dedicated to the conscientious pursuit of their profession, and thus desiring to merit the high regard of the entire medical profession and the respect of the general public which they serve, do pledge themselves to strive always to:

A. render service with full respect for the dignity of humanity;

B. respect confidential information obtained through employment unless legally authorized or required by responsible performance of duty to divulge such information;

C. uphold the honor and high principles of the profession and accept its disciplines;

D. seek to continually improve the knowledge and skills of medical assistants for the benefit of patients and professional colleagues;

E. participate in additional service activities aimed toward improving the health and well-being of the community.

AAMA Creed

I believe in the principles and purposes of the profession of medical assisting.
I endeavor to be more effective.
I aspire to render greater service.
I protect the confidence entrusted to me.
I am dedicated to the care and well-being of all people.
I am loyal to my employer.
I am true to the ethics of my profession.
I am strengthened by compassion, courage, and faith.

FIGURE 3–4   AAMA Code of Ethics (Copyright by the American Association of Medical Assistants. Revised 2001. Reprinted with permission)

SOCIAL POLICY ISSUES

The term **social policy** refers to rules or guidelines that make the world a better place in which to live. Each nation develops its own social policy by taking into consideration the religion(s) of the people, its culture, history, technology, demographics, ethics, and other related issues. In Hindu societies, for instance, women are required to cover their faces and assume a secondary role, whereas women in the United States play prominent roles in all spheres, with laws protecting their equal status and treatment. Each society must develop its own social policy from the values, customs, and constraints of its circumstances.

Some of the most difficult social policy issues in the United States concern medical ethics. To illustrate, consider these questions. Is artificial insemination by an anonymous donor ethical? Is releasing medical information about some patients ethical, for example, patients who have AIDS and may have infected others in the community? Is prescribing birth control devices for teenagers or performing abortions without their parents' permission ethical for a physician? The answers to these questions are complex and cannot be answered simply. Leaders of the medical profession refer to the ethics codes of their profession, legal statutes, and historical precedents as they try to set guidelines for the future.

The Judicial Council of the American Medical Association publishes an interpretation of the AMA Principles of Medical Ethics called

---

Current Opinions of the Judicial Council of the American Medical Association. Revised periodically to address current thinking or new issues, *Current Opinions* provides direction for physicians about responsible professional behavior. Although *Current Opinions* is not the only guide to ethical professional behavior, it provides a basis for understanding what is considered ethical and unethical in our society. Individual physicians' opinions about social issues may differ from those expressed in *Current Opinions* and are explored in the next section.

Abortion

Today the term **abortion** is commonly used to mean **induced** abortion, the intentional and deliberate ending of a pregnancy. Actually, abortion may be spontaneous or nondeliberate and result from natural causes. The term is properly used to describe any termination of pregnancy during the first three months. Whether induced or spontaneous, abortion results in the death of the embryo or fetus.

Abortion is a controversial subject. Churches have spoken out on this issue; many women's rights groups have taken a strong position in favor of abortion; and others concerned with the moral questions surrounding abortion have debated the issue both publicly and privately. The controversy involves two important questions: (1) Should a woman be permitted to have an abortion by law and under what circumstances? (2) To what extent should the law protect the unborn child's right to life?

The term **pro-choice** describes the position of a person who thinks that abortion is proper under some circumstances and that it should be a matter of personal choice. Pro-choice advocates believe that abortion is acceptable if a woman's life or health will be endangered by pregnancy or if there is evidence that the child will be born with a serious mental or physical defect. They also approve of abortion when pregnancy results from rape.

The terms **pro-life** and antiabortion describe the position of a person who thinks that abortion is always wrong. Groups who are against abortion believe that abortion is an unjustified killing of an unborn child, based on the idea that life begins when sperm fertilizes an egg. They argue that legal abortion will increase the incidence of irresponsible sex and lead to disrespect for human life. Antiabortion activists often picket abortion clinics and are seen on the news for their activities. Physicians and their staffs have been wounded and even murdered by individuals opposed to abortion.

In 1973, the United States Supreme Court legalized abortion performed during the first three months of pregnancy. Provision was made for individual states to regulate abortion to protect the mother's health after the first three months. Physicians are not prohibited from performing an abortion in accordance with good medical practice and under circumstances that do not violate the law. Although you as a medical assistant will not be directly involved in decisions involving abortions for patients, you should be aware of the stress and concern faced by patients and physicians, especially if you work for an obstetrician/gynecologist or a surgeon. You should be supportive, understanding, nonjudgmental, and noncritical of their decisions.

Abuse of Children, Elderly Persons, and Others at Risk

Physicians *are required by law* to report suspected cases of child abuse and abuse of elderly persons or others. This may represent a dilemma for the doctor because the abused person may deny being harmed to protect the abuser. Fearful of losing their parents, children may say their injuries came from a fall or another accident, and, afraid of the repercussions if they confide in the physician, elderly people may deny that their injuries were inflicted by someone else.

The incidence of physical violence is increasing, with many cases going unreported. The law clearly says that suspected cases of abuse must be reported, obligating the physician and medical staff to protect the patient even though the patient may not wish to cooperate.

Allocation of Health Resources

The health care environment is constantly changing because of the introduction of new technologies and treatments. A few years ago, individuals with rare heart, lung or liver disorders were poor candidates for transplant surgery. Now, new antirejection drugs make transplants a safer option.

Because a shortage of donor organs exists, the decision to allocate limited health care resources must be made fairly. According to *Current Opinions*, limited health care resources should be given to patients who are most likely to be treated successfully or who will have long-term benefits. A patient's social worth or relative worth to society should not determine whether the patient is denied or given preference in receiving scarce health care treatment or resources.

Although regional and state organ banks have protocols to determine who is next in line for available organs, controversy still occurs. Pennsylvania's Governor Robert Casey received a heart–liver transplant after being on a waiting list for less than twenty-four hours. Many people, including other potential transplant patients who had been waiting for over a year, questioned whether priority treatment had been given to the governor. The medical center that performed the transplant said no priority was accorded the governor, indicating that Casey's was the first name on a special list for patients needing *dual-organ* transplants. Dual-organ transplants routinely were performed before single-organ transplants at this facility.

The question of rationing health care based on age or overwhelming odds against survival surfaces in such diverse cases as Baby Faye, an infant who received a baboon's heart transplant, and Mrs. Helga Wanglie, an elderly woman with irreversible brain damage. Baby Faye did not live, and Mrs. Wanglie was hospitalized for two years at a cost of $800,000, when the hospital lost a suit to terminate her care. As technology continues to advance and the elderly population of the United States grows, physicians are faced with many legal and ethical questions regarding the allocation of resources and the division of responsibility among individuals, medical institutions, and the government.

In Vitro Fertilization

In vitro fertilization, or fertilization "in glass," is a scientific development in which an egg and sperm unite in an artificial environment outside the woman's body. The embryo is then transferred to the mother's reproductive system to develop normally. In vitro fertilization allows couples to conceive and bear a child even though they previously have been unable to do so. The children conceived in vitro are sometimes called "test tube babies."

Ethical issues surround in vitro fertilization. For example, Mrs. Arlette Schweitzer gave birth to twins fertilized in vitro with her daughter's eggs and her son-in-law's sperm. The daughter had been born without a uterus, and the mother volunteered to carry her daughter's babies to birth. The physician who participates in this method of reproduction is bound by the highest ethical standards and must follow the Principles of Medical Ethics strictly.

Capital Punishment

A physician may have an opinion as an individual about whether capital punishment is right or wrong. However, as a member of a profession dedicated to preserving life, a physician should not participate in an execution although it may be legally authorized by the court system.

Clinical Investigation

New medical procedures and drugs for treating disease and introduced only after many years of clinical research and experimentation on animals. After a procedure or drug is deemed safe for humans, the federal Food and Drug Administration may approve clinical investigation and experimentation of these procedures or drugs on people. With the hope of controlling the AIDS epidemic, many new drugs and treatment protocols have been approved more rapidly than usual.

A physician may participate in clinical investigation and experimentation only if the study is scientifically valid. The physician has a responsibility to keep the patient's interests above the need for research and must not perform any procedures without the consent of the patient or the patient's representative. Participation is considered coercive and involuntary if the participant is pressured into the activity.

Fetal Research Guidelines

Research on fetuses is acceptable when the research is part of a valid scientific study, when it has been preceded by research on animals, and when it involves no monetary payment for fetal material. The issues of fetal research, fetal stem cell research, and fetal cloning go to the heart of medical ethics. On one side of the argument are those who predict that fetal research — particularly stem cell research — holds great promise for the prevention and treatment of previously untreatable diseases. On the other side are those who say that to create life (a fetus) only to destroy it in the name of research is wrong.

Government policy on fetal research, including stem cell research and cloning, has wavered over the years and over presidential administrations, reflecting the difficulty of the ethical issues the research raises. Stem cells, depending on how they are modified, have the potential to grow into any of the body's tissues or organs, and they have the ability to regenerate themselves indefinitely. Although stem cells can be harvested from adult cells, placentas, and umbilical cord remainders, scientists believe that the embryonic cells offer the best hope for useful research results.

Stem cells, it is anticipated, will be used to treat juvenile diabetes, Alzheimer disease, spinal cord injuries, and Parkinson disease, which already is being treated in a process using fetal tissue. Cloning human embryos to create an unlimited supply of stem cells has been discussed, but both public polls and votes in Congress indicate a desire to ban the cloning of human embryos for any purpose.

With one exception, federal funds are prohibited for use in stem cell research. The exception is a pool of sixty genetically diverse stem cell lines being used for medical research, including federally funded research. Because these stem cell lines were created privately from embryos subsequently destroyed, and because they were in existence at the time of the ban on federal funds for genetic research, they are exempt from the ban.

The physician should demonstrate the same degree of care for the fetus in research as for any other fetus in a nonresearch setting. This includes arranging for the proper consent of the mother or the fetus's representative. In treating a fetus, the physician must use the simplest and safest treatment.

Genetic Counseling and Genetic Engineering

Genetics is the study of genes and their role in illness and disease. Over 2,000 genetically related disorders have been identified, including Down syndrome, sickle cell anemia, and multiple sclerosis. Researchers are currently participating in a worldwide gene mapping study. Mapping assists researchers in determining which specific gene is missing or damaged in certain diseases and disorders.

Genetic Counseling

Prospective parents may request screening before conception to predict the likelihood of bearing a child with a gene disorder. After conception, **in utero** gene testing is performed on the fetus through ultrasound, amniocentesis, and fetoscopy to determine the fetus's condition.

Genetic counseling is available to individuals who may be at risk of having certain illnesses or diseases. A Columbia University researcher successfully located the gene that causes Huntington disease. When her mother was diagnosed with Huntington disease, Wexler learned she had a 50% chance of inheriting the illness, which leads to severe brain damage and death. Due largely to Wexler's global research effort, tests are now available to determine whether or not individuals carry the disease.

Physicians engaged in genetic counseling have an ethical responsibility to provide parents with complete information for making a decision about childbearing. This presents a dilemma for physicians who oppose contraception, sterilization, or abortion, because the parents faced with a genetic defect in the fetus may request an abortion based on their own beliefs. In such cases, the physicians may decide to refer the parents to another doctor.

Genetic Engineering

Genetic engineering, or altering of genes, is one of the most advanced, complex, and controversial of all contemporary social issues. In genetic engineering, a gene is isolated and replaced, or its components are rearranged to form a mutant gene that may reduce or eliminate the chances of a person's developing a particular disease. For example, researchers are trying to isolate a gene that appears in people with Alzheimer disease, which affects more than 2.5 million people in the United States. Identification will help scientists find a cure for this disease.

Scientists have also mapped the approximate location of the genes responsible for manic depression, which afflicts two million Americans; neurofibromatosis, or elephant man's disease, which affects 100,000; and cystic fibrosis, the most common genetic killer of young people. Other diseases, such as heart disease, arteriosclerosis, diabetes, and cancer, which are strongly influenced by hereditary or genetic factors, are drawing attention, and many of the mysteries surrounding these diseases will surely be illuminated through genetic study.

One of the most exciting breakthroughs came when scientists finally identified the gene responsible for muscular dystrophy, which affects more than 50,000 Americans. After the initial discovery, it took only nine months for scientists to discover the protein missing in Duchenne, the most common childhood dystrophy. Following these discoveries, there is hope that patients with muscular dystrophy will be cured in the future. For the present, the rate of deterioration caused by the disease will be slowed.

If and when genetic engineering allows gene replacement to treat human disorders, physicians must make certain that Judicial Council guidelines on clinical investigation are followed, along with the usual and customary standards of medical practice. The full procedure should be discussed with the patient and written consent obtained. The procedure must be in conformance with other standards outlined in the Judicial Council.

Organ Transplantation Guidelines

Transplants of the heart, lungs, kidney, and liver offer patients with organ disorders a chance at life that was not possible only a few years ago.

Yet in any organ transplant procedure, the physician must protect the rights of both the donor and the recipient. This means disclosing all known risks and possible hazards to both parties. The physician's interest in advancing scientific knowledge must always be secondary to concern for the patient. A transplant should be performed only if other therapy has been ineffective. When a vital organ is transplanted, the donor's death must be certified by a physician other than the recipient's physician. Because few organs are available and the waiting list is long, tissue matches may identify several patients who are eligible for a transplant. Ethical guidelines with clear priority standards must be followed.

Quality of Life

The physician's primary responsibility always is to do what is best for the patient. Therefore, quality of life becomes an important factor in determining the treatment for newborns with serious deformities, critically injured accident victims, and patients suffering from terminal illnesses. If prolonging life would result in inhumane or unconscionable treatment, withholding or removing life support systems is ethical. Normal care of the patient should be continued after life support systems are removed.

Withholding treatment is such a controversial social issue that physicians and hospitals are reluctant sometimes to remove life support systems. Faced with the threat of a medical malpractice lawsuit, a hospital or physician may take a less controversial course and continue extraordinary treatment although the patient is living in a vegetative state. In recent years, families of permanently comatose patients have gone to court to force hospitals or physicians to withhold treatment. These cases usually take years to settle in court and cost the family a great deal in legal fees and personal agony. Even so, the outcome may be to continue treatment.

One such case in Massachusetts was Brophy vs. New England Sinai Hospital. The patient, Brophy, who was in an irreversible coma after suffering an aneurysm, remained alive only because a feeding tube was surgically implanted in his stomach. The family asked the hospital to remove the tube and let Brophy die; however, the hospital refused, even though the court ruled that this was acceptable procedure. The court acknowledged the hospital's right and allowed the family to move the patient to another facility that eventually granted the family's request.

Society seems to have grown more comfortable with allowing terminally ill patients to die. Since 1986, the AMA holds that discontinuing or withholding life-prolonging medical treatment, including food and water, for the terminally ill is not unethical (Figure 3–5). In June 1987, the New Jersey Supreme Court issued three landmark decisions that allowed patients who were in a near-vegetative state to refuse life-sustaining medical treatment, even though they were neither terminally ill nor elderly. In each case, the patient's request to be allowed to die was granted. State laws vary on providing nutrition to a comatose patient, therefore, court rulings in one state may not apply in other states. Many similar cases have worked through the court systems in other states.

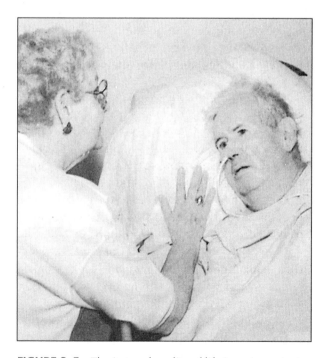

FIGURE 3–5 The issue of quality of life is an important factor in determining who should receive medical resources.

Terminal Illness

Physicians are bound to both prolong life and to relieve suffering. When one obligation conflicts with the other, the physician, patient, and family together may resolve the matter. The physician may not intentionally cause death; but with informed consent, the physician may cause or omit treatment to allow a terminally ill patient to die. Do Not Resuscitate (DNR) orders are common in facilities that treat elderly patients. These orders clearly state that when the lungs or heart stop the patient will not be subjected to an aggressive attempt to restart them. No matter what the age of the patient, the physician is ethically bound to alleviate severe pain for the comfort of the patient. In the recent past, a few doctors gained notoriety by assisting in suicides of terminally ill patients. This type of assistance is viewed as unethical by most U.S. medical professionals, although assisted suicide has been decriminalized in the Netherlands.

HIV Testing

The threat of AIDS has resulted in a requirement that individuals be tested for the human immunodeficiency virus (HIV) before joining the military and as a prerequisite for some jobs. Physicians must ensure that HIV testing is conducted in a way that respects the patient's rights and ensures patient confidentiality. Therefore, they should secure the patient's informed consent before testing for HIV. Because of the need for pretest counseling and the potential consequences of an HIV test on an individual's job, housing, insurability, and social relationships, the consent should be specific for HIV testing. In addition to protecting patients' rights, health care workers also have the responsibility of self-protection. It is recommended that universal precautions and body fluid precautions be used for all patients, especially when the infection status of the patient is unknown.

Drug and Substance Abuse

Drug abuse is one of the major factors in the rise in health care costs because physicians and hospitals must provide long-term care not only to drug addicts, but also to those injured during drug-related crime, the battered spouses of addicts, and babies born to drug-addicted mothers. Drug users are also susceptible to many serious infections, including hepatitis and HIV. Often, other complications develop, requiring surgery. Although drug users are more likely to be infected with HIV and to place the surgical team at great risk, it is considered unethical to deny treatment to a known drug user. In some states, however, denial of treatment may not be illegal.

Physicians are required to follow established standards and should not be influenced by financial considerations in prescribing drugs. Although doctors may dispense drugs from their offices, patients have the right to obtain and fill prescriptions wherever they wish. Physicians, must be alert, however, to the patient who is attempting to obtain prescription drugs for resale, or other illegal use.

Because physicians and their staffs have access to drug and prescription forms, care must be exercised to prevent abuse within the office. Proper inventory control is important in preventing improper usage. Physicians, because of their easy access, are in a tempting position to abuse drugs. Physicians cannot ethically or legally practice medicine while under the influence of a controlled substance, alcohol, or other chemical agent. If, as a medical assistant, you become aware of a substance abuse problem in your office, you must bring the problem to the attention of your employer. If your employer is the abuser, seek advice from an individual whose judgment you respect on how to report the abuse. Many local or state medical societies have resources to assist an impaired physician in receiving help to overcome a substance abuse problem.

Costs

Concern for the patient's care should be the physician's primary consideration. Nevertheless, the physician may participate in policy-making decisions concerning health care costs, either as a member of a professional group or as a private citizen. Health care reforms are being discussed widely by physicians who anticipate that their incomes will be affected.

Unnecessary Services and Worthless Services

Physicians cannot ethically provide or prescribe unnecessary services or treatments in unnecessary facilities. The physician is compelled to ask privately: "Is this additional diagnostic test (which adds to my practice's income) necessary for my patient's treatment?" "Does this patient really need to be rechecked in two weeks (when I will receive an additional fee)?" "Should I transfer this patient to the nursing home (which I partially own) or is treatment at home sufficient?" Furthermore, a physician should not provide services that reputable physicians would regard as worthless. Such services might include knee surgery for a patient whose knee will heal if left alone or eye surgery for a patient who has no hope of recovering sight.

As a medical assistant, usually you will not have the medical background or knowledge to determine when a physician is supplying unnecessary or worthless services. However, if clear-cut patterns of unethical service exist, you probably can detect them. For example, the physician who routinely sends patients for a second opinion to a relative who is also a physician may be crossing the boundaries of ethical behavior. A physician who recalls patients several times for minor medical problems may be increasing the practice's income at the patients' expense.

Providing unnecessary services is not only unethical but also may be illegal. The federal government is concerned about the amount of fraud and abuse in the health care system. According to one General Accounting Office report, health care fraud and abuse account for more than $10 billion a year. Under the False Claims Act, it is illegal to bill for services not provided, overbill for the care provided, or bill for "assembly line" care, such as performing a urinalysis for every patient. Under the antikickback statute, physicians cannot legally receive any type of payment, in cash or in kind, for the referral of a patient. In the past, the physician usually was the only person held responsible for fraud or abuse. Today, the medical assistant who knowingly and willingly participates in providing unnecessary services is also at risk to be prosecuted.

1. After freezing the husband's sperm, a couple decides to divorce. The wife sues to maintain the sperm, as she would like to become pregnant in the future. The husband countersues to destroy the sperm, citing legal and financial obligations. Who do you think is right? Why?
2. A wealthy person creates an infomercial for cable TV to plead for a liver transplant for his small son. Parents in another city offer to donate the liver of their child who has been killed in an automobile accident. Should the child of the wealthy parents receive the liver ahead of other children who may need it more?
3. Under what circumstances do you think patients should be tested for HIV?

COMPUTERS AND ETHICS

Computer technologies allow medical information to be accumulated in large quantities and retrieved quickly; however, the potential for unauthorized access to patient information is increased. Protection of patient confidentiality in a computerized world is a growing concern (Figure 3–6).

Confidentiality and Computers

Computer technology poses a threat to patient confidentiality unless medical records are properly secured. Computer "hackers," or people with the ability to break into a computer's files from a remote location, have invaded the central storage of some of the country's most sophisticated computer installations. Although many of these hackers are amateurs testing their ability to break into a computer's code, their activities are illegal and should be reported when discovered. When a hospital computer is invaded and the hacker looks at medical records, patient privacy is violated. Because medical records show personal as well as medical information, a hacker can gain a variety of confidential information. This kind of crime is not yet widespread, however, computer piracy offers some fairly dramatic opportunities for the hacker with a vivid imagination. Consider

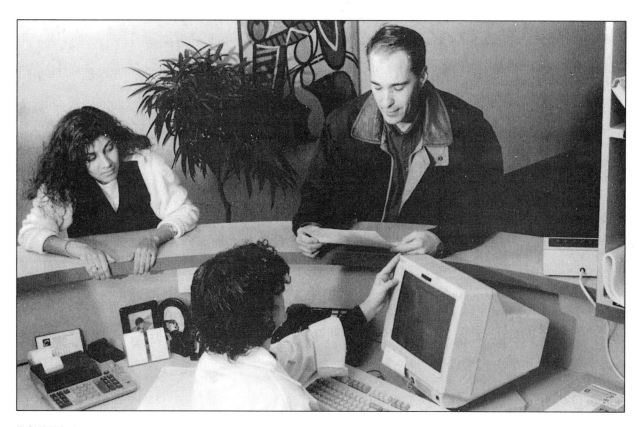

FIGURE 3–6 Keeping computer records secure is essential for patient confidentiality.

the criminal who wishes to use negative or potentially injurious medical information to bribe a judge undergoing treatment for alcoholism or to bribe a political candidate who had psychiatric treatment in the past.

If you are working in a large computer center and you discover suspicious activity within patient records or accounts, you must report your suspicions immediately to the person in authority. After you have worked in a medical facility for several months, you will learn the charges for certain procedures and treatments. An account that has been changed to reflect lower charges will catch your attention and should be reported. For example, several incor-

rect charges in the same patient's account over a period of time should raise your suspicions. On a simpler note, patient confidentiality is threatened when a medical secretary leaves the desk but allows the computer screen to remain visible to patients or office visitors.

AMA Position on Computer Security

The AMA has adopted guidelines for patient records in computer databases. Although these guidelines focus on computer services, many are relevant for private practices as well. AMA guidelines are given in Figure 3–7.

E-5.07 Confidentiality: Computers.

The utmost effort and care must be taken to protect the confidentiality of all medical records, including computerized medical records.

The guidelines below are offered to assist physicians and computer service organizations in maintaining the confidentiality of information in medical records when that information is shared in computerized data bases:

(1) Confidential medical information should be entered into the computer-based patient record only by authorized personnel. Additions to the record should be time and date stamped, and the person making the additions should be identified in the record.

(2) The patient and physician should be advised about the existence of computerized data bases in which medical information concerning the patient is stored. Such information should be communicated to the physician and patient prior to the physician's release of the medical information to the entity or entities maintaining the computer data bases. All individuals and organizations with some form of access to the computerized data bases, and the level of access permitted, should be specifically identified in advance. Full disclosure of this information to the patient is necessary in obtaining informed consent to treatment. Patient data should be assigned to a security level appropriate for the data's degree of sensitivity, which should be used to control who has access to the information.

(3) The physician and patient should be notified of the distribution of all reports reflecting identifiable patient data prior to distribution of the reports by the computer facility. There should be approval by the patient and notification of the physician prior to the release of patient-identifiable clinical and administrative data to individuals or organizations external to the medical care environment. Such information should not be released without the express permission of the patient.

(4) The dissemination of confidential medical data should be limited to only those individuals or agencies with a bona fide use for the data. Only the data necessary for the bona fide use should be released. Patient identifiers should be omitted when appropriate. Release of confidential medical information from the data base should be confined to the specific purpose for which the information is requested and limited to the specific time frame requested. All such organizations or individuals should be advised that authorized release of data to them does not authorize their further release of the data to additional individuals or organizations, or subsequent use of the data for other purposes.

FIGURE 3–7 AMA position on computer-based records (Reprinted with permission from the American Medical Association Web site, copyright 2002.) *(continues)*

(5) Procedures for adding to or changing data on the computerized data base should indicate individuals authorized to make changes, time periods in which changes take place, and those individuals who will be informed about changes in the data from the medical records.

(6) Procedures for purging the computerized data base of archaic or inaccurate data should be established and the patient and physician should be notified before and after the data has been purged. There should be no mixing of a physician's computerized patient records with those of other computer service bureau clients. In addition, procedures should be developed to protect against inadvertent mixing of individual reports or segments thereof.

(7) The computerized medical data base should be on-line to the computer terminal only when authorized computer programs requiring the medical data are being used. Individuals and organizations external to the clinical facility should not be provided on-line access to a computerized data base containing identifiable data from medical records concerning patients. Access to the computerized data base should be controlled through security measures such as passwords, encryption (encoding) of information, and scannable badges or other user identification.

(8) Back-up systems and other mechanisms should be in place to prevent data loss and downtime as a result of hardware or software failure.

(9) Security: (a) Stringent security procedures should be in place to prevent unauthorized access to computer-based patient records. Personnel audit procedures should be developed to establish a record in the event of unauthorized disclosure of medical data. Terminated or former employees in the data processing environment should have no access to data from the medical records concerning patients.

(b) Upon termination of computer services for a physician, those computer files maintained for the physician should be physically turned over to the physician. They may be destroyed (erased) only if it is established that the physician has another copy (in some form). In the event of file erasure, the computer service bureau should verify in writing to the physician that the erasure has taken place. (IV) Issued prior to April 1977; Updated June 1994 and June 1998.

FIGURE 3–7   (continued)

THE MEDICAL ASSISTANT'S ROLE IN ETHICAL ISSUES

Medical assistants who suspect a physician of unethical behavior face a difficult dilemma. To accuse the physician will almost certainly result in job termination, and the accusation may be inappropriate and unfair, especially if it is based on a difference in philosophy of what is ethical. After you begin work as a medical assistant you should not make negative statements about a physician's ethics unless you have verifiable evidence of unethical behavior. If you and the physician disagree on what is ethical, you should look for employment with another practice. If, however, you possess information that conclusively shows unethical behavior, you should report your concerns to another physician who knows the local customs for policing physicians' ethics. Because you can destroy the reputation of a physician by assuming knowledge you do not have or interpreting medical situations incorrectly, you should allow another professional with the appropriate medical background to pursue the matter.

Appropriate Patient Charges

You will also be faced with ethical issues not directly related to the social issues discussed in this chapter. For example, physicians often charge patients for long-distance telephone calls related to a case, such as a consultation with a physician in another city or a return call to a patient who is out of town. You must make sure that nonpatient-related long-distance calls are not charged to patient accounts.

Physicians' fees represent another ethical area involving the medical assistant. Most physicians charge for office visits based on the amount of time spent with the patient. Some physicians identify the type of visit on the patient's charge slip, but others expect the medical assistant to complete this information based on the reason for the visit and the medical assistant's knowledge of the physician's procedures. You may face ethical dilemmas from time to time about the correct charge. If so, make sure that both the patient and the practice are treated fairly.

Ethical issues that are harder to describe but just as important to the medical assistant involve sensitivity to people's feelings. Courteous behavior toward elderly, handicapped, or anxious patients; honesty with other staff members; respect for patients' privacy when undressing, and related issues occur almost daily. No one can tell you how to act in each situation; however, your personal sense of ethics and service to your profession can help you act responsibly. A medical assistant's ethics must be impeccable because nothing can destroy a career faster than the appearance of unethical behavior.

Confidentiality

Maintaining confidentiality of patient information is one of the biggest challenges for any medical office, and the problem grows more complex in a small town or when the medical staff and patients live in the same neighborhood. In upcoming chapters, you will learn about the legal issues of confidentiality, about maintaining private patient records, and about ensuring confidentiality of information when filing insurance claims.

As a medical assistant, you must ensure patient confidentiality by keeping to yourself any personal or medical information you learn at work. Your obligation is legal as well as moral, and you could be charged with breach of confidentiality if you share information that becomes part of a court proceeding.

A good rule of thumb is: Share patient information with other staff members only when doing so will provide better health services for the patient.

One potential source for releasing information unintentionally is over the telephone. The following guidelines will help you circumvent this troublesome problem.

- Always take patient phone calls in private, away from other patients.
- Close the doors to open hallways when taking a patient call.
- If your voice projects, lower your volume when other patients are nearby.
- Do not use a patient's name during a telephone conversation if it might be heard by passers-by.

INTERNET ACTIVITIES

1. Log on to http://www.cnn.com. When the CNN home page appears, select HEALTH from the index box. After the health screen appears, enter the Keyword Bioethics. Select from the list of articles that appear, and critique an article of your choice about bioethics. Indicate the issues on which you agree or disagree with the author.
2. Go to the Journal of Medical Bioethics Web site at http://jme.bmjjournals.com. Choose the Top 10 Papers and read about an ethics issue of particular interest to you. Identify one aspect of the issue that is probably unknown to the general population and write a newspaper-type article on the issue.

STUDENT STUDY CHECKLIST

Workbook

1. Complete Chapter 3 exercises in the workbook.
2. Complete Chapter 3 simulations in the workbook that access the CD-ROM in the back of the book.

Administrative Skills CD-ROM

1. Go to the Library on the CD-ROM and play the interactive games for Chapter 3.
2. Go to the Library on the CD-ROM and complete the crossword puzzle.

REFERENCES

A Patient's Bill of Rights. Chicago, IL: American Hospital Association, 1992.

American Association of Medical Assistants Bylaws. Chicago: American Association of Medical Assistants.

American Association for Medical Transcription Bylaws. Modesto, CA: American Association for Medical Transcription.

American Journal of Bioethics, vol. 2, no. 1, entire issue. University of Pennsylvania Center for Bioethics and the MIT press, April 2002.

Current Opinions of the Judicial Council of the American Medical Association, Chicago: American Medical Association, 2002.

Journal of Medical Ethics, April, 2002 entire issue. BMJ Publishing of the BMA.

Policies of the American Medical Association related to computer-based records and electronic medical records, AMA Web site.

Spice, Byron. "Ethics Dilemma Restricts Embryonic Stem Cell Research." *Pittsburgh Post-Gazette,* March 26, 2001.

White House Press Release, remarks of the president on stem cell research, Office of the Press Secretary, August 9, 2001, The Bush Ranch, Crawford, TX.

CHAPTER ACTIVITIES

PERFORMANCE-BASED ACTIVITIES

1. Choose a social policy issue you believe will probably become more important in the future. Debate the issue with another member of the class. Name the point of view you will debate, either pro or con, and list in the chart below the points you will make.

Ethical Issues Debate

Position Statement   Points To Be Made
"I believe . . .   "Why . . .

1. _____
2. _____
3. _____
4. _____
5. _____
6. _____

2. Study a report on genetic engineering research from a general news periodical published within the last two years. Summarize the research and discuss the social, ethical, and medical implications.

Genetic Engineering Research

Name of Report _____

Publication _____ Date _____ Page _____

Research Summary

Implications

   Social

   Ethical

   Medical

3. Develop a set of confidentiality guidelines to be given to interns who work for a medical practice. Think about the challenges that an intern might face, such as wishing to share information with friends. Write the guideline, then prepare one or two sentences to explain to the intern why the guideline is important.

Confidentiality Guidelines for Medical Assistant Interns

Guideline 1: _____

_____

Guideline 2: _____

_____

Guideline 3: _____

_____

Guideline 4: _____

_____

Guideline 5: _____

_____

4. Develop an ethical situation in which a medical assistant might become involved, and role-play the scene with another class member.

EXPANDING YOUR THINKING

1. In what situations do you think violating patient confidentiality is the ethical choice?

2. A prison psychiatrist informs the police chief of a parolee's hometown that she thought the parolee represented a danger to society. Do you agree with this action? Why or why not?

3. In what ways might your professional ethics conflict with your personal beliefs?

4. A member of the medical staff is an avid gambler and has been known to incur large gambling debts. In what ways might this situation create a professional dilemma?

5. A neighbor of yours is a patient of your practice. A mutual friend has noticed that this person has recently lost a great deal of weight and asks you if this person has AIDS. What do you reply?

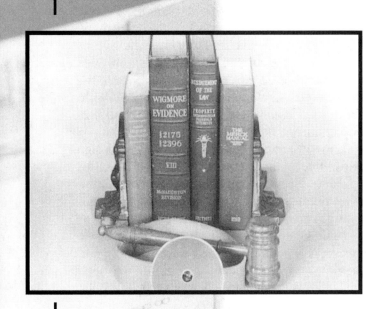

CHAPTER 4

Medical Law

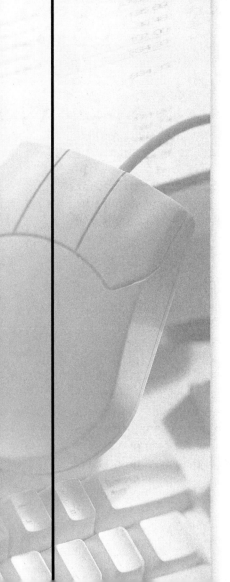

KANSAS CITY, KANSAS

This is a large and successful internal medical practice where things often get hectic. Even though circumstances and instinct tell me to hurry, I've learned to slow down. When I rush, it's easier to make mistakes. That's what happened to Kathy, one of the MAs who works here.

About a month ago, Carlos Hernandez came in with a bad rash on his back. The doctor treated the rash, told Mr. Hernandez to return in two weeks for a follow-up appointment, and asked Kathy to give the patient some samples of a medication to treat the rash. In her rush to take care of Mr. Hernandez and move on to a half dozen other tasks, Kathy pulled the wrong bottled lotion and gave it to him.

Two days later Mr. Hernandez was back. His back was blistered and peeling, and he was in pain. The doctor took one look at the wound and asked Mr. Hernandez to call home and ask his wife to read the label of the medication we had dispensed. Realizing her mistake, Kathy turned red, began to cry, and apologized profusely. The doctor apologized to Mr. Hernandez also and then walked to the supply room to personally pull the correct medication.

Now Mr. Hernandez's back has healed, but it is scarred, and he is threatening a lawsuit. He doesn't think he should have to pay for the treatment. That seems reasonable since he just did what the medical office said, but he also wants to collect for pain and suffering.

The doctor seems to have done the right thing; he ordered the correct medication and gave appropriate instructions. That leaves Kathy at fault. Chances are Mr. Hernandez will sue the practice and the doctor, and he may name Kathy in the suit. She is terribly concerned that she will spend years paying for a plastic surgery bill. I'm not sure what will happen, but

I know everyone in the office is on high alert to give patients the right medications. In this business, mistakes can be costly.

Hector Rabine
Medical Assistant

PERFORMANCE-BASED COMPETENCIES

After completing this chapter, you should be able to:
1. Determine needs for documentation and report and document accurately.
2. Advise patients on their rights regarding advance directives.
3. Trace a malpractice claim from its inception through settlement or trial.
4. Use appropriate guidelines when releasing records or information.
5. Follow policy for disposing of controlled substances.
6. Use appropriate guidelines in terminating medical treatment by means of a withdrawal letter.

VOCABULARY

Advance directives Patient's wishes regarding future treatment if the patient is incapacitated.
Civil law Rights and obligations that people have toward one another, usually concerned with a wrong or injury one person inflicts on another.
Criminal law Rights and obligations people have toward society.
Drug schedules Categories of drugs divided according to their potential for abuse.
Good Samaritan laws Laws that protect the physician and other health care professionals who assist people in unusual emergency situations.
Informed consent Law that states a patient must be given medical information about risk before undergoing a procedure.
Malfeasance Wrongful treatment of a patient.
Misfeasance Lawful treatment performed in the wrong way.
Nonfeasance Failure to act when duty requires.

Medical law is becoming increasingly complicated and controversial as technology advances. Physicians today can offer treatments that only five years ago were considered impossible. We learn of organ transplants, experimental drugs, and newly developed medical procedures almost daily. But, because not all medical breakthroughs are in humanity's best interests, standards of acceptable practice must be established and legally enforced to protect patients. Genetic engineering, for example, is considered by many experts to be a positive step toward finding cures for many diseases; in the wrong hands, however, gene mutations could cause great damage to the human race. As evidence of this, during World War II Adolf Hitler tried to create a super race of people through genetic engineering. Fortunately, Nazi scientists did not have the ability to design their perfect human being, nor do we have this capability for the time being. Researchers can, however, alter a gene's characteristics. Both public and for-profit organizations are working as fast as they can to complete the human genome map, which is the first step toward more far-reaching genetic science. Therefore, we need laws to control potentially dangerous genetic engineering experimentation. We also need laws to protect us from negligent or unscrupulous physicians.

STATE MEDICAL PRACTICE ACTS

Medicine, nursing, dentistry, and other professional health care occupations are regulated by laws in the fifty states. These laws, known collectively as the Medical Practice Acts, specify the training set standards of competence, identify the tasks, and stipulate the category of patients that doctors, nurses, and others may treat. Licensure, license renewal, and license revocation or suspension are also established by the states. Because each state sets its own laws, the standards vary from state to state. As a medical assistant, you need to know about the laws of the state in which your practice is located, so you can coordinate the license renewals for the professionals with whom you work. For example, if you previously worked as a medical assistant in California and then moved to Iowa, you cannot assume the licensing requirements for physicians are the same in both states. Your employer will rely on you to be knowledgeable about the laws of your state.

Licensure

Physicians, nurses, dentists, pharmacists, and certain other health care professionals must be licensed to practice their professions (Figure 4–1). Two primary reasons exist for licensing: (1) to protect the public, and (2) to protect the profession. A license means that the practitioner has met some minimum standard and is qualified and capable of providing medical service to the public. Bogus or phony physicians are uncommon; however, occasionally we hear stories about physicians who have continued to practice medicine after losing their licenses. When these people are caught, they are charged with a crime and are usually fined and jailed. Reputable physicians usually frame their licenses and display them prominently in their offices. Although licensing requirements are not uniform across the country, there are considerable similarities. Typical requirements for physicians include graduation from an accredited medical school, completed residency, good moral character, and successful completion of the Federal Licensing Examination. Each state's medical board sets licensing requirements, approves and administers the written examination, and issues licenses

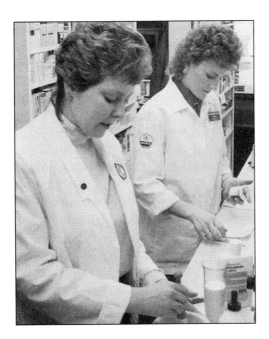

FIGURE 4–1 Pharmacists are among the health care professionals who must be licensed to practice their profession. (Courtesy of the Michigan Pharmacists Association and the Michigan Society of Pharmacy Technicians)

to physicians, nurses, dentists, pharmacists, and other specified by the board. To practice in another state, a medical practitioner must meet its requirements and be granted a license. Reciprocity agreements between states with the same licensing requirements allow licenses to be granted to residents who move from one state to the other. Licensing is not required for medical assistants.

Medical practitioners who work for a federal government medical unit are not required to obtain a license from the state in which they practice. For example, an Army, Navy, or Air Force physician who practices in many different states during the course of a military career does not need a license from each state. Nor is a license required for a research physician who does not practice medicine.

Renewal of License

Periodic renewal of a practitioner's license is required by all states. For physicians, successfully completing a minimum amount of continuing education is necessary before a license can be renewed. Continuing education requirements may be met through course work, professional reading, teaching, and self-instruction.

A physician may ask the medical assistant to maintain a file that documents the necessary professional activity for license renewal. This continuing education file should be current and well organized. If this is your responsibility as a medical assistant, you should be sure that all certificates, receipts, and other documents related to professional activity are clearly identified and stored together.

Revocation or Suspension of License

The privilege of practicing medicine may be taken away from a physician who (1) is convicted of a crime, (2) engages in unprofessional conduct, or (3) is repeatedly negligent because of personal or professional incapacity. Crimes committed by unethical physicians include overprescribing or abusing narcotic drugs, sexually abusing patients, and engaging in other illegal activities. In a Pennsylvania case, a physician was charged with repeatedly fondling female patients while they were under mild anesthesia. After the first patient made a charge against the physician, others stepped forward to make the same claim. The case was proved, and the physician was fined, imprisoned, and his license suspended.

Physicians who practice obstetrics and gynecology are especially vulnerable to charges of sexual misconduct, and they take preventive measures so that their examinations cannot be misinterpreted or misrepresented. There are two reasons an obstetrician/gynecologist (OB/GYN), either male or female, calls a female nurse to the examining room during a woman's pelvic examination: (1) The patient is less likely to be embarrassed with another woman in the room, and (2) The patient will have difficulty proving sexual misconduct by the physician if a witness was present.

Unprofessional conduct refers to falsification of records, splitting fees with another physician for patient referrals, accepting gifts from pharmacies for referring patients, and engaging in advertising that misleads the patient, for example, advertising cosmetic surgery that promises certain results. A physician may be incapacitated personally or professionally because of alcohol or drug abuse, a physical injury, mental instability, or insanity. As a medical assistant, you are responsible for reporting to the licensing agency any physician who cannot function because of drug or alcohol addiction or any other problem that affects his competency.

A physician's license cannot be revoked or suspended without due process of law. This means that the state board bringing the charge must give the physician adequate notice of the charge, provide sound evidence for the charge, and allow a hearing at which the physician may be represented by legal counsel. The board then investigates and dismisses the charge or prosecutes the physician and makes a judgment.

Because nurses, medical assistants, and other allied health professionals, unlike physicians, are usually full-time employees, they do not have the same rights of due process as physicians unless specified in an employment contract. If no employment contract exists, they may be discharged for "good cause," "bad cause," or "no cause at all." Their employment is "at will,"

which means that the person can be terminated by the employer without reason. An employee who thinks that his or her termination is due to race or sex discrimination can file a complaint with the appropriate state or federal agency.

IN YOUR OPINION

1. What improprieties or crimes committed by your employer would cause you to bring charges?
2. What are the advantages and disadvantages of individual states developing their own licensing guidelines?
3. What conflicts of emotion do you think a medical assistant working for an alcoholic or drug-addicted physician might experience?

THE PHYSICIAN AND THE LAW

Litigation has become an increasingly popular method of resolving conflicts between patients and their physicians. Physicians in high-risk specialties are either quitting their practices or reducing their patient load to guard against the possibility of being sued.

Physicians must be concerned about a variety of legal matters. As a medical assistant, you can assist the physician by (1) becoming familiar with the laws of your state; (2) compiling a file of all the dates for federal, state, and local forms, including license renewal; (3) maintaining complete and up-to-date patient records, and (4) keeping a proper inventory of all drugs received and dispensed (Figure 4–2).

Federal, state, and local laws establish the rules by which our society is governed. The law outlines a person's rights and obligations and sets penalties for those who violate the rules. The law is divided into two parts: (1) private or civil law, which is concerned with the rights and obligations people have toward one another, for example, a physician's responsibility to treat patients according to accepted procedures; and (2) public or criminal law, which refers to the rights and obligations people have to live within the laws of society.

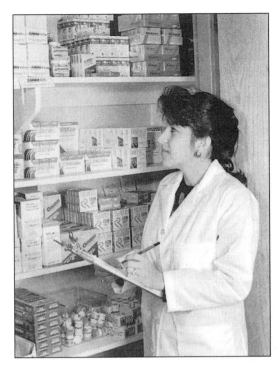

FIGURE 4–2 A medical assistant may be responsible for keeping an inventory of the drugs received and dispensed.

Civil Law

Most legal cases involving physicians are based on civil law. The branch of civil law that usually applies to medical cases is called **tort law**. It is concerned with a wrong or injury one person inflicts on another and the remedies available to the injured party.

A physician who is suspected of violating the law is subject to civil or criminal prosecution or both. If the physician is found guilty in a civil case, the physician or the physician's insurance company will likely have to pay monetary damages. For a criminal offense, the physician may be imprisoned.

Medical Malpractice/Professional Liability Insurance

A patient who thinks that a physician was negligent in diagnosing or treating an illness or accident may file a medical malpractice claim and, if the case is proved, recover monetary damages from the physician or the physician's insurance carrier. The number of malpractice, or professional liability, suits against physicians has risen dramatically since the 1960s, especially for those in high-risk specialties. The number of claims has risen more than 100% in the last decade.

Large monetary damages awarded in some cases have driven up the cost of malpractice insurance for physicians. The cost of insurance coverage at $10,000 to $100,000 per year is so prohibitive that some physicians have changed their specialty to one with a lower risk of being sued. Other doctors have become self-insured, meaning they cover their own malpractice court awards. This is highly risky. Obstetricians and gynecologists, for example, are often the target of malpractice lawsuits, and some have stopped delivering babies. Many insurance companies now refuse to offer medical malpractice coverage because of the large payments they are required to make when a jury has decided against the insured physician.

Medical professional liability is estimated to account for more than 15% of total expenditures for physicians' services. These costs include professional liability insurance premiums, costs of defensive medicine, such as additional x-rays, and losses not covered by liability insurance. Ultimately, these costs must be passed along to the patient in the form of higher fees for physicians' services.

A survey of physicians by the American Medical Association (AMA) found that one-third of U.S. physicians identify professional liability as medicine's primary problem. Physicians are practicing **defensive medicine** in an attempt to prevent lawsuits. In cases where one laboratory or diagnostic test might have been required previously, a physician may now ask for additional tests to confirm a diagnosis or treatment. A physician may ask a patient to return for additional visits to follow the progress of recovery. Each additional test, return visit, or other defensive measure increases the patient's medical costs. The AMA, along with local medical associations, private physicians, and other groups concerned about the spiraling cost of medical care, are seeking solutions to the problem of professional liability.

Medical Malpractice Claims

The concept of **negligence** is basic to any medical malpractice claim. The patient or other plaintiff must prove that the plaintiff was harmed in some way by the physician's or other health practitioner's failure to act. The plaintiff must prove failure to meet two standards of care: (1) what is considered normal care in the patient's geographic area, and (2) the care that another physician or health care professional would have shown in the same circumstances.

Negligence may be claimed when an incorrect procedure is performed (**malfeasance**), when a mistaken diagnosis is made, or when an improper treatment has been used (**misfeasance**). A patient may also claim negligence when a condition calls for treatment that the physician failed to provide; for example, when a medical condition is serious enough to warrant a specialist's advice which the primary care physician failed to get (**nonfeasance**). The following cases are examples of negligence.

Malfeasance

Dr. Sanchez, a radiologist, fails to see a tumor on a patient's liver while reading the patient's ultrasound. He reports to the primary care physician that the ultrasound shows no irregularities. When the patient continues to complain of pain, the primary care physician conducts further tests that reveal a tumor. Even after surgery, the patient does not regain his health and dies two years later. The family, which was harmed by the death, has legal grounds for a malpractice (tort) claim against Dr. Sanchez.

Misfeasance

Holly David, a high school star basketball player, breaks her arm in a fall during a game. Dr. Chung, an orthopedist, sets the arm and puts it in a cast. When the cast is removed, Holly discovers that she can no longer shoot baskets successfully. An x-ray reveals that the break healed improperly because Dr. Chung did not set the arm correctly. Holly is harmed because she can no longer qualify for a four-year basketball scholarship to a major university. She has grounds for a malpractice suit against Dr. Chung.

Malpractice by the Physician's Staff

Physicians are liable and can be sued for the actions of their medical employees while the employees are on duty. For this reason, most physicians carry, as a part of their professional liability insurance, additional coverage for the clinical and office staff. The following case illustrates an employee's action for which the physician would be held responsible.

A patient, Mr. Senker, comes to the office for treatment of a gash in his forehead. The physician treats the head and instructs the medical assistant to give the patient a sample of a particular ointment. The medical assistant picks up the wrong sample and gives it to Mr. Senker who uses the sample on his head for two weeks. Mr. Senker's head becomes inflamed and infected. When he returns to the physician in great pain, the medical assistant's mistake is discovered. As a result of the error, Mr. Senker undergoes plastic surgery and several weeks of additional pain. He has a tort claim against the physician because he suffered a wrong or injury as a result of the medical assistant's mistake. The medical assistant can also be sued, but since the physician's assets and insurance coverage are likely to be greater than the medical assistant's, the physician will bear the brunt of the suit.

A medical assistant or other employee of a medical office should never rely fully on the physician's insurance to provide for professional liability coverage because all employees are held responsible for their own professional conduct. A medical assistant, nurse, laboratory technician, medical technologist, or other employee can be held personally or jointly liable with the physician for medical malpractice. An especially dangerous situation exists when an employee is charged with practicing medicine without a license. This can happen innocently when an employee, who desires to be helpful, suggests medication or treatment for a patient. If the patient becomes ill or harmed as a result of the advice, the employee can be sued, both as an employee of the physician and as an individual. It is important, therefore, that you as a medical assistant never give the impression you are recommending a treatment or a medication. The following example illustrates a case in which a well-meaning medical assistant can be sued for practicing medicine without a license.

A young, inexperienced mother calls the pediatrician's office to ask the doctor about her son's high fever following the flu. When she discovers the physician is out of the office, she asks the medical assistant who answers the telephone what she should do. The medical assistant, who knows the physician usually prescribes aspirin or acetaminophen to reduce fever, suggests that the mother give one of the two medications to her son. When the mother asks if either medication will be all right, the medical assistant replies, "Yes." A week later the mother calls the office crying that her son is experiencing a seizure following severe vomiting in the morning. After giving the child emergency treatment, the physician diagnoses Reye's syndrome, a condition sometimes attributed to taking aspirin following the flu. The medical assistant and the physician can be sued because the medical assistant practiced medicine without a license by recommending that the child be given aspirin.

To be fully protected for professional liability, you should purchase a professional liability insurance policy as soon as you become employed in a medical office. This insurance can be purchased from the American Association of Medical Assistants (AAMA) for approximately $100 annually; the alternative, no protection, can cost thousands of dollars if you are sued.

Preventing Malpractice Claims

The best way to protect against medical malpractice lawsuits is to avoid situations that can lead to malpractice charges. The physician, nurses, medical assistant, and other medical staff should understand the two primary methods of reducing malpractice claims: **informed consent** and accurate medical records.

Informed Consent

A patient may consent to procedures for diagnosis and treatment, which relieves the physician of liability if the procedure fails or causes damage. A patient's consent may be oral, written, or implied by the actions of the patient, although most physicians and hospitals require the patient to sign a consent form before undergoing procedures that are considered risky in any way.

Informed consent, as created by the courts, is a doctrine stating that before consenting to undergo a procedure, a patient must be told

(1) the reason for the procedure, (2) how the procedure will be performed, (3) the risks to the patient, including the possibility of bodily harm or death, (4) the benefits of the procedure, and (5) possible problems after recovery. The assumption is that before a patient can consent to a procedure, its implications must be clear. There are four reasons that a patient's informed consent is necessary:

1. Patients are not knowledgeable about medical science.
2. An adult of sound mind has the right to determine whether or not to submit to medical treatment.
3. To be effective, the patient's consent must be informed consent.
4. The patient depends on the physician for information to make a reasoned decision about treatment.

A physician is legally required to disclose risks that might occur during a procedure. The modern legal interpretation is that informed consent is a duty of health practitioners and that the lack of informed consent is negligence. The courts use the term **material risk** to establish what risks should be disclosed, meaning that a risk should be explained if a reasonable person would consider it important. For example, the risk of death or injury during a cardiac catheterization should be disclosed; however, the risks associated with stitching a cut finger are not considered serious enough to merit a physician's disclosing them. Informed consent is given before surgery, experimental procedures, the administration of experimental drugs, or other treatments involving risk to the patient. For example, if you awoke one morning with a severe pain in your right side and, after visiting the physician, learned you required an emergency appendectomy, the surgery would not be performed unless you (assuming you are of legal age) or your parent or guardian signed a consent form.

Consent forms signed by the patient prior to receiving a treatment or procedure document that the patient has been fully informed of potential risk. Physicians and hospitals routinely require consent forms as a means of protecting themselves from claims. The consent form should be specific and provide enough detail for the patient to understand fully what she is signing.

The physician will rely on you as a medical assistant to organize and coordinate the signing of all consent forms. This is an important responsibility, because these forms would be required as documentation in a lawsuit. Although a missing form might never be noticed, a multimillion dollar malpractice lawsuit could hinge on evidence of a patient's informed consent.

To compile the necessary consent forms, the medical assistant must understand the procedures and treatments the patient will undergo. The physician usually supplies the names of the procedures and treatments; then the medical assistant determines which forms will be needed. If any question exists about the necessity for a form, the medical assistant should consult the physician. Refer to Figure 4–3 for an example of an informed consent form.

Even routine forms in the patient's medical records are important if a malpractice claim is filed. The patient's record is evidence that a physician tested and treated a patient thoroughly. Because no physician or medical assistant's memory can recall the circumstances of all treatments, only the documentation is valid proof that the physician followed the standard of care considered normal in the circumstances and, therefore, was not negligent in treating the patient.

Follow these procedures to ensure that informed consent is always obtained:

1. Keep an adequate supply of consent forms.
2. Compile consent forms for each patient as needed before the patient arrives at the office.
3. Type a list of all consent forms needed and ask the physician to check the list for accuracy. Leave a blank line for the physician's check mark (✔).
4. Put all consent forms for an individual patient in a folder.
5. Review the forms with the patient, explaining the purpose of each form fully.
6. Ask the patient to sign and date all forms; then check the forms to be sure they are completed in full.
7. File the forms in the patient's medical record.

Medical Records

Besides informed consent, the most valuable preventive measure in reducing malpractice claims is maintaining documented medical records for each patient. Because medical records can be used as evidence during a malpractice court case, they should be complete, accurate, and up to date at all times. they should include (1) consent forms for procedures or treatments the physician has performed; (2) copies of all medical histories, laboratory reports, the physician's notes, and consulting physicians' reports; (3) a list of all medications prescribed and dispensed from the office; (4) permission forms authorizing the physician to release information about the patient; (5) miscellaneous medical information; and (6) records from any government-funded program, such as Medicare or Medicaid, in which the patient participates.

If the physician withdraws from the case for any reason, a **physician-withdrawal letter** should be sent to the patient, and a copy of the letter should be stored in the patient's file. A common reason physicians withdraw from cases is the patient's failure to cooperate with treatment; for example, a refusal to take a prescribed drug. Other reasons include a patient's move to another geographic area or a patient's doctor shopping, that is, going back and forth to a series of doctors for the same symptoms. Figure 4–4 shows examples of physician-withdrawal letters. (*Note*: This letter should be sent by registered or certified mail with return receipt requested.)

Advance Directives

A health care advance directive is a document in which patients give instructions about their health care if, in the future, they cannot speak for themselves. Health care advance directives have two parts:

1. They give someone — a spouse, child, or other person — the power to make health care decisions for the patient and describe the limits of the power or authority the agent will have.
2. They also give instructions about the kind of health care a patient does or does not want.

In the second part of the statement, patients can provide specific instructions about their

Acknowledgment of Informed Consent
for Surgical or Medical Procedures

I hereby indicate that I have given consent to _____Dr. Tarik Maneurse_____ (insert doctor's name), with associates or assistants of her choice, to perform the following surgical, diagnostic, and or medical procedure (including without limit anesthesia, x-rays, or laboratory tests) on myself _____Alena Sanchez_____ my _____ (cross out inappropriate description of patient):

Cesarean section _____

_____

_____

Name of Procedure(s)

I hereby indicate that in giving this consent the nature and purpose of the procedure; what the procedure is expected to accomplish; alternate means of therapy, if any; and reasonably known risks, complications, and discomfort have been explained to me by the above named doctor.

I understand that during the course of the above described procedure, unforeseen conditions may be revealed that make advisable an extension of this procedure or the use of a different procedure. I hereby authorize the above named doctor(s) to carry out any extension or to perform any other procedure that in the doctor's judgment is advisable for my well-being if circumstances make it impossible or, in the doctor's opinion, medically undesirable, to obtain my specific consent to such extension or other procedure. The authority granted under this paragraph shall extend to treating all conditions that require treatment and are not known to the above named doctors at the time the procedure is commenced.

I am aware that the practice of medicine and surgery is not an exact science and that the possibility and nature of results or complications cannot be anticipated with complete accuracy. I acknowledge that no guarantees, express or implied, have been made as to the results of the above described procedure or any cure.

I consent to the admittance of observers and to the photographing or televising of the surgical, diagnostic, and or medical procedure to be performed, including appropriate portions of my body provided my named or identity is not revealed by the pictures or by the descriptive texts accompanying them.

Date _____September 10, 2002_____

Time _____7:30_____ (AM) PM

_____*Jane Andress*_____
WITNESS

_____*Alena Sanchez*_____
SIGNATURE OF PATIENT

_____
SIGNATURE OF PARENT (WHERE REQUIRED)

_____
SIGNATURE OF OTHER PERSON WITH
LEGAL AUTHORITY (WHERE REQUIRED)

FIGURE 4–3 Consent form signed by patient

health care, including a statement about organ donation.

Federal law requires all states and most health care facilities to give information to patients about their rights to make decisions about their health care. The law, known as the Patient Self-Determination Act, is intended to make sure that all adult patients know what their rights are in controlling their health care decisions and understand how to use advance directives to protect those rights.

Form 1a

Date: _____

Dear _____:

I will no longer be able to provide medical care to (you/your children). If you require medical care within the next ____ days I will be available, but in no event longer than ____ days.

To assist you in continuing to receive medical care for (you/your children), we will make records available to a new physician as soon as you authorize us to send them to that physician.

Sincerely,

_____, M.D.

Form 1b

_____   Date: _____

Dear _____:

I find it necessary to inform you that I am withdrawing from further professional attendance on you since you have persisted in refusing to follow my medical advice and treatment. Since your condition requires medical attention, I suggest that you place yourself under the care of another physician without delay. If you desire, I shall be available to attend you for a reasonable time after you receive this letter, but in no event for more than ____ days.

This should give you ample time to select a physician of your choice from the many competent practitioners in this city. With your authorization, I will make available to this physician your case history and information regarding the diagnosis and treatment you have received from me.

Very truly yours,

_____, M.D.

FIGURE 4–4   Physician-withdrawal letter

Written directives are usually either a living will or a durable power of attorney for health care. Most hospitals provide advance directive forms, eliminating the necessity of having an attorney draw up the document. However, patients may want to discuss advance directives with an attorney.

Living Wills   A traditional living will is a simple document in which a patient explains what kind of life-prolonging medical care is acceptable if the patient is terminally ill.

Power of Attorney   In a Health Care Power of Attorney, also known as a Durable Power of Attorney, the patient appoints someone else to make medical treatment decisions if the patient is unable to make them. Many health care directives combine and expand the traditional Living Will and the Health Care Power of Attorney into a single document as shown in Figure 4–5. Instructions can be given about any treatment wanted or to be avoided. Unlike a living will, a durable power of attorney may apply when a patient has any serious medical condition, not only a terminal illness. Refer to Chapter 3 for additional information on a durable power of attorney as an ethical issue.

Criminal Law

Criminal law involves a wrong to society and is usually punishable by imprisonment, perhaps combined with a fine. A physician found guilty of a criminal offense is usually censured by or expelled from membership in the AMA or the local medical society. On the other hand, a physician who is acquitted by a court of law may still face disciplinary action from a medical society.

Illegal Acts by a Physician

In an imperfect world, physicians can be guilty of wrongdoing. Because physicians are faced with many temptations, some slip into criminal activities for which they must be prosecuted. The physician who evades taxes, dispenses illegal drugs, abuses drugs, or sexually assaults or physically harms a patient will be convicted of the crime if discovered. Physicians can also be involved in other crimes.

Health Care Declaration and Power of Attorney of

_____

A. Health Care Declaration

I, _____ of _____ County, Pennsylvania, being of sound mind, willfully and voluntarily make this declaration to be followed if I become incompetent. This dedication reflects my firm and settled commitment to refuse life-sustaining treatment under the circumstances indicated below.

1. If I should be in a terminal condition or in a state of permanent unconsciousness, I direct my attending physician to withhold or withdraw life-sustaining treatment that serves only to prolong the process of my dying.

2. If I am in the condition described above, I direct that treatment be limited to measures to keep me comfortable and to relieve pain, including any pain that might occur by withholding or withdrawing life-sustaining treatment.

In addition, if I am in the condition described above, I feel especially strongly about the following forms of treatment:

I ( ) do ( ) do not want cardiac resuscitation.

I ( ) do ( ) do not want mechanical respiration.

I ( ) do ( ) do not want tube feeding or any other invasive form of nutrition (food) or hydration (water).

I ( ) do ( ) do not want blood or blood products.

I ( ) do ( ) do not want any form of surgery or invasive diagnostic tests.

I ( ) do ( ) do not want kidney dialysis.

I ( ) do ( ) do not want antibiotics.

I realize that if I do not specifically indicate my preference regarding any of the forms of treatment listed above, I may receive that form of treatment.

Other Instructions:

I hereby designate _____ [name and address of surrogate]

(Tel. No. _____) as my surrogate to make medical treatment decisions for me if I should be incompetent and in a terminal condition or in a state of permanent unconsciousness.

If the surrogate designated above is, for any reason, unable to serve, I designate as substitute surrogate to serve: [name and address]

(Telephone No. _____)

My surrogate or substitute surrogate ( ) is ( ) is not authorized to withhold tube feeding or any other artificial or invasive form of nutrition (food) or hydration (water).

FIGURE 4–5   Health care declaration and power of attorney _(continues)_

B. Power of Attorney:

In addition to the declaration and appointments made above, I, _____
hereby appoint the surrogate and substitute surrogate named above, in the order listed, my attorney-in-fact for health care for me and in my name to:

1. Authorize my admission to a medical, nursing, residential, or similar facility, enter into agreements for my care, and authorize medical and surgical procedures; consent to, withhold consent from, waive, and terminate any and all medical and surgical procedures on my behalf, including, without limitation, the administration of drugs and the withholding of tube feeding of any other artificial or invasive form of nutrition (food) or hydration (water).

2. Have access and to authorize access for others to any and all medical information and records of mine and all related information concerning me.

3. Authorize the payment of all bills for my health and medical care, to have access to and completed insurance and other health record forms, applications, certifications, and other documentation.

4. Make all medical treatment decisions for me if I should be incompetent or unable to make them or to communicate such medical decisions for myself.

This Health Care Declaration and Power of Attorney shall not be affected by my subsequent disability or incapacity.

Should any specific direction in this Health Care Declaration and Power of Attorney be held to be invalid, such invalidity shall not offset other directions of this document which can be effected without the invalid direction.

I made this declaration on the _____ day of _____ 20_____.

Declarant's signature: _____
 NAME

Declarant's address:

The declarant (or the person who on behalf of and at the direction of the declarant) knowingly and voluntarily signed this writing by signature or mark in my presence.

Witness's signature: _____

Witness's printed name: _____

Witness's address:

Witness's signature: _____

Witness's printed name: _____

Witness's address:

FIGURE 4–5 *(continued)*

The Medical Assistant's Responsibility for Reporting Crimes

Most physicians and other medical professionals are moral people who never commit a crime. However, if, as a medical assistant, you learn that a physician or other office employee has committed a crime, you must report the crime to the authorities. A medical assistant who does not report a crime can be prosecuted as an accessory.

IN YOUR OPINION

1. Under what circumstances do you think it is fair for a patient to bring a malpractice suit?
2. In settings in which nurses, doctors, medical assistants, medical technologists, and other staff have access to patient records, who should be held accountable for missing documents?
3. Is the monthly premium for professional liability insurance for a new medical assistant a worthwhile expense or a waste of money? Explain.

CONFIDENTIALITY

The law protects the patient's right of confidentiality, which means that employees of medical offices, hospitals, and other health care facilities are legally bound to keep all patient information confidential unless the law requires disclosure. The patient should feel free to provide complete information to the doctor without fearing that it will be revealed to others.

Certain news is a matter of public record, and the physician must report this information immediately. Information of this kind includes births, deaths, accidents, and police cases.

Patient–Physician Relationship

The legal concept of **privilege of patient confidentiality** guarantees that the medical information a patient gives a physician will be held in greatest confidence, by both the physician and the physician's employees. The contents of the medical records must also be safeguarded and held in complete confidentiality. The privilege of releasing information belongs to the patient, not to the physician.

The privilege of patient confidentiality assures patients that their records will be kept in complete privacy, even in court, unless they give written permission. However, if the patient waives the privilege of confidentiality, the physician may be required to testify in a court case. If the patient consents, the physician may discuss the patient's history, diagnosis, treatment, and prognosis with the patient's lawyer. Here is an illustration of the way the privilege of patient confidentiality works:

Alexander Onegin reveals his past alcoholism to his physician during an examination for an injury suffered while on the job. When Mr. Onegin files a workers' compensation claim, the employer suspects alcohol as a factor in the injury. The employer contacts Mr. Onegin's physician and asks about the patient's drinking habits. The privilege of patient confidentiality protects Mr. Onegin's privacy, and the information cannot be shared. The physician may be expected to provide *medical* details regarding the accident on a worker's compensation claim form.

Exception to the Patient–Physician Privilege

The **exception to the physician–patient privilege** protects society against harmful acts by or against the patient. For example, if an angry patient threatens to stab another person and shows the physician the knife that will be used, the physician is ethically and legally required to report the threat to authorities.

Physicians are also required to report gunshot wounds, rapes, stabbings, and other crimes against patients and to provide information that they believe will be helpful in solving the crime. However, only the physician may provide this information.

The medical assistant and other medical office employees are responsible for reporting to the physician any unusual cases that may involve a crime. These include suspected cases of child abuse, abuse against the elderly, and related crimes. If a parent waiting with a child in the lobby is verbally and physically abusive, as a medical assistant you should report this information to the physician immediately. If a patient who is bleeding profusely is brought to the office by another person who disappears, you should inform the physician so that the patient can be questioned about the circumstances of the injury. Here is another example of a situation that the medical assistant should report:

The medical assistant sees an elderly patient being brought into the office by a person who is apparently a relative. The patient is crying, and the relative is talking in a harsh manner. When the patient reaches up to touch the relative, the patient is given a sharp slap on the hand and shoved into a seat. This pattern of behavior, which the medical assistant considers abusive, continues until the relative accompanies the patient into the examining room. The relative is "all smiles" during the physician's examination of the elderly patient. The medical assistant has an ethical responsibility to call the doctor aside and report the behavior seen in the reception area.

The news media may ask for information about patients involved in accidents or about patients who are in the public eye, for example, movie stars, sports stars, politicians, community leaders, and others. A physician may not discuss a patient's medical condition, disease, or illness with the press without the patient's permission. However, information in the public domain, such as the patient's name, address, age, sex, and race, can be provided without the patient's consent, as can general information about an accident, such as the body part involved. Internal injuries and the patient's state of consciousness when brought to the hospital may be reported, but the physician may not state that a patient attempted suicide, that a patient was intoxicated or using drugs, or that a moral wrong was involved. The physician may make a general statement about the patient's condition. Furthermore, only the attending physician may make a statement about a patient's diagnosis or prognosis. As a medical assistant, you should refer all questions of this nature to the physician.

(Telephone rings)

Caller: This is CNN calling. We've just heard that the senator's son took a drug overdose and has been brought to your office. Is that true?

Medical Assistant: I can't answer any questions about private patients.

Caller: Just tell me if the senator's son is in your office now, so I can come take some pictures.

Medical Assistant: I can't release that information. I will not be able to help you.

Patient Confidentiality and Insurance Companies

History, diagnosis, prognosis, treatment or service, and fee information acquired during the physician–patient relationship may be disclosed to an insurance company only if the patient provides written consent. Insurance companies generally include a statement of permission on their claim forms that the patient signs, granting the medical office the authority to release information to the insurance company. Without full documentation of diagnosis, treatment, and service, the insurance company will not pay benefits on a claim. Hospitals must also have written permission before releasing information about a patient.

Item 12 of the insurance claim form illustrated in Figure 4–6 shows the patient's signature giving permission to release medical information to the insurance carrier.

Medical Assistant's Responsibility for Confidentiality

Except for insurance forms, which the medical assistant completes with the physician's permission, any information released about a patient should come only from the physician. Many doctors consider confidentiality to be the most desirable character trait that a medical assistant can possess. In addition to moral concerns for confidentiality, physicians are legally responsible for the actions of their employees during the

APPROVED OMB-0938-0008

CARRIER

| | PICA | **HEALTH INSURANCE CLAIM FORM** | PICA | |

1. MEDICARE	MEDICAID	CHAMPUS	CHAMPVA	GROUP HEALTH PLAN (SSN or ID)	FECA BLK LUNG (SSN)	OTHER (ID)	1a. INSURED'S I.D. NUMBER (FOR PROGRAM IN ITEM 1)
(Medicare #)	(Medicaid #)	(Sponsor's SSN)	(VA File #)	☒			331-26-9648

2. PATIENT'S NAME (Last Name, First Name, Middle Initial)
Stoner, Jay G.

3. PATIENT'S BIRTH DATE MM 04 DD 03 YY —   SEX M ☒ F

4. INSURED'S NAME (Last Name, First Name, Middle Initial)
Stoner, James B.

5. PATIENT'S ADDRESS (No., Street)
401 N. Broad Street

6. PATIENT RELATIONSHIP TO INSURED
Self ☐ Spouse ☐ Child ☒ Other ☐

7. INSURED'S ADDRESS (No., Street)
same as Item 5

CITY **Rockford** STATE **IL**

8. PATIENT STATUS
Single ☐ Married ☐ Other ☐
Employed ☐ Full-Time Student ☒ Part-Time Student ☐

CITY STATE

ZIP CODE **61111-0136** TELEPHONE (Include Area Code) **(312) 555-3894**

ZIP CODE TELEPHONE (INCLUDE AREA CODE) **(312) 555-3894**

9. OTHER INSURED'S NAME (Last Name, First Name, Middle Initial)
DNA

10. IS PATIENT'S CONDITION RELATED TO:

11. INSURED'S POLICY GROUP OR FECA NUMBER
4324-8965

a. OTHER INSURED'S POLICY OR GROUP NUMBER
DNA

a. EMPLOYMENT? (CURRENT OR PREVIOUS)
YES ☐ NO ☒

a. INSURED'S DATE OF BIRTH MM 01 DD 15 YY —   SEX M ☒ F ☐

b. OTHER INSURED'S DATE OF BIRTH MM DD YY   SEX M ☐ F ☐

b. AUTO ACCIDENT? PLACE (State)
YES ☐ NO ☒

b. EMPLOYER'S NAME OR SCHOOL NAME
Grayson Agency

c. EMPLOYER'S NAME OR SCHOOL NAME

c. OTHER ACCIDENT?
YES ☐ NO ☒

c. INSURANCE PLAN NAME OR PROGRAM NAME
Statewide Insurance

d. INSURANCE PLAN NAME OR PROGRAM NAME

10d. RESERVED FOR LOCAL USE

d. IS THERE ANOTHER HEALTH BENEFIT PLAN?
YES ☐ NO ☒ If yes, return to and complete item 9 a-d.

READ BACK OF FORM BEFORE COMPLETING & SIGNING THIS FORM.
12. PATIENT'S OR AUTHORIZED PERSON'S SIGNATURE I authorize the release of any medical or other information necessary to process this claim. I also request payment of government benefits either to myself or to the party who accepts assignment below.

SIGNED *James B. Stone* DATE **5/21/—**

13. INSURED'S OR AUTHORIZED PERSON'S SIGNATURE I authorize payment of medical benefits to the undersigned physician or supplier for services described below.

SIGNED *James B. Stone*

14. DATE OF CURRENT: MM DD YY   ILLNESS (First symptom) OR INJURY (Accident) OR PREGNANCY(LMP)

15. IF PATIENT HAS HAD SAME OR SIMILAR ILLNESS. GIVE FIRST DATE MM DD YY

16. DATES PATIENT UNABLE TO WORK IN CURRENT OCCUPATION FROM MM DD YY TO MM DD YY

17. NAME OF REFERRING PHYSICIAN OR OTHER SOURCE

17a. I.D. NUMBER OF REFERRING PHYSICIAN

18. HOSPITALIZATION DATES RELATED TO CURRENT SERVICES FROM MM DD YY TO MM DD YY

19. RESERVED FOR LOCAL USE

20. OUTSIDE LAB? $ CHARGES
YES ☐ NO ☐

21. DIAGNOSIS OR NATURE OF ILLNESS OR INJURY. (RELATE ITEMS 1,2,3 OR 4 TO ITEM 24E BY LINE)
1. ⌞___.__⌟   3. ⌞___.__⌟
2. ⌞___.__⌟   4. ⌞___.__⌟

22. MEDICAID RESUBMISSION CODE ORIGINAL REF. NO.

23. PRIOR AUTHORIZATION NUMBER

24.	A DATE(S) OF SERVICE						B Place of Service	C Type of Service	D PROCEDURES, SERVICES, OR SUPPLIES (Explain Unusual Circumstances) CPT/HCPCS MODIFIER	E DIAGNOSIS CODE	F $ CHARGES	G DAYS OR UNITS	H EPSDT Family Plan	I EMG	J COB	K RESERVED FOR LOCAL USE
	From MM	DD	YY	To MM	DD	YY										
1																
2																
3																
4																
5																
6																

25. FEDERAL TAX I.D. NUMBER SSN ☐ EIN ☐

26. PATIENT'S ACCOUNT NO.

27. ACCEPT ASSIGNMENT? (For govt. claims, see back) YES ☐ NO ☐

28. TOTAL CHARGE $

29. AMOUNT PAID $

30. BALANCE DUE $

31. SIGNATURE OF PHYSICIAN OR SUPPLIER INCLUDING DEGREES OR CREDENTIALS (I certify that the statements on the reverse apply to this bill and are made a part thereof.)

SIGNED DATE

32. NAME AND ADDRESS OF FACILITY WHERE SERVICES WERE RENDERED (If other than home or office)

33. PHYSICIAN'S, SUPPLIER'S BILLING NAME, ADDRESS, ZIP CODE & PHONE #

PIN# GRP#

(APPROVED BY AMA COUNCIL ON MEDICAL SERVICE 8/88) **PLEASE PRINT OR TYPE**

FORM HCFA-1500 (U2) (12-90)
FORM OWCP-1500 FORM RRB-1500

PATIENT AND INSURED INFORMATION

PHYSICIAN OR SUPPLIER INFORMATION

FIGURE 4–6 Insurance form giving permission to release medical information

course of duty. A physician can be sued if an employee releases confidential information. Consider this situation:

A medical assistant tells a friend who works for a Fortune 500 company that the company CEO is being treated by the physician, a psychiatrist, for alcoholism. The friend, unable to keep this information to himself, tells another person at work. Soon the grapevine has passed the story along to many employees, and someone leaks it to the news media. The negative publicity seriously reduces the value of a new stock offering. The fortune 500 company traces the source of the story to the medical assistant, who loses his job as a result. The president has grounds for a lawsuit against the physician and the medical assistant.

Personal information that patients supply is also confidential, even though it may not be of a medical nature, and should not be released or discussed with anyone outside the office. Information falling into this category includes a patient's age, number of marriages, number of children, and similar facts. Information can be released inadvertently if the medical office staff is not cautious. An employee who speaks too loudly while visitors are in the reception area may reveal confidential information. Similarly, an employee who tends to "talk too much" may divulge confidential information unintentionally. Carelessly released information can cause ethical and legal problems for the physician and for the employee who released it. A good rule to follow is: Never talk about patients except with the professional medical staff.

Sometimes a husband, wife, friend, child, or employer of a patient may ask about a patient's condition. Although these questions are legitimate expressions of concern, a medical assistant should not provide information about the patient. Instead, the inquiry should be referred to the physician, as in this example:

A man who accompanies his wife to the gynecologist's office waits in the reception area while his wife talks with the physician. The husband tells the medical assistant that he believes his wife is pregnant but that she won't confirm the pregnancy. As her husband, he feels it is his right to know whether he is going to be a father, and he asks the medical assistant to check his wife's medical record. A medical assistant must keep confidential all information about the patient. The fact that the concerned person is the patient's husband has no bearing on the patient's right to confidentiality.

IN YOUR OPINION

1. What can you as a medical assistant do to guard against inadvertently releasing information about a patient?
2. If a medical assistant and nurse in an open office discuss a patient's answers to medical questions, how might they break the rule of patient confidentiality?
3. What advice regarding confidentiality would you give a new medical assistant?

TELECOMMUNICATIONS AND CONFIDENTIALITY

Advancing technology has improved health care by reducing the time between testing and diagnosis and treatment, but it has created complex confidentiality problems. Fax machines and e-mail, especially, offer a challenge to patient privacy.

Fax Machines

Although fax machines need to be near or in the central office, they should be sheltered by a partition or covering that provides privacy. The fax machine should not be located in a central area where unauthorized personnel can view documents. Before sending any document by fax, be sure it will not violate confidentiality, obtain permission to transmit it by fax, and attach a cover sheet with strict instructions that the information is for the recipient only. A recommended fax cover sheet is shown in Figure 4–7.

E-mail

Electronic mail is deceptive because it leaves the impression that only a machine will see the content of a message. However, e-mail is vulnerable

Cardiology Associates, P.C.

201 Medical Arts Building
Lakewood, NJ 08701

....
FAX TRANSMITTAL COVER SHEET
....

*Confidential Information
for Named Recipient
Only*

TO:

FROM:

DATE:

NUMBER OF PAGES, INCLUDING THIS PAGE:

FAX NUMBER:

FIGURE 4–7   Confidential fax cover sheet

to viewing by unorthodox computer users who enjoy breaking into computer networks. Nothing that is transmitted by e-mail can be considered totally confidential; therefore, always obtain permission before sending any confidential information electronically through a computer network and designate the message "Confidential — To be read by addressee only."

CONFIDENTIALITY AGREEMENTS

All medical offices should develop and execute confidentiality agreements with physicians, nurses, employees, interns, staff, computer consultants, and any others who might have an opportunity to gain access to patient information.

It is especially important to inform individuals who do not have a health care background of the requirement for strict adherence to confidentiality policies. By signing a confidentiality agreement, an individual enters into a legal contract. Figure 4–8 shows a confidentiality agreement.

THE PHYSICIAN IN COURT

Physicians are usually called to court for one of two reasons: (1) as the defendant in a lawsuit or (2) as an expert witness in a case. These situations may involve a variety of circumstances.

Physician as Defendant

When a malpractice claim is made against a physician or other health care professional,

SAMPLE ACCESS AND CONFIDENTIALITY AGREEMENT
(Physician/Employee/Volunteer/Student)

As an physician/nurse/employee/volunteer/student with access to medical images and reports from (HEALTHCARE ENTITY), you will have access to what this agreement refers to as "confidential information." The purpose of this agreement is to help you understand your duty regarding confidential information. Confidential information includes patient information, medical images, and reports. You may learn of or have access to some or all of this confidential information through a computer system or through your employment activities. Confidential information is valuable and sensitive and is protected by law and by strict (HEALTHCARE ENTITY) policies. The intent of these laws and policies is to ensure that confidential information will remain confidential — that is, that it will be used only as necessary to provide authorized patient care. As a physician/employee/volunteer/student, you are required to conduct yourself in strict conformance to applicable laws and (HEALTHCARE ENTITY) policies governing confidential information. Your principal obligations in this area are explained below. You are required to read and to abide by these duties. The violation of any of these duties will subject you to discipline, which might include, but is not limited to, termination of employment and to legal liability.

Accordingly, as a condition of and in consideration of your access to confidential information, you promise that:

1. You will use confidential information only as needed to perform your legitimate duties as a physician/employee/volunteer/student receiving information from (HEALTHCARE ENTITY). This means, among other things, that:
   A. You will only access confidential information for which you have a need to know; and
   B. You will not in any way divulge, copy, release, sell, loan, review, alter, or destroy any confidential information except as properly authorized by (HEALTHCARE ENTITY).
   C. You will not misuse confidential information or carelessly care for confidential information.
2. You will safeguard and will not disclose your access code or any other authorization you have that allows you to access confidential information.
3. You accept responsibility for all activities undertaken using your access code and other authorization.
4. You will report activities by any individual or entity that you suspect may compromise the confidentiality of confidential information. Reports made in good faith about suspect activities will be held in confidence to the extent permitted by law, including the name of the individual reporting the activities.
5. You understand that your obligations under this Agreement will continue after termination of your employment. You understand that your privileges hereunder are subject to periodic review, revision, and if appropriate, renewal.
6. You understand that you have no right or ownership interest in any confidential information referred to in this Agreement. (HEALTHCARE ENTITY) may at any time revoke your access code, other authorization, or access to confidential information. At all times during your employment, you will safeguard and retain the confidentiality of all confidential information.
7. You will be responsible for your misuse or wrongful disclosure of confidential information and for your failure to safeguard your access code or other authorization access to confidential information. You understand that your failure to comply with this Agreement may also result in your loss of employment and other legal liability.

_____
Physician/Employee/Volunteer/Student Signature and Date

_____
Printed Name

FIGURE 4–8   Confidentiality agreement

the person being sued files the claim with his professional liability insurance carrier. The carrier may decide that the claim is invalid and refuse to make any settlement, or it may offer the patient a sum of money to settle the claim out of court. The patient can accept the offer, try to negotiate a higher settlement figure or counter offer with the carrier, or file a lawsuit that ultimately will end in a trial if the carrier and the patient cannot agree on a figure.

Settlement of Claims

Many malpractice lawsuits never go to trial because the insurance company and the patient agree on damages. The insurance carrier pays the patient and the patient drops the case against the physician. Sometimes negotiations continue while a trial is in session; if the two parties agree to a settlement during the trial, the case is dropped.

When an agreement between the patient and insurance carrier cannot be reached, the carrier hires an attorney to defend the physician or health care professional (Figure 4–9). The attor-

ney reviews the patient's medical record and talks with the physician, patient, medical assistant, and any other principals involved in the case. After thoroughly reviewing the facts, the attorney answers the charge through legal documents filed with the court.

Court Papers

The patient is the plaintiff in a malpractice lawsuit, and the physician is the defendant. The burden of proof is on the plaintiff to show that the physician was negligent; the physician must show that the plaintiff's accusation is false. Because the outcome of many malpractice lawsuits depends on the contents of the patient's medical record, complete and up-to-date records are crucial.

Summons and Complaint

If the physician is sued, a legal summons and complaint will be mailed or hand delivered to the physician by a member of the local sheriff's department. These documents may be left with

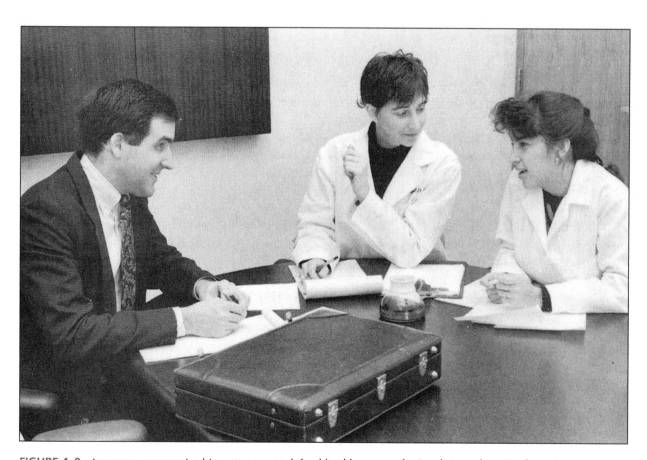

FIGURE 4–9 Insurance companies hire attorneys to defend health care professionals in malpractice lawsuits.

the medical assistant if the physician is unavailable. They are extremely important and must be given to the physician immediately. Failure by the physician to answer the summons could result in a default judgment, that is, a judgment against the physician because no answer was made. Figure 4–10 illustrates a legal summons, and Figure 4–11 illustrates a complaint. You should become familiar with the appearance of these documents so you can recognize them if they are delivered to your office.

The physician notifies the attorney and insurance company at once if a summons and complaint are received. If the physician and the professional liability carrier believe that no malpractice was involved or if they cannot agree with the plaintiff on a settlement, the case goes to trial. During the trial, all parties involved in the lawsuit give evidence. Expert witnesses, including other physicians and related experts may be called by the plaintiff to attest to the physician's negligence. The insurance carrier then presents expert witnesses to defend the physician's position.

After several days, weeks, or months of trial, during which negotiations for settlement may continue among the lawyers for the plaintiff and defendant, a judge or jury decides the physician's innocence or guilt. If the physician is found guilty, the judge or jury sets monetary damages, and the malpractice carrier pays the patient up to the limits set by the physician's insurance policy. The physician must personally pay any difference between the policy limits and the damages set by the judge or jury. The court may also dismiss the suit if the plaintiff fails to establish a cause of action against the doctor, or if the plaintiff's argument against the physician is not strong enough.

NAME AND ADDRESS OF ATTORNEY	TELEPHONE NO:	FOR COURT USE ONLY
JUENGERT AND WATSON 1043 Peachtree Street Atlanta, GA 30033–4161 ATTORNEY FOR (Name) Plaintiff	404-555-4925	

Insert name of court, judicial district or branch court, if any, and Post Office and Street Address:

FULTON COUNTY DISTRICT COURT

Capitol Square, SW

Atlanta, GA 30334–4161

PLAINTIFF

ARNOLD RIFKEN

BERNICE RIFKIN

DEFENDANT

ERROL DUPLESSIS, M.D.

BEAU GIRARD, M.D.

SUMMONS	CASE NUMBER

FIGURE 4–10 Legal summons

NO. 430219.

PLAINTIFFS, Arnold Rifkin   I IN THE DISTRICT COURT

        Bernice Rifkin

vs.

DEFENDANTS, Errol DuPlessis, M.D.   I OF FULTON COUNTY, GEORGIA

        Beau Girardf, M.D.   I 5th JUDICIAL DISTRICT

                    PLAINTIFFS' ORIGINAL PETITION

TO THE HONORABLE JUDGE OF SAID COURT:

    COME NOW ARNOLD RIFKIN AND BERNICE RIFKIN, hereinafter styled
Plaintiffs, complaining of ERROL DUPLESSIS, M.D. and BEAU GIRARD, M.D.
hereinafter styled Defendants, and for cause of action would show to the
Court as follows:

                              I.

    This is a suit for wrongful death under Articles 4671 et. seq. of the
Revised Civil Statutes of Georgia, and plaintiff BERNICE RIFKIN is the
surviving mother of JEREMY RIFKIN deceased. Plaintiff, ARNOLD RIFKIN, is
the father of JEREMY RIFKIN deceased. Said JEREMY RIFKIN, plaintiff's
deceased 3-month old minor son, left no will and there was no administration on his estate and no necessity therefor. Plaintiffs are responsible
for the debts of the estate of their deceased son, including funeral
expenses.

                              II.

JEREMY RIFKIN was wrongfully killed as hereinafter described, but did not
die instantly; he experienced conscious pain and suffering, for which he
would have been entitled to recover damages; and the cause of action for
damages of conscious pain and suffering prior to his death survived, and
on his death accrued to his heirs at law under Article 5525 of the
Revised Civil Statutes of the State of Georgia.

FIGURE 4–11 Legal complaint

Physician and Medical Assistant as Witnesses

Physicians may also be called as witnesses in court cases, either against themselves or as expert witnesses in other cases. Sometimes the physician must appear in the courtroom, or the physician may provide testimony through a **deposition**. A deposition is a sworn statement given by a party to a lawsuit before the suit goes to trial. During a deposition, which may be given at the attorney's office or in some other location, an attorney asks the witness questions. The witness's answers are recorded by a stenographer or court reporter who keyboards the proceedings in final form and notarizes it.

As a medical assistant, you may be asked to give a deposition. If this happens, tell the facts as you know them, without changing them in any way. When you are unsure of answers to any questions, say so. It is better to give no answer than to given an incorrect answer that might cause greater difficulty at a later time.

GOOD SAMARITAN LAWS

Good Samaritan laws protect the physician and other health care professionals who help people in unusual emergency situations. This includes (1) the physician who stops at the scene of an automobile accident to offer aid; (2) the doctor who amputates the fingers of a man when he catches them in a boat motor; (3) the paramedic who treats a fire victim while off duty; and (4) other medical practitioners who treat emergencies that would result in death if aid were not offered. Good Samaritan laws in all fifty states protect medical practitioners from fear of reprisal when they offer emergency care. Generally, these laws cover practitioners who provide treatment within their area of expertise. However, each state has different laws, so you should check the law in your state to determine the extent of liability for medical practitioners who assist people in an emergency.

THE PHYSICIAN AND CONTROLLED SUBSTANCES

The Controlled Substances Act regulates the dispensing of drugs from medical offices. Physicians who dispense narcotic drugs are required to maintain complete and detailed records because of the potential for abuse. Less detail is required for nonnarcotic drugs. Generally, the medical assistant is responsible for keeping records of all drugs dispensed.

Narcotic Drug Records

Narcotic drugs that are dispensed from a medical office fall into a special category of importance. Because drug abuse has become a major problem today, all drugs must be monitored properly. Theft of drugs can be overlooked if the medical assistant does not follow strict recording procedures for the physician's drug file.

Procedures for Monitoring Dispensed Drugs

1. Record the date and time the drug was dispensed.
2. Record the name and address of the patient to whom the drug was dispensed.
3. Record the name and quantity of the drug dispensed.
4. Record the method of dispensing.
5. Explain the reason the drug was given.

An example of a narcotic record is shown in Figure 4–12.

Drug Security

Narcotic drugs should be secured in a locked cabinet at all times; the keys to the cabinet should be held only by the physician, and possibly the nurse. Prescription pads and drug samples should also be locked, so they cannot be stolen by visitors or disreputable staff members. The physician can be held liable if safe measures are not used to store narcotic drugs.

Federal drug enforcement officers have the right to inspect a physician's office and drug records if suspicion of dispensing abuse exists. If improper storage or record keeping is found, the physician may lose the right to dispense and prescribe drugs.

As a medical assistant, you must be sure that controlled substances are kept safely and disposed of in accordance with the law. If you have any concerns about the way drugs are stored, dispensed, or discarded, you should report them to the physician immediately.

Narcotic Record					
DATE	TIME	NAME OF PATIENT	DRUG	QUANTITY	EXPLANATION
4/6/—	2 PM	Pamela Ohlberg 202 W. 18th Street, Nashville, TN	Percodan	5.0 mg	postoperative
4/10/—	10 AM	Erik Gladding 8504 Green Hills Pike, Nashville, TN	Ergostat	2 mg	migraine headaches

FIGURE 4–12 Narcotic record

DRUG SCHEDULES

Narcotic and nonnarcotic drugs are divided into five categories or schedules, depending on their potential for abuse. These schedules and some examples of drugs in each category are listed below.

Schedule I

Drugs listed in Schedule I have a high potential for abuse. They are not legitimately used in the United States for treating patients; however, with special permission, Schedule I drugs may be used for research.

Examples: Heroin, LSD, hashish, and marijuana

Schedule II

Schedule II drugs have a high potential for abuse and may lead to psychological or physical dependence. Unlike Schedule I drugs, however, they have been accepted for medical use in the United States. Schedule II drugs can be dispensed only with a prescription signed by a physician; telephone prescriptions are not acceptable.

Examples: Demeral, morphine, codeine, Dilaudid, methadone, cocaine, and Ritalin

Schedule III

The potential for abuse is lower with Schedule III drugs. Although use of the drugs is accepted in the United States, a moderate degree of physical or psychological dependence may result from abuse. Schedule III drugs can be dispensed with either a written or telephone prescription.

Examples: Tylenol No. 3 with codeine, Fiorinal, phenobarbital, paregoric, and Butisol

Schedule IV

Schedule IV drugs have low potential for abuse and are accepted for medical use in the United States. Abuse may lead to limited physical or psychological dependence. Prescriptions for Schedule IV drugs may be written by a nurse or medical assistant as long as the physician signs the prescription. Refills can be approved by the medical assistant as long as the physician is consulted.

Examples: Valium, Librium, and Tranxene

Schedule V

The potential for abuse of Schedule V drugs is low. These drugs are accepted for medical use in the United States and can be purchased without a prescription. Abuse may lead to a more limited physical or psychological dependence than will abuse of Schedule IV drugs.

Examples: Donnagel PG, Robitussin AC, and Lomotil

IN YOUR OPINION

1. In giving a deposition, if a medical assistant has an opinion but no concrete proof of wrongdoing by a physician-employer, what should the medical assistant do?
2. Log on to the Internet and enter the keywords "Good Samaritan Laws" into a search engine such as Google. Compare the Good Samaritan Laws in two states. How are they alike? Different?
3. If a medical assistant discovers narcotic drugs missing from the office supply cabinet on several occasions and tells the physician, who does nothing, what steps should the medical assistant take?

INTERNET ACTIVITY

Log on to the AMA Web site at http://www.ama-assn.org and determine the professional liability insurance requirements for physicians in your state. If your state is not listed, determine the requirements in a nearby state. Briefly summarize the requirements.

STUDENT STUDY CHECKLIST

Workbook

1. Complete Chapter 4 exercises in the workbook.
2. Complete Chapter 4 simulations in the workbook that access the CD–ROM in the back of the book.

Administrative Skills CD-ROM

1. Go to the Library on the CD–ROM and play the interactive games for Chapter 4.

REFERENCES

American Academy of Pediatrics Web site: Report of Committee on Medical Liability Web site at http://www.aap.org/visit/coml.htm, 2002.

"A Medical Liability White Paper," Physician Insurers Association of America Web site at http://www.thepiaa.org/publications/telewhitepaper.html, 2002.

Annas, John D., with Alex London, and Bonnie Steinbock. *Ethical Issues in Modern Medicine*, 6th ed. New York: McGraw-Hill, 2002.

"Introduction to Health Care Directives," American Association of Retired Persons at the AMA Web site http://www.ama-assn.org, 1995.

"What to Consider When Someone Else is Responsible for Your Insurance," AMA Web site at http//:www.ama-assn.org/ama/pub/article/2431-283b.html.

CHAPTER ACTIVITIES

PERFORMANCE-BASED ACTIVITIES

1. Create a dialogue with an elderly patient who has asked you to explain advance directives and their purpose. Print your dialogue.

2. Make a chart tracing the development of a medical malpractice claim from its origination by the patient through trial.

Route of a Medical Malpractice Claim

1. _____

2. _____

3. _____

4. _____

5. _____

6. _____

7. _____

8. _____

3. Interview three medical assistants in your area. Ask what security procedures they follow for drugs kept in the office. Write a paper recommending what you consider to be the best procedure.

EXPANDING YOUR THINKING

1. List at least three ways in which you can help yourself remember not to talk about patients outside of the office.

2. Do you think there should be a limit on the amount of damages a person suing for malpractice can be awarded? Why or why not?

3. What are some ways in which you, a medical assistant, can prevent the wrong medication from being dispensed?

4. What record-keeping practices can help safeguard your office against malpractice claims?

5. Some well-respected experts believe that the availability of drugs should not be regulated by law. Do you agree? Why or why not? Debate this topic with a classmate.

PART II

Patient Relations

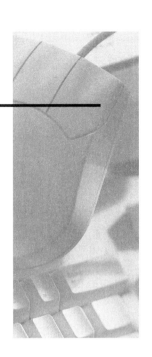

For most medical assistants, working with patients is a favorite responsibility. Developing positive relationships with patients will depend on your interpersonal skills, communication techniques, and confidence. Remember that the success of the practice and your career is directly tied to high quality service and caring attitudes. Beginning with the patient's first visit and during all successive appointments, you should put yourself in the patient's place. In addition to their physical discomforts, patients may be anxious. They need to be shown empathy and concern.

As a medical assistant, you will learn how to contact people and information sources all over the world with a single click of the mouse. You must remember, however, not to let technology form a barrier between you and the patient. The human touch supplemented by technological support is the balance you hope to achieve.

The next three chapters focus on your relationship with patients. The chapters on patient interaction, scheduling, and telephoning offer concrete suggestions for forming relationships with patients, coordinating patient visits, and for placing and taking telephone calls.

CHAPTER 5

Interacting with Patients

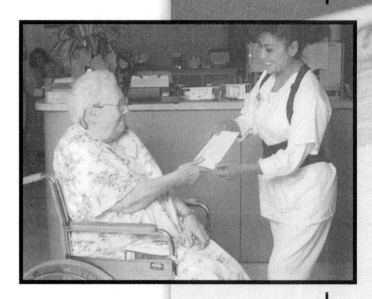

WHITEHALL, NEW YORK

Winter is definitely worse than summer, and summer keeps us pretty busy. I'm a medical assistant in a good-sized practice for a small town, rotating through different responsibilities including working the front desk. For a rural setting, we get a lot of activity.

One day late last fall during hunting season, it had started snowing early and kept on going. There had been some fender benders and our examination rooms were full. In came three hunters, all dressed in a curious combination of camouflage and fluorescent outfits, and one of them with a bad cut in the thigh. His friends had applied a compress that had contained the bleeding. I explained that there would be a wait and told them why; I've found out that when people understand why there's a hold-up, they're a lot calmer about accepting it. I had the wounded man elevate his leg.

Then, a man came in with his 3-year old son. The son was crying and his hand was swollen. I let the man know that I would be with him in a minute. He was frantic. A window he'd been working on, stripping off old paint, had slammed down on the boy's hand. I had to explain to him that the only thing we could do right away was to get an x-ray. I said I would schedule him as soon as possible.

It's difficult when everything happens at once and you have to make decisions about what comes first. But it's part of the pressure that makes this work exciting and rewarding—even if it is exhausting sometimes. One of the biggest rewards, I think, is on days like today, when there are a lot of people in real need, competing for assistance, and I'm able to manage them so that they all get taken care of in turn and no one gets upset. It isn't easy. And it doesn't always work out. But I've learned to handle things most of the time.

Allyson Carmichael
Medical Assistant

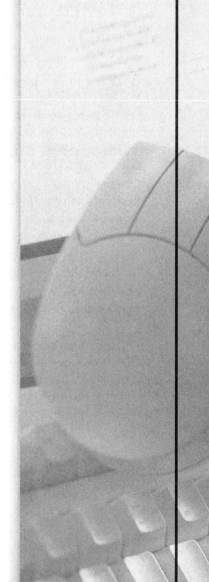

After completing this chapter, you should be able to:
1. Compare and contrast appropriate and inappropriate behaviors for a medical assistant interacting with patients.
2. Demonstrate nonverbal behaviors you can use to show that you are listening to the patients.
3. Prioritize interpersonal skills necessary for a medical assistant when dealing with patients.
4. Analyze the effect of excessive paperwork and record keeping on a medical assistant's relationships with patients.
5. Establish guidelines for a well-managed reception area.
6. Compare and contrast the procedures for handling a walk-in emergency patient and a call-in emergency patient.

VOCABULARY

Active listening   Conscious attention to the speaker, asking open-ended questions that elicit additional information, and using verbal and nonverbal skills to provide feedback.

Anxiety   An intense feeling of dread or worry; fear of a situation or of the unknown.

Burnout   The physical and mental letdown that occurs after a period of stress, intensity, or overwork.

Culturally diverse   Representing a variety of traditions, language, and customs.

Disabled   Unable to participate at the normal level because of a physical or mental weakness or incapacitation.

Empathy   Mentally putting oneself in another's situation.

Feedback   Responses that provide direction.

Interpersonal   From one person to another.

Nonverbal communication   The signals humans send out without speaking, including facial expressions, gestures, posture, and appearance.

Tact   Diplomacy in handling difficult situations.

Have you ever been shopping in a grocery store and felt that the checkout clerk did not know that you were there? The checker was so busy having a personal conversation with another checker that the two of you did not even make eye contact! How did that make you feel?

On the other hand, have you ever had a shopping experience in which the salesperson gave you time and personal attention and told you about your choices without patronizing or rushing you? How did that make you feel about that store and that purchase?

Patients are customers too — customers of medical goods and services. Sometimes they are anxious because they or their family members are ill. They may also be upset because of the confusing nature of medical terminology and baffling regulations about insurance procedures. As with any other customer, you want patients to feel confident they are receiving high-quality service from caring people.

A medical assistant, often the receptionist who answers the telephone or greets visitors, provides the first impression of a medical office. Because the first impression sets the tone for future relationships, as a medical assistant your role is very important. You must make certain that the patient feels good about the first visit and will be comfortable about returning.

INTERPERSONAL COMMUNICATION

The term **interpersonal** communication refers to interaction between or among people. It is the way we relate to one another, the way we listen, and the way we look when we are listening. It is how we reassure and offer comfort in stressful situations and how we help people feel good about themselves. More people lose their jobs because of poor interpersonal skills than because of poor technical skills. A medical assistant who maintained an "A" average in school, knows the office routine perfectly, and possesses excellent technical skills, but will not succeed without good interpersonal skills.

Studies completed by the American Medical Association show that most medical malpractice suits could have been avoided if patients had felt they were listened to and that their questions were answered. Your attitude, speech, and behavior are vital components of the caring, professional climate that is part of the service your office provides to its medical customers.

This chapter discusses several behaviors necessary for good interpersonal relations in the medical office. Your employer hires not only your medical and office skills, but also your behavior at the workplace. As you read this chapter, think about words and attitudes that will ensure you deserve your paycheck.

Concern for the Patient

To put patients at ease, smile, greet them courteously, and treat them with respect. Use the patient's full name, "Mrs. Stevenson" instead of "Mary." Add a few words of greeting to make the person more comfortable. Remember, most people are not in the doctor's office because they want to be there. They have no desire to be ill or injured, their normal routine is interrupted, and they are in an unfamiliar environment where they feel out of control.

Concern for patients shows through your tone of voice, words, and actions (Figure 5–1). Because emotional sensitivity is higher when a person is sick, patients may be offended by an attitude, manner, or remark that would be completely normal in other circumstances, or they may read more into your words than you intended. You should:

1. Choose your words carefully
2. Use a soothing tone of voice
3. Display a professional manner

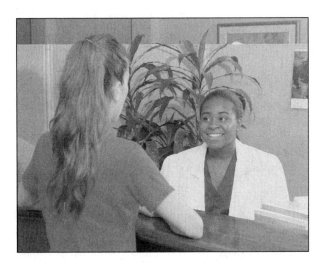

FIGURE 5–1 Smiling not only makes patients feel more comfortable, but also conveys a positive attitude.

In the following examples, consider how the words and actions demonstrate that the medical assistant cares for the patient.

"Mrs. Guiterrez, how nice to see you today. I'm sorry it's so wet out. Would you like me to hang your raincoat in the hallway?"

Important Points: (1) The medical assistant makes Mrs. Guiterrez feel that her comfort is important. (2) The medical assistant assumes partial responsibility for the coat and acknowledges that Mrs. Guiterrez has had to come out in bad weather. This establishes an "I'm sorry for your inconvenience" attitude that will carry over to other aspects of the patient's care.

"Good morning, Mr. Akkim. How is Elena's throat? The flu season has been very bad this year. She's still coughing a lot? The doctor will want to hear that."

Important Points: (1) The medical assistant tells the patient through words and tone of voice, "I care about you." (2) The medical assistant remembers the patient's problem, which makes the person feel important. (3) The medical assistant reassures the patient about the care she will receive.

"Hello, Ms. Costanzo. It's been a long time since we've seen you. You must have been taking good care of yourself! Has a year really passed since your last examination? I'm glad to see you again."

Important Points: (1) The medical assistant pays Ms. Costanzo a compliment by suggesting that her good health is the result of her own actions. (2) The medical assistant implies "I like you" by saying "I am glad to see you again."

Listening

Perhaps even more important than what you say to patients is how well you listen to them. Listening shows respect for patients as human beings, not just as purchasers of medical service. You show patients that you are listening by facing them and making good eye contact, and by setting aside all other work while speaking with them. Have you ever tried to talk with someone who was shuffling through papers on a desk? Although the person might have said, "Go on, I'm listening," you probably did not feel you had the person's complete attention. Patients will know, too, when you are not listening attentively because you will be missing, or seeming to miss, the point or concern they are raising. A crowded waiting room is a very distracting environment, and you may be unable to give patients your full attention right at the moment they arrive. When this is the case, acknowledge a patient's presence by saying, "Hello, Mr. Faust, we are very busy today. Please have a seat, and I will be with you right away." Make eye contact from time to time to let him know you have not forgotten him.

Empathy

Empathy refers to understanding another's feelings and responding to those feelings sensitively. Empathy means putting yourself mentally in another's place. An emphatic medical assistant understands and offers comfort when a patient is anxious or in pain. Empathy is also important when dealing with relatives and friends of patients because they are worried, too. Consider the medical assistant's behavior in the following two situations. Does the medical assistant communicate empathy?

"Mrs. Robinette, I know how concerned you are about your mother's condition. The doctor will be able to tell you more about what you both can expect as she recovers."

Important Points: (1) The medical assistant tries to reassure the daughter. (2) The medical assistant does not make promises about the condition improving quickly.

(Interaction with a child.) "Don't worry, Raphael, if you can't give us a urine sample right now. You can try again before you leave the office. If that doesn't work, we'll give you a plastic container you can take home. Your mom can bring your sample back tomorrow."

Important Points: (1) The medical assistant tries to set the child at ease and does not embarrass him because he is unable to provide a urine sample immediately. (2) The medical assistant gives the child an alternative to providing a sample at the office, which relieves the child's stress.

You may not like every patient you meet. But remember, you are paid to treat them courteously and professionally, not to like them.

Tact

Tact means being careful about how you communicate so people will not become offended or upset. A tactful person is diplomatic and uses good judgment when working with other people. Most of us would not ask a friend, "Are you pregnant, or have you just gained a lot of weight?," or "Simone seems awfully small for her age. Are you sure she's all right?" In a medical office, the situations requiring tact are less personal but just as important. The patient who owes the physician money must be tactfully reminded to pay; the person who disturbs the reception area by talking loudly should be asked tactfully to speak more quietly; and the child who enters the treatment area often to go to the bathroom should be requested to remain in the reception area.

Most people know the difference between tact and tactlessness and strive to be tactful. Medical assistants who do not understand the effect of tactless comments and actions may jeopardize their jobs. Consider this situation. Did the medical assistant handle the following situation tactfully?

| Patient: | These insurance companies are robber barons. I paid my insurance every month for thirty years, and now the company won't cover my wife's operation. |
| Medical Assistant: | It can be very frustrating when you are not used to the insurance paperwork. Is there anything about your coverage that you do not understand? |

Important Points: (1) The medical assistant validates the patient's feelings by acknowledging them and offers to help explain the paperwork. (2) The medical assistant remains in control and does not make unprofessional remarks about insurance companies.

"I'll leave the room while you undress, Ms. Trolinger. Please remove your slacks and cover yourself from the waist down with this sheet (or gown). The doctor needs to check your abdomen and pelvis. You may wear your shirt."

Important Points: (1) The medical assistant is aware of the patient's modesty and leaves the room while the patient undresses. (2) The medical assistant provides explicit instructions about which clothes should be removed. (3) The medical assistant tells the patient the type of examination to expect.

Patience

Perhaps no human relations skill is as important to a medical assistant as patience. Being patient means that you do not show anger or irritation, even when patients are angry and irritable. Patients do not want to be sick; they do not want to wait; they do not want to incur large expenses for health care; they do not want to be frustrated by confusing paperwork or worried by unfamiliar medical terminology. They are likely to be bothered by any or all of the above when you see them and may sound angry or rude when actually they are frightened. You, as a medical assistant, cannot make them well, pay their bills, or take away all of their fears. What you can do is greet them calmly and courteously, listen attentively, and treat them with patience (Figure 5–2). Their anger is not directed at you, although it may seem so at times.

Patience often involves waiting — for people to undress or dress, give you information, or pay their bill. You may want to hurry them, interrupt their sentences, or speed things up so you can move on to the next task. When you feel yourself becoming impatient, maintain your self-control, breathe deeply, smile, and look for realistic ways to remedy the problem. Consider these situations.

The reception area is crowded because an obstetrics patient in labor required the physician's services at 8 AM at the hospital, and the doctor has not arrived at the office yet. Although waiting patients were understanding and gracious when they heard about the emergency, they are complaining to one another now about the delay, and several are irritable. One patient asks if she can be placed ahead of others.

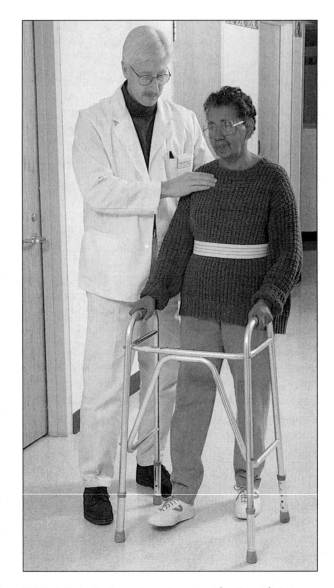

FIGURE 5-2 Patience is an important human relations skill for a medical assistant.

"Mrs. Parella, I'm sorry you've been delayed. Only three people remain ahead of you; and they too want to leave. Your wait will not be much longer, at most thirty minutes. You may reschedule the appointment if you like, or if you have errands close by, perhaps you could do a few chores, and come back in about thirty minutes."

Important Points: (1) The medical assistant recognizes that the patient's point is valid and that the wait has been long. (2) The medical assistant tries to give the patient a time frame for any additional wait and offers an alternative to waiting. (3) The medical assistant does not place this patient ahead of others.

(Interaction with an elderly person.) "Mr. Nuyen, we'll take all the time you need to walk down this hall slowly; we're not in any hurry. Would you like to hold my arm?"

Important Points: (1) The medical assistant recognizes that the elderly patient has difficulty walking but attempts to put him at ease by implying, "It's all right to walk slowly." (2) The medical assistant gives the patient the option of an arm to hold but does not insist, recognizing that the patient may prefer to walk without help.

Efficiency and impatience should not be confused. Efficiency means making good use of available time, whereas impatience refers to being rushed or hurried. You may feel conflict as you try to complete your paperwork and office chores and still give patients the time and courtesy they require. Review the list in Figure 5–3 to determine whether you are susceptible to impatient behavior. If you are susceptible, work to reduce your impatience.

Impatient Behavior

Rushing patients

Thinking that patients are slow

Finishing a patient's sentences

Interrupting people

Feeling stressed

Thinking ahead to what you will say

Feeling the urgency of time

Planning too far in advance

Skipping lunch or eating too fast at lunch

Looking at a clock often

Trying to do two things at once

Answering questions curtly

Taking on too many projects

FIGURE 5–3 Impatient behaviors

IMPORTANCE OF VERBAL AND NONVERBAL COMMUNICATION

The words that come out of our mouths are known collectively as oral or verbal communication, but we all have many other ways of expressing thoughts and feelings. Messages that are not written and do not use spoken words are called **nonverbal communication**. Consider the following examples:

"I'm not angry," the patient says, but her mouth is tight, her shoulders tense, and she stalks out of the room. What nonverbal message does she deliver? Does it agree with her oral communication?

"You're such a bad boy," a father tells his infant, smiling tenderly and tickling the baby's tummy. What is the father's real message?

When working with patients, you must be careful that your verbal and nonverbal communications send the same message and that both forms are appropriate to the circumstances; otherwise, you may confuse, hurt, or offend someone. Consider the following situation. Do you think the medical assistant's verbal and nonverbal messages agree?

The medical assistant is explaining office policy and procedures to a new patient. The assistant does not make eye contact with the patient, and her tone of voice is bored and flat.

"We strive to maintain a friendly, caring environment for all of our patients and always listen to questions and concerns."

How likely is the new patient to have questions and concerns? Does the medical assistant's communication convey a real sense of caring?

Verbal Communication

Verbal communication refers to spoken messages and includes face-to-face encounters, announcements, questions, offhand remarks, telephone conversations, gossip, and other forms of spoken communication. Successful communication depends on correct word choice and on the listener's understanding of what you say.

Many factors influence the communication process and affect understanding between communicators, including level of education, economic status, prior experiences, and cultural heritage (Figure 5–4). Because no universal meaning for words exists in people's minds, each person defines words based on the influencing factors. The greater the difference in backgrounds between communicators, the more difficulty they may encounter in understanding each other.

A patient who complains of a high fever may mean a temperature of 100°, but the medical assistant may think of a "high" fever as anything above 102°. If you advise a patient that the doctor is a "few minutes" behind schedule, your internal clock — the way you measure time — may be different from the patient's. The patient who expects to see the physician in ten or fifteen minutes may become angry at having to wait thirty or forty-five minutes. In each of these examples, you should be specific and avoid making general remarks. You should ask the patient the actual temperature degrees and pro-

vide an estimate of the length of the wait by saying, "Dr. Papastamou is about thirty minutes behind schedule."

As a medical assistant, you must be particularly careful about using technical or medical terms beyond the scope of the patient's understanding. Some people use technical words to impress the listener or to prove their superior knowledge. New employees or recent graduates, especially, may feel more important by using big words to show how smart they are. If you are confident of your education, you will recognize that use of medical words does not necessarily demonstrate knowledge, and you should not display your vocabulary at the expense of a patient's understanding or comfort. Consider this example.

"Mrs. Riser, here's a pamphlet on Lou Gehrig's disease that Dr. Valenti asked me to give you. It will help you understand your husband's illness. You'll notice from the pamphlet that weakness of the hand muscles is an early symptom."

This medical assistant knows that the patient will not understand medical language and uses layman's language to discuss the medical condition. A less informed medical assistant might have communicated in the following manner:

"Mrs. Riser, here's a pamphlet on amyotrophic lateral sclerosis that Dr. Valenti asked me to give you. The etiology of this disease is unknown; however, the pamphlet will help you understand your husband's illness. You'll notice from the pamphlet that atrophy of the hand muscles is an early symptom."

Nonverbal Communication

Nonverbal communication refers to messages sent without words or in addition to words. It includes facial expressions, touch, tone of voice, listening, eye contact, gestures, appearance, manner, time, body language, and silence (Figure 5–5). Every person sends and receives hundreds of nonverbal messages daily. They enhance the communication process and should be used by both the sender and the receiver to confirm verbal messages.

Nonverbal communication is important to any relationship, and this is especially true with

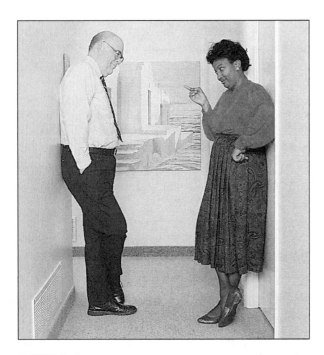

FIGURE 5–4 Communication is an important element in relationships.

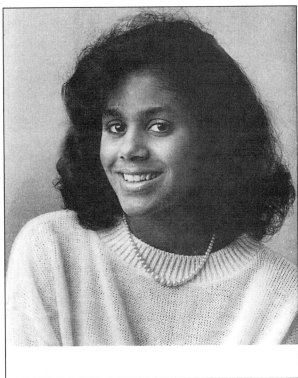

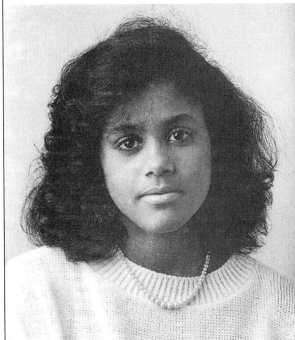

FIGURE 5–5 Facial expressions provide clues about how someone feels physically and emotionally.

people who are sick, uncomfortable, or anxious. If you are working with a diverse population of patients from many different backgrounds and cultures, touching the patient is not appropriate. This is a sign of disrespect. Your competence in using and interpreting nonverbal behavior will determine the degree of success you enjoy in your relationships with others. Several important nonverbal behaviors are explained in Figure 5–6.

Facial Expression

Appropriate Medical Assistant Facial Expression
- Response
- Alert
- Good eye contact

Revealing Patient Facial Expression
- Eyes looking away or down
- Frowning or sad expression
- Stare or unfocused look
- Thankful glance

Touch

Appropriate Medical Assistant Touch
- Firm handshake
- Light touch on arm or shoulder
- Guiding touch on elbow

Revealing Patient Touch
- Demanding grasp
- Grateful pat
- Attention-getting tap

Posture

Appropriate Medical Assistant Posture
- Upright
- Facing speaker
- "Open" posture; arms unfolded
- Relaxed, few distracting movements

Revealing Patient Posture
- Limping or otherwise showing pain
- "Closed" posture, feeling threatened
- Slumping, weary

Tone of Voice

Appropriate Tone of Voice for Medical Assistant
- Pleasant, clear

Revealing Patient Tone of Voice
- Sad
- Worried
- Fearful
- Bewildered

FIGURE 5–6 Nonverbal behavior

Feedback

Feedback refers to the response to a communication and may be verbal or nonverbal, positive or negative. Feedback is important when working with patients because it provides clues about the patient's health that the person may not articulate. As a medical assistant, you should be alert to patient feedback and use it to determine whether the patient's verbal and nonverbal messages agree. For example, the patient who replies, "Not really," and shrugs when the medical assistant asks, "Do you experience chest pain often?" may really mean "I experience chest pain enough that it bothers me, but I am frightened to talk about it." The answer, "Not really," therefore may mean, "Yes." The shoulder shrug represents nonverbal feedback and should alert the medical assistant to ask additional questions: "When is the last time you experienced chest pain?" "How long did it last?" and "When was the time prior to the last time? Tell me about that time." The patient's posture, hand gestures, eye movement, and tone of voice are important clues to how the patient is feeling.

COMPUTERS AND RELATIONSHIPS WITH PATIENTS

Complex tasks involving mountains of data make computers indispensable in modern medical offices. Computer software can organize and maintain patient records, reduce appointment scheduling conflicts, bill patients, complete insurance forms, and perform a wide variety of other time-saving duties. The disadvantages of software are apparent when computerization reduces the interaction between the medical staff and patients or complicates interpersonal relationships.

You may get caught up in the task you are trying to complete on a computer and forget to make proper eye contact with patients (Figure 5–7). One good rule is to be out of sight of patients if you are busy with paperwork and record keeping, especially if the waiting area is full and many people are waiting in line. Speak with your office manager about such an arrangement.

Because the use of computers in medical offices has increased and taken over many of the

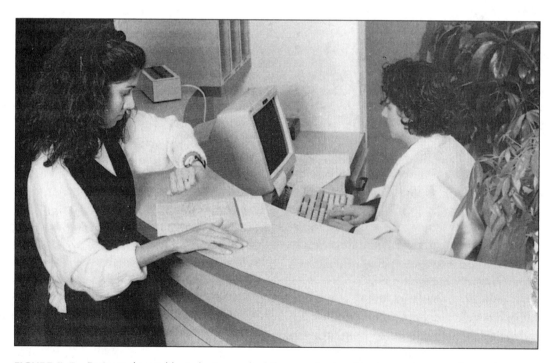

FIGURE 5–7   Patients do not like to be ignored while a medical assistant completes another task.

clerical tasks previously assigned to medical assistants, you may work with patients on a one-to-one basis less frequently. You must continue to show empathy and understanding for each patient's individual problems. For example, the patient who questions a billing statement and insists that he mailed a check to cover a previous balance is rightly concerned about a possible lost check. As a medical assistant, you should review the patient's account immediately to determine whether a check was received and, if so, when it was received. Do not rely on the excuse of "computer error." The last thing a patient wants to hear is about your internal office problems.

In a medical office where a patient's **anxiety** level is related to a physical condition, even insignificant computer errors become magnified and may cause extreme stress. You should be careful to avoid computer errors when possible and correct them if they do occur.

Although you may spend much of your time at a computer keyboard, make sure that you always greet patients with a warm "hello" and spend a minute or so in a brief "good-bye" when the patient pays for the day's services. If you have time to chat with a patient, stand, so you and the patient are on the same face-to-face level. Whether you are seated at your computer station or standing, maintain eye contact as you take part in each conversation.

Several Do's and Don'ts for the medical assistant who uses computers are listed here. Can you add others to this list?

1. *Do not* allow the computer to interfere with your relationship with patients.
2. *Do not* key data into a computer at the same time you talk with patients either in person or on the telephone.
3. *Do not* blame a computer for human errors.
4. *Do not* assume that mistakes will be eliminated when a computer is used. If computer input is flawed, a mistake will occur.
5. *Do not* allow patients to feel that they are merely accounts; they are people.
6. *Do not* refer to patients as numbers, for example, Patient No. 1602, or by their diagnosis, "the diabetic in 4."

7. *Do not* ask patients to wait several weeks for a computer correction of a billing or related problem.
8. *Do not* allow computerization to reduce your level of service to patients. If a patient makes a special request, follow up on it manually if the computer software does not allow the request, for example, by typing a special billing for a particular month.
9. *Do not* send impersonal, computerized form letters to patients.

IN YOUR OPINION

1. A patient storms into the outer office and pushes his way to the front of the line. Several other patients look alarmed. What verbal and nonverbal behaviors can you exhibit to defuse this situation?
2. Should a medical assistant pay more attention to verbal or nonverbal communication if a patient sends conflicting messages? Why?
3. How can a medical assistant reduce patient frustration over difficult paperwork and computer record keeping?

MANAGING PATIENT ACTIVITIES

A medical assistant manages many different patient activities each day. The effectiveness with which you accomplish these tasks will depend on your organizational and interpersonal skills.

Managing the Reception Area or Lobby

Managing the reception area or lobby is a constant challenge, especially during high traffic times. Because the reception area offers patients a comfortable place to rest while they wait to see the doctor and also provides the medical assistant with a means for monitoring patient traffic, you will be responsible for maintaining a gracious and tranquil environment. This means you must eliminate noisy play or running among children and ask patients to chat quietly. Patients weeping or in obvious distress should be taken to a private office.

> "Mr. Markham, you are in great distress; we've set aside a place in the office for our patients who need privacy. Let me show you the way."
>
> **Important Points:** (1) The medical assistant shows compassion. (2) The medical assistant suggests an alternative seating area.

Reception Area Appearance

Because the appearance of the reception area conveys a message about the organization of the medical office, it should be clean and inviting. Follow these procedures to create an attractive, pleasant place for patients to wait:

1. Arrange magazines in an orderly manner in a central location where they can be located easily. Discard magazines when they become outdated or tattered.
2. Discard dead or unattractive plants.
3. Reorganize children's toys several times during the day. Encourage children to keep toys within the area designated for play.
4. Arrange seating so that patients can chat, but make sure a few chairs provide privacy for patients who do not wish to socialize.
5. Use lighting to create a warm effect and provide a good reading light near magazine stands and chairs.
6. Straighten crooked lamp shades.
7. Play soft and soothing music to create a relaxing atmosphere (Figure 5–8).

Orderly Flow of Patient Traffic

If possible, you should have an unobstructed view of the lobby entrance and the entrance to the examining area from your desk. Attach a bell or other device at the lobby entrance if you cannot see it clearly, so you will know when a patient arrives. Check periodically to see that seating is available for everyone. Follow these procedures:

1. Answer the telephone before the third ring, if possible. An unanswered telephone is annoying both to patients waiting in the lobby and to the caller.

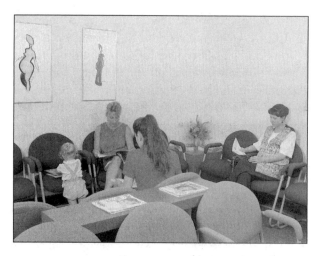

FIGURE 5–8 The appearance of the reception area communicates a message about the medical office.

2. Complete the checkout procedure for patients who are ready to leave before registering new arrivals. (This procedure is discussed in detail in the following chapters.)
3. Ask arriving patients to sign the registration pad. Then suggest they take a seat until you have completed all checkouts. Call the patients back individually to the registration desk when other traffic has slowed.

Greeting Patients

Greet patients immediately when they walk into the office. If you are busy with a task that cannot be interrupted, stop long enough to say, "Hello, Mrs. _____, I'll be with you in just a minute." Finish your task quickly or find a logical stopping place; then give your full attention to the patient. If you are talking on the telephone, acknowledge the patient's arrival with a friendly nod and a smile. Finish your conversation as quickly as possible. Then help the arriving patient. Never wait more than one minute to greet a patient.

> *Medical assistant who is conducting a telephone conversation with another person gives a friendly smile and a welcoming nod when a patient arrives at the office. After finishing the telephone conversation, the medical assistant greets the patient:*
>
> "Good morning, Mr. Longdon, how are you this morning? I hope you're feeling better."

Established Patients

Established patients know the office routine and usually sit and read or chat with other patients after checking in. They generally do not require a great deal of attention after they have registered with the receptionist; however, you should be alert to any special problems and help as needed. In the following example, an alert medical assistant makes the patient more comfortable.

An elderly patient on crutches is brought to the physician by her son who must return to work. The patient looks confused and anxious as the lobby fills with other patients. The assistant asks,

"Mrs. Allenton, would you like to sit in Dr. Brader's office while you wait? I'll bring a magazine in for you to read and you can call the nurse if you need anything. I think you may be more comfortable in the doctor's office."

Important Points: (1) The medical assistant recognizes that the crowded lobby and the long wait may bother the patient. (2) The medical assistant tries to relieve the patient's stress by moving her away from other patients.

New Patients

New patients require instruction in the registration procedure and office routine. Follow these procedures to orient new patients to the medical office:

1. Ask each new patient to sign the register; then give the person a pen or pencil and a patient information questionnaire. If the new patient is illiterate or speaks English as a second language, ask the questions from the form; give the patient ample time to respond; and then fill in the answers yourself.
2. Give new patients a pamphlet describing the office's billing practice, payment policy, business hours, telephone policies, and after-hours emergency procedures. Explain the policies if a pamphlet is not available.
3. Provide the names of all doctors sharing the practice and the names of the hospitals where the primary care physician is affiliated.
4. Ask patients if they have questions, and answer them completely.
5. Show the patient where to sit when registration is complete. Point out the magazines

and the water fountain and say that the physician will see the patient shortly.
6. Give the room number and ask the patient to follow you or the nurse to the treatment area.

A student at the local high school, a recent immigrant who lives with his single mother and brothers and sisters, has been referred to the medical office by the physical education teacher who senses that the teenager's recent absences may be due to an untreated physical problem. The medical assistant recognizes that the student has trouble with English.

"I need to ask you some questions for the doctor's records, so he can treat you. I will ask each question slowly. You tell me the answer, and I will write it on this form for the doctor to study." *(After completing the form.)* "Come with me, and I will show you where the doctor's office is located. He will want to talk with you before he examines you."

Important Points: (1) The medical assistant explains why the questions are being asked. (2) The medical assistant walks with the patient to the doctor's office.

DISCUSSING FINANCES AND BILLING

Discussing finances with patients may feel awkward at first, particularly with patients who have difficulty paying their bills. Yet the ability of the practice to pay employees, suppliers, the landlord, and others depends on steady income from patients. You should maintain a relationship with patients that encourages open discussion about finances and billing. After all, it is in the best interest of the patient and the doctor that you clarify with patients how their bill will be handled.

Importance of the First Visit

The best opportunity to discuss finances and billing is at the patient's first visit. You should provide the patient with a written copy of the practice's payment policy and then orally review the policy, explaining any unfamiliar terms. If the patient has questions, answer them fully. A patient's frown or an uncertain or skeptical look are examples of body language that should alert you to review and clarify the payment policy.

"Ms. Klavens, Dr. Becca requires payment at the completion of medical services. In the case of your surgery, the total fee will be $1,260." *(The patient states that her insurance company will be responsible for paying the fee. The medical assistant acknowledges the patient's insurance and explains that the patient must pay the physician first and then collect from the insurance company.)*

"Our policy is to ask the patient to pay the doctor's fee at the time of service; then you can file a claim with your insurance company for reimbursement. I will show you how to complete the insurance form if you like." *(The medical assistant notices that the patient is moving nervously in her chair as if she wants to speak but is uncertain.)*

"If you prefer, we can create a financial contract that allows you to pay a portion of the fee each month. A small finance charge will be added as a part of the contract."

Insurance Company Payments

Although most patients are covered by health insurance, the patient or the patient's guardian is responsible for payment of the account when the insurance does not pay. Patients may think the insurance company will pay the entire physician's fee, but this is not always true. Private insurance and government-funded programs, such as Medicare, do not pay the total cost for many medical procedures. Therefore, you must explain to patients their responsibility to pay the balance of the bill. In the initial conversation to explain billing, be sure the patient understands the payment procedures. This will reduce future misunderstandings.

Medical Assistant: Mr. Carberry, many insurance companies pay only a portion of your claim. Usually, you are responsible for paying a deductible amount of approximately 20%. That is why you were not reimbursed in full for Dr. Giuiella's fees.

Patient: These darned insurance companies, you think you're covered and then you're not. How would you like to explain that, young lady? How am I supposed to make heads or tails of this insurance lingo? Doctors, insurance companies, they're all in it together.

Medical Assistant: I can certainly see why you are upset. Is there someone at your company who can explain these forms to you? Or would you like me to make an appointment for you with our financial aid assistant?

HANDLING EMERGENCIES

Emergencies will severely test your interpersonal skills. You may feel upset personally, while also feeling responsible for keeping a calm atmosphere for the other patients. In addition to interrupting the daily schedule, walk-in emergency patients raise the anxiety level of people waiting in the reception area. Call-in emergency patients force the staff to change its daily schedule, and sometimes the physician may have to leave the office to attend the emergency.

Recognizing an Emergency

An emergency is clearly apparent when a patient bleeds profusely, appears catatonic, shakes violently, is short of breath, complains of chest pains, or demonstrates any other symptoms that indicate severe illness. However, emergencies that are not as easy to identify, such as internal bleeding, blood clots, or allergic reactions, are potentially more harmful because if left untreated, they become life-threatening. In addition, some acute illnesses, such as strep throat accompanied by a high fever, are considered emergencies by the patient, but do not actually represent an illness for which the physician should be interrupted.

The difficult responsibility of screening emergency calls goes to the medical assistant who greets patients and answers the telephone. If you have a question about whether an apparent emergency is real, you should alert the physician immediately. You do not have the medical background or the authority to determine what is an emergency and what is not. To attempt to make this decision is practicing medicine without a license and can be the basis for a malpractice lawsuit (see Chapter 4).

Whether an emergency patient arrives at the medical office or the emergency is telephoned, certain problems represent serious, potentially life-threatening situations and must receive priority status. Figure 5–9 lists examples of life-threatening emergencies.

Obtaining Specific Information about Call-in Emergency Patients

Emergencies reported by telephone are difficult to identify because you cannot see the patient, yet you must obtain enough information to determine whether the physician should be interrupted. If a telephone caller is hysterical, crying, or too excited to provide precise information, ask the caller to put another person on the line if possible.

You can increase the efficient handling of an emergency by remaining calm and composed. Before emergencies arise, ask the physician to help you prepare a list of questions to ask in specific situations, such as a heart attack or premature labor. Then ask the questions on the list each time you receive an emergency call. Several general questions are provided in the following list. Discuss these with your employer and add others appropriate for the medical specialty.

1. The name of the patient and the relationship of the caller? (Wife, mother, brother, friend, passerby?)
2. The nature of the emergency? (What happened?)
3. When the emergency occurred? (What time? Today?)
4. The extent of the emergency? (How bad?)
5. The patient's symptoms? (Is the patient bleeding? Profusely?)
6. Treatment provided? (What has been done for the patient?)
7. Has an ambulance been called? (Will the patient receive treatment from a rescue team?)
8. The name of the patient's physician? (Is your employer the patient's primary care physician?)

The situations described here demonstrate the proper method for screening emergency calls. If a caller indicates that an emergency is taking place, alert the physician immediately.

Medical Emergencies

Heart attack

Drug overdose

Profuse bleeding from a head or chest wound

Damage to eye

Allergic reactions (such as to a bee sting or to food)

Poisoning

Burns

Suicidal behavior

Premature labor

Foreign objects in windpipe

Extreme fever in adults

Gunshot wound

Car accident

FIGURE 5–9 Emergency medical situations

Caller:	I need to talk to the doctor right away. I'm five months pregnant, and I think I'm in labor.
Medical Assistant:	What is your name, please?
Caller:	Amelia Greene, but I need to talk to Dr. Moskowitz.

Medical Assistant: I will get Dr. Moskowitz, but I need to be able to tell her your symptoms. Are you in pain?

Caller: I have awful stomach cramps.

Medical Assistant: Do you have back pain?

Caller: No, not really, but the stomach pains make me hurt all over.

Medical Assistant: Are you spotting blood?

Caller: No.

Medical Assistant: Have you lost any clear fluid from your vagina?

Caller: No.

Medical Assistant: Do you have a fever?

Caller: I didn't take my temperature, but I don't feel hot.

Medical Assistant: Is this your first pregnancy?

Caller: Yes.

Medical Assistant: When did you eat last?

Caller: I had lunch with a friend about three hours ago.

Medical Assistant: Did your pains start before or after lunch?

Caller: After lunch.

Medical Assistant: What did you eat for lunch?

Caller: Pizza.

Medical Assistant: What telephone number are you calling from?

Caller: 555-4580. Are you getting Dr. Moskowitz?

Medical Assistant: Dr. Moskowitz is treating another patient, but she should be finished in about five minutes. I will tell her about your symptoms immediately, and she will call you back.

The medical assistant in this situation used a list of questions prepared in advance by the physician. The medical assistant may suspect that the patient is suffering stomach cramps from lunch, but does not have the medical background or the authority to make such a decision. The physician is notified immediately because this problem represents a potential emergency.

Caller: My baby isn't breathing! Give me the doctor!

Medical Assistant: I'm sorry, I can't understand you. Say that again.

Caller: I want to talk to Dr. Petty! Right now!

Medical Assistant: Is someone with you? I can't understand you. Please put another person on the phone.

Neighbor: This is Myra Broadhurst.

Medical Assistant: What is your relationship to the patient?

Caller: I'm a neighbor. I live next door.

Medical Assistant: What is the patient's name and the problem?

Neighbor: It's Matthew Johnson, he's 8 months old, and he's having a convulsion.

Medical Assistant: What are Matthew's symptoms?

Neighbor: He's been sick for about four days, and today he's been listless. About ten minutes ago he cried out; then he went stiff, and now he's motionless. I think he's still breathing.

Medical Assistant: What is the baby's temperature?

Neighbor: He's had a high fever for two days; just about an hour ago it was 105 degrees.

Medical Assistant: Do you have a car to take the baby to the hospital emergency room?

Neighbor: Yes.

Medical Assistant: Hold on just a minute while I get Dr. Petty.

This is an obvious emergency that the medical assistant recognizes should be referred to the physician. However, the medical assistant obtains specific information for the physician before interrupting another patient's treatment.

Arranging for Emergency Medical Care

Immediate treatment should be provided for life-threatening emergencies. Follow these procedures for maximum efficiency in dealing with emergency patients:

1. As soon as an emergency patient appears, alert the physician and take the person to an examining room.
2. For emergencies reported by telephone, ask the physician whether the emergency patient should be brought to the office or taken directly to the hospital.
3. If the physician is out of the office briefly, ask the nurse what to do.
4. If both the physician and nurse are unavailable, tell the patient to go directly to a hospital emergency room.
5. After patients are referred to the hospital emergency room, call the emergency room to alert the staff that the patient is on the way. Give a description of the medical problem so the staff can prepare for the patient's examination. Locate the physician and provide full details about the emergency.
6. If the patient is an accident victim, call the police and provide the address of the accident. The dispatcher will send a rescue unit to the scene and alert the nearest emergency room that a patient is on the way. Once the patient has stabilized, a private ambulance can transport the person to any hospital the primary care physician designates.

Reassuring Family and Waiting Patients

The medical assistant's responsibility does not end when the emergency patient receives treatment. You must reassure family members, who will be frightened, and other persons who witnessed the arrival of the emergency patient. To reduce confusion, take family members to a private room where they will not interfere with the physician's examination or further upset patients in the reception area. Check back often to answer the family's questions.

Advise patients waiting in the reception area that the emergency patient is being treated. Tell them you will let them know as soon as possible the length of delay in the physician's schedule. Some patients will ask questions about the emergency that are too private to share. Tactfully field these questions.

Curious Patient: What happened to that man who was bleeding?

Medical Assistant: He was in an accident.

Curious Patient: What kind of accident? That looked like a gunshot wound.

Medical Assistant: I don't know the details.

IN YOUR OPINION

1. How can the medical assistant ensure a welcoming, uncluttered atmosphere in the waiting area, especially during busy times like flu season?
2. What are the most important things for the medical assistant to determine when answering an emergency call?
3. What would you do with a first-time patient who does not speak English very well, or read it at all, and who does not understand the payment terms?

INTERNET ACTIVITIES

Go to the *Nurse Week* magazine Web site at http://www.nurseweek.com. At the Search box, enter *How to work with patients of all ages*. When the article with this title or an article of a similar title appears, read the recommendations for dealing with different types of patients. Summarize the article briefly.

STUDENT STUDY CHECKLIST

Workbook

1. Complete Chapter 5 exercises in the workbook.
2. Complete Chapter 5 simulations in the workbook that access the CD-ROM in the book.

Administrative CD-ROM

1. Go to the Library and play the interactive games for Chapter 5.
2. Go to the Patient Reception area of the office on the CD-ROM, take the tour, and complete the exercises.
3. What can be done in a reception area to make it patient-friendly? If you were designing and staffing a reception area for a medical office, list the attributes you would want in the office and the staff.

REFERENCES

Career Solutions Training Group. *The Quick Skills Series: Attitude and Self-Esteem.* Cincinnati, OH: South-Western, 2001.

Career Solutions Training Group. *The Quick Skills Series: Listening.* Cincinnati, OH: South-Western, 2000.

Career Solutions Training Group. *The Quick Skills Series: Handling Conflict.* Cincinnati, OH: South-Western, 2000.

Humphrey, Doris. *Pediatric Associates, P.C.* Cincinnati, OH: South-Western, 1997.

Lindh, Wilberta Q., Marilyn S. Pooler, and Carol D. Tamparo. *Administrative Medical Assisting,* 2nd ed. Clifton Park, NY: Delmar Learning, 2002.

CHAPTER ACTIVITIES

PERFORMANCE-BASED ACTIVITIES

1. Go to Google.com or another search engine and enter the key words Medical Office Furniture. From the list of several vendors of medical office equipment, review the e-catalogs and identify the furniture that would be needed to outfit the reception area of a new medical office.

   _____

   _____

   _____

   _____

2. Identify communication behaviors that would be appropriate among your family and friends but would be considered unprofessional in a medical office.

   _____

   _____

   _____

   _____

3. Discuss your communication style with a classmate. Ask for a list of (1) your communication characteristics that would be most helpful in a medical office and (2) a list of your communications characteristics that you need to change before working with patients and medical professionals.

   _____

   _____

   _____

   _____

4. An emergency situation affects each of the following: other medical assistants, nurses, doctors, waiting patients. Write a short paper describing how you can assist each.

5. Establish guidelines for communication, including words and actions, when dealing with a bewildered, elderly, or foreign-born patient.

6. Develop and print the dialogue you would have with a patient angry over confusing claim forms. Role-play the dialogue with a classmate.

EXPANDING YOUR THINKING

1. Which situation would you give priority?

   a. A ringing phone or an arriving patient?

   b. A patient with a question or a patient ready to pay a bill?

   c. Retrieving a file for a doctor or updating a computer record?

   d. A messy waiting area or a late report?

e. An arriving elderly patient or an arriving mother with infant?

f. An angry patient or a weeping patient?

2. What could you say or do in each of the following situations to exemplify professional behavior?

a. A patient is flirting with you.

b. A child is throwing toys, and the child's mother does not seem to notice.

c. A patient refuses to pay a bill.

d. A patient wants to talk about a sick family member, and you have other pressing duties.

e. A patient claims that he has been charged for services not provided.

3. What questions would you ask if you received each of the following emergency phone calls?

a. "There's been a fire . . ."

b. "My child fell off her bike."

c. "There's been a diving accident at the quarry."

d. "My mother has been asleep all day, and I can't wake her."

e. "My husband was shoveling snow, and he collapsed."

CHAPTER 6

Telecommunications

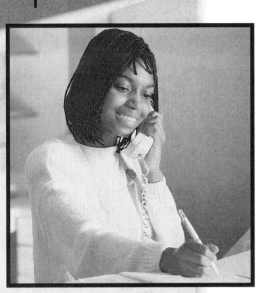

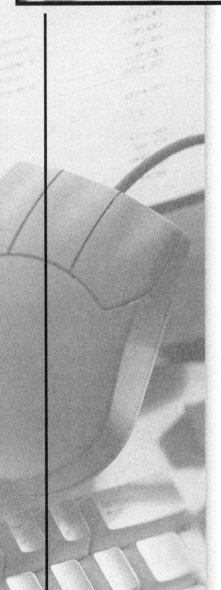

MUNCIE, INDIANA

I'm amazed at how telecommunications has affected our work in this midsized group practice. Fifty years ago the staff was using rotary phones, making long-distance calls through operators, just getting used to dictating machines, and marveling at the first electric typewriters. Calculating machines were large and loud, capable of annoying you for minutes as they chugged mechanically through their calculations.

Now, I routinely set up and place multistate long-distance conference calls, send facsimiles — faxes — over telephone lines to insurance companies all across the country, manage the doctors' beeper and pager systems, and coordinate our office answering service. Our computers are networked, so all of us are constantly updating central files, as well as using the Internet to send e-mail and attachments or locating a research document for one of the doctors.

Fifty years from now? Who knows? Maybe we'll have computer chips embedded in our earlobes that will allow us to connect directly, on voice command, to other people, or businesses, or computers. Maybe we'll be our own telephones. Anyway, what we have right now is more than enough for me. Learning all the systems, knowing when to use which, and discovering how to do two or three operations at once takes a little time. But once I got the rhythm of it all, it was amazing how much I could accomplish.

Christian Stoudt
Medical Assistant

PERFORMANCE-BASED COMPETENCIES

After completing this chapter, you should be able to:

1. Originate and respond to business telephone calls.
2. Formulate appropriate telephone greetings for a medical office.
3. Compare the advantages and disadvantages of station-to-station, person-to-person, direct-dialed, and operator-assisted calls.
4. Discriminate between instances in which putting a caller on "hold" is acceptable and those in which it is unacceptable.
5. Outline eight pieces of information needed for a callback message.
6. Prepare a fax message.

VOCABULARY

Answering service   Twenty-four-hour service that answers phones for a fee.

Callback   A message that requires a return call.

Cellular phone   Portable telephone that operates by means of batteries, independent of any fixed location.

Conference call   A single call that allows several individuals—perhaps in different cities—to participate. Even the most inexpensive office telephone systems usually provide a feature that allows a medical office assistant to connect up to three or four individuals to one call.

DDD   Direct Distance Dialing; placing long-distance calls directly, without intervention of an operator.

E-mail   Electronic mail routed through a computer network allows persons at different computer terminals around the world to write messages for others on the network.

Fax   Facsimile transmission of documents by telephone line from one location to another.

Hold   Telephone function that allows a call to be kept waiting on the line.

Modem   Hardware that connects your computer, via phone lines, to other computers and to the Internet.

Reversed charges   Collect call.

Screening   Evaluation of a call for proper referral.

Time zone   Geographic area identified by its time of day in relation to time in other parts of the country or world.

Videoconference   A conference that connects participants in various locations through telephone lines, a video camera, and computer hookups. Videoconferences are often substituted for costly in-person conferences that would require participants to travel long distances.

Voice mail   Voice messages that are left in an answering system when the office staff is not available to take a call personally.

Most physicians are rarely out of phone reach. The telephone links patients with the physician at all times by (1) ringing the medical office when a patient dials the correct number, (2) switching calls automatically to an **answering service** or answering machine when the office is closed, and (3) forwarding calls to a consulting physician when the primary care physician is unavailable. Telephone communication allows local and long-distance business transactions to be conducted quickly and efficiently. Long-distance service expands the local calling area to more than 500 billion telephones nationally and internationally. The convenience and communication capability of such a vast network is immense, allowing a person in one part of the world to talk to another in a matter of minutes. The computer in your office will probably have a **modem**, allowing you and other members of your office team to send and receive records, to access databases, and to tap medical resources worldwide using telephone connections.

Communicating by telephone will consume a major portion of your day as a medical assistant. Effective, courteous telephone communication will make you a valued asset in any medical environment. Whether a telephone conversation is about a patient's health, an appointment, a billing problem, or some other matter, each conversation is unique and must be handled in a professional manner. You will learn to handle multiple calls, some of which will be urgent. Your interviewing and analytical skills will help you determine rapidly (1) the nature of the call, (2) the urgency of the call, and (3) how to direct or respond to the call. Time is a scarce resource in the medical office, and your thoughtful, intelligent handling of telephone communications will improve efficiency.

ANSWERING THE TELEPHONE

The first contact most people have with the medical office is by telephone with the medical assistant. Your telephone manner and tone of voice will create the first impression. You must speak clearly and slowly, give your full attention to the caller, and use good human relations skills (Figure 6–1).

Telephone Turnoffs — I

Do not use slang in conversations at the medical office. Although casual language may be acceptable in personal conversations, you are labeled as unprofessional when you use slang in business conversations. Words such as "hi" instead of "hello" or "yeah" instead of "yes" are typical examples of slang. You should also avoid technical language, because patients feel uncomfortable if they do not understand the terminology used.

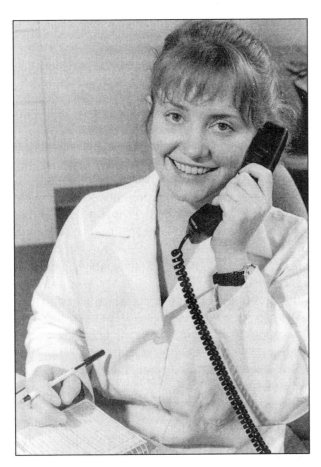

FIGURE 6–1 Good telephone communication skills are essential for a medical assistant.

Telephone Turnoffs — II

Have you ever placed a call that was answered by someone who spoke so quickly you were not sure whether you had called the right number? Or perhaps the person answered with a false cheeriness that you found annoying or spoke so loudly that it hurt your ears? Because patients react negatively to annoying greetings, you should analyze your telephone answering manner and eliminate any behaviors that could be considered irritating or unprofessional.

Answer the telephone as soon as possible but no later than the third ring. Use a sincere, warm greeting that communicates good will. Your office should have a standard greeting, used by everyone who routinely answers the phone. This helps patients recognize that they have reached the right number. In a small practice of one or two physicians, you may use the physicians' names, a cordial greeting of "Good morning" or "Good afternoon," followed by "May I help you?" Identifying yourself is unnecessary.

Group practices may be large. Using all the names is time-consuming as well as confusing to the patient. A shortened greeting giving the corporate name or identifying the medical practice is acceptable. Use greetings such as these:

"Good morning, Dr. Suarez' office. May I help you?"

"Drs. Gladding and Squires. How may I help you?"

"Doctor's office. How may I help you?"

"Allied Medical Services. How may I help you?"

The "Hold" Function

Holding refers to the telephone's capability to keep a call waiting on one line while a second call is on another line. The two callers do not hear one another's conversations. When a call is placed on **hold**, it blocks the telephone line, making the line unavailable to incoming and outgoing calls. Asking a person to hold is often necessary, as you will usually need to retrieve a schedule or record to respond to the caller's need. You should use the "hold" function when the person being called cannot come to the telephone immediately or when the person answering the telephone is busy with another call. Do not abuse "hold" by using the function too frequently or by keeping callers waiting for long periods.

Recipient of the Call Is Not Immediately Available

When the recipient of a call will be available within several minutes, you may ask the caller to hold. Before placing a caller on hold, ask the person's permission and give the reason for the delay. Then check back at thirty-second intervals. If the recipient of the call cannot answer within one minute, take a **callback** message and telephone number so the line can be freed for another call. The policy in some medical offices is to ask for a callback message first and to place the caller on hold only if the person specifically requests, as this example shows:

Medical Assistant:	Family Medical Associates. How may I help you?
Caller:	This is Ken Oja. Dr. Ozick told me to call this morning about my son's fever.
Medical Assistant:	Dr. Ozick is on another line, Mr. Oja. May I take your number and have her return your call?
Caller:	I'd rather hold, if you don't mind.
Medical Assistant:	That's fine. I'll check back with you shortly.
	(A half minute passes.)
Medical Assistant:	Mr. Oja, Dr. Ozick is still on another line. Do you want to continue holding or would you prefer she call you back?
Caller:	I still want to hold.
Medical Assistant:	Fine. I'll put you on hold again.
	(Another half minute passes.)
Medical Assistant:	Mr. Oja, Dr. Ozick is taking much longer than I expected. I'm not sure when she will be finished. If you will give me your number, I'll give her the message and she will call you as soon as she is available.
Caller:	All right. My number is 555-2129.
Medical Assistant:	Thank you. Good-bye.
Caller:	Good-bye.

The Person Answering the Telephone Is Talking on Another Line

On busy days, you will juggle telephone calls constantly, and some calls must be placed on hold. When holding is necessary, *ask the caller's permission before pressing the hold button.* Take a callback message if you cannot return to the line in one minute, and remember that time will seem much shorter to you, fielding calls, than it does to the person waiting on the other end of the line. Never answer a ringing phone with the words "Hold" or "Hold, please" before giving the caller an opportunity to speak. This practice is rude and some people will hang up rather than wait.

Medical Assistant:	Good morning, Pediatric Specialties. May I help you?
Caller:	This is Gina Flynt. I'd like to make an appointment.
Medical Assistant:	Ms. Flynt, I'm on another line. May I call you back shortly?
Caller:	May I hold?
Medical Assistant:	My other call may take several minutes. I would rather call you back.
Caller:	Okay, I'm at 555-1314.
Medical Assistant:	Thank you. I'll speak with you shortly.

Abuses of the Hold Function

When the hold function is abused, it creates a negative impression for the office and for the person who answers the telephone. Basic good manners and business sense dictate when hold should be used. A list of Dos and Don'ts for holding is given in Figure 6–2. You may be able to add to the list from your personal calling experience.

SCREENING CALLS

Most of the calls to a medical office are from people who wish to make appointments. Other calls are from patients seeking information, sales representatives, or insurance claim handlers. As a medical assistant you will screen all incoming calls and handle most of them yourself.

Hold Function Etiquette

Do	Don't
Ask the caller's permission before putting a line on hold.	Put a line on hold until the caller states a reason for the call.
Check back with the caller frequently.	Leave a caller suspended on the line for several minutes.
Ask for a callback message and number.	Put several lines on hold at the same time.
Remember for whom the caller is holding.	Ask, "Whom are you calling?"
Push the correct button for the line to be held.	Cut a caller off because of carelessness.
Return the call and apologize if you cut someone off by mistake.	Be rude or flippant about cutting a caller off.

FIGURE 6–2 Hold function etiquette

The physician personally takes very few telephone calls. Calls you should direct to the physician fall into five major categories:

1. Emergencies
2. Calls from other physicians
3. Patients who wish to talk to the physician personally
4. The physician's family
5. Business calls you think should be referred to your employer (Figure 6–3).

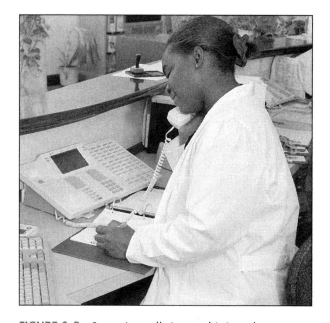

FIGURE 6–3 Screening calls is a sophisticated process.

The only people who should be routed to the physician immediately are emergency callers, other physicians, and family members the physician has identified. Because family callers are a matter of personal preference, you should ask the physician to explain the policy on family calls. Patients who do not have a medical emergency and important business callers should be asked to leave a telephone number. The doctor will return the call at a convenient time later in the day. The patient who is concerned about a reaction to a medication and the physician's attorney are other examples of people who should be allowed to speak to the physician personally, depending on office policy. Some telephone calls are difficult to screen because the caller says that the physician asked to be telephoned or that the matter is personal business. If callers refuse to leave their name or telephone number, suggest they write or **e-mail** the medical office. Remember, callers with legitimate business do not mind leaving their names.

Unless an emergency is involved, physicians rarely take telephone calls. You should take a message and a callback number for calls that the physician is to return and suggest an approximate time of day when the call will be returned. Physicians generally set aside special times of the day, such as after lunch or in the late afternoon, for making callbacks.

Procedures for Screening Calls

1. Ask the person's name and the reason for the call.
2. Ask questions that clarify the reason for the call.
3. Handle the call personally if you can.
4. Transfer the call to another staff member when appropriate.
5. Get the details for a callback message if the physician should return the call.

Typical Screening Situations

Incoming Call — To Make an Appointment

Medical Assistant: Dr. Reber's office. Good morning.

Caller: I need to speak with Dr. Reber.

Medical Assistant: Dr. Reber is with a patient right now. May I ask who is calling?

Caller: This is Samuel Chapman.

Medical Assistant: Are you a patient of Dr. Reber's?

Caller: Yes.

Medical Assistant: Would you like to make an appointment, Mr. Chapman?

Caller: Yes, I would.

(Continue with conversation by scheduling an appointment.)

Incoming Call — To Discuss a Medical Condition

Medical Assistant: Dr. Mooring's office. May I help you?

Caller: I'd like to talk to Dr. Mooring.

Medical Assistant: Dr. Mooring is not available at the moment. May I ask who is calling, please?

Caller: This is Su Kim.

Medical Assistant: Are you a patient of Dr. Mooring's?

Caller: Yes.

Medical Assistant: Would you like to make an appointment, Ms. Kim?

Caller: No, I need to speak with the doctor.

Medical Assistant: Is your question about a medical problem?

Caller: Yes.

Medical Assistant: If you will tell me your symptoms, I will check with the nurse who is available.

Caller: Well, it's my son, Ling. Last night, he vomited several times. This morning, he has diarrhea, a sore throat, and a fever. He's diabetic, and I wondered if I should bring him in.

Medical Assistant: Ms. Kim, I'm sure Dr. Mooring will want to check Ling. Can you come in this afternoon at either 3:30 or 4:30?

Caller: I can come at 3:30.

(Continue by making appointment.)

Incoming Call — Referral to a Consulting Physician

Medical Assistant: Dr. Avellino's office. May I help you?

Caller: I'd like to talk to Dr. Avelino.

Medical Assistant: Dr. Avelino is in surgery. May I ask who is calling?

Caller: This is Tanya Tyrell.

Medical Assistant: Are you a patient of Dr. Avelino's?

Caller: Yes.

Medical Assistant: Do you need an appointment, Ms. Tyrell?

Caller: No, I'd like to talk to Dr. Avelino.

Medical Assistant: Is your call about a medical problem?

Caller: Yes.

Medical Assistant: If you will tell me your symptoms, I will check with the nurse who is available.

Caller: Well, I think I might have broken my foot at hockey practice yesterday, and I wanted Dr. Avelino to check it.

Medical Assistant: Ms. Tyrell, Dr. Avelino will want you to see an orthopedist. He refers all our patients to Dr. Amy Rodriguez, who is in our same building. Dr. Rodriguez's telephone number is 555-8923. After checking your foot, Dr. Rodriguez will send a report to Dr. Avelino.

Caller: Thank you. I wasn't sure whom I should see.

Incoming Call — For Billing Charges and Insurance Information

Medical Assistant: Dr. Wilton's office. May I help you?

Caller: This is Elvia Alvarez with United Mutual Insurance Company. I need information about the charges for one of your patients.

Medical Assistant: Ms. Alvarez, I will transfer your call to Joycelyn Chambers, who is in charge of insurance payments for our office.

Incoming Call — "Personal Business"

Medical Assistant: Good morning, Dr. Darryl's office. May I help you?

Caller: Dr. Darryl, please.

Medical Assistant: I'm sorry, Dr. Darryl is unavailable. May I ask who is calling?

Caller: This is a personal call. I'm a friend of his.

Medical Assistant: Dr. Darryl usually returns calls at the end of the day. If you will leave your name and number, I will ask him to return your call.

Caller: It's Rolfe Dijon at 555-7892.

Incoming Call — About a New Doctors' Building

Medical Assistant: Dr. Duprey's office. May I help you?

Caller: I'd like to talk to Dr. Duprey.

Medical Assistant: I'm sorry, Dr. Duprey is with a patient at the moment. May I ask who is calling?

Caller: This is Alice Russell.

Medical Assistant: Are you a patient, Ms. Russell?

Caller: No.

Medical Assistant: May I ask why you are calling?

Caller: I'd like to speak to Dr. Duprey about a new professional building we have almost completed. Many physicians in the city are relocating because of the choice location.

Medical Assistant: Ms. Russell, I'll transfer you to our office manager, who will take the details and give the information to Dr. Duprey.

Caller: I'd rather talk to Dr. Duprey.

Medical Assistant: I regret that will not be possible. May I transfer you?

Incoming Call — Refusal to Speak to Anyone but Physician

Medical Assistant: Rosemont Medical. May I help you?

Caller: I'd like to talk to Dr. Lesnick.

Medical Assistant: Dr. Lesnick is not available right now. May I ask who is calling?

Caller: This is Lance Clark.

Medical Assistant: Are you a patient of Dr. Lesnick's?

Caller: Yes.

Medical Assistant: Would you like to make an appointment, Mr. Clark?

Caller: No, I'd like to talk to Dr. Lesnick.

Medical Assistant: Is your call about a medical problem?

Caller: Yes.

Medical Assistant: If you will tell me your symptoms, I will check with the nurse who is available.

Caller: No, I just want to talk to the doctor.

Medical Assistant: May I ask if your problem is an emergency?

Caller: It's not an emergency.

Medical Assistant: Dr. Lesnick usually returns her calls after seeing her last patient before lunch. That will be between 12:30 and 1:00 PM. If you will give me your number, I'll ask her to call.

(Continue by taking the telephone number. Put the message on the physician's desk immediately with a note that the patient wanted to speak only to the doctor.)

Taking Messages

Physicians and nurses do not routinely answer telephone calls; therefore, you will take callback messages frequently.

Procedures for Taking Callback Messages

1. Write the date and time of the call.
2. Write the name of the person who was called.
3. Ask the caller's name and telephone number.
4. Ask whether the caller will telephone again.
5. Write the complete message (Figure 6–4).

Be sure to ask for specifics if the message is unclear. Add your initials as the person who took the call. Figure 6–5 illustrates a telephone message pad. Some medical offices use carbon-coated telephone message pages, so a record of all incoming calls is available.

Special Screening Procedures

Patients often call physicians for advice about medication, dosage, prescriptions, side effects, symptoms, or recovery. In **screening** calls per-

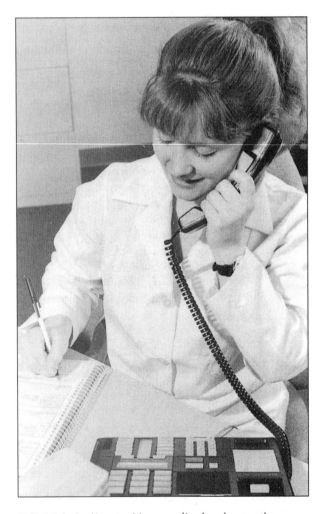

FIGURE 6–4 Keep writing supplies handy near the telephone.

IMPORTANT MESSAGE

TO ___Dr. Margehon___

DATE ___5/2/0–___   TIME ___9:15___ (AM) PM

WHILE YOU WERE OUT

M ___Joseph Petriccione, President___

OF ___Chamber of Commerce___

Area Code & Exchange ___215-555-7164___

TELEPHONED		PLEASE CALL	X
CALLED TO SEE YOU		WILL CALL AGAIN	
WANTS TO SEE YOU		URGENT	
	RETURNED YOUR CALL		

Message ___Needs to know how much time___
___to schedule for your presentation___
___on medical malpractice___

Operator ___Al Paige___

FIGURE 6–5 Telephone message pad

taining to a medical condition, ask questions that will help the patient give a complete explanation. Two typical situations that require in-depth screening are calls about prescriptions and calls about an illness. You must follow special procedures for screening these calls. Review the procedures and the screening situation. Then compare the callback form left for the physician in Figure 6–6.

Procedures for Prescription Refill Requests

Ask:

1. Name of the patient
2. Name of the medication
3. Length of time the patient has taken the medication
4. Patient's symptoms
5. Patient's age and weight, if a child
6. Name and telephone number of the patient's pharmacy
7. Patient's telephone number

NAME *Shana Grimwade*	PHONE	DX *Graves' Disease*		
DATE *6/10* TIME *9:00* DR	/ EXAM			TELEPHONE CONVERSATION RECORD

FROM TO *Dr. Midori Chisara*   RETURN PHONE # WILL CALL BACK *(215) 555-0101*   RETURN TIME *4:00*

MESSAGE CC/HC *Patient's medication will run out before we can give her an appointment for a routine checkup. She requests a refill.*

PHARMACY *Gateway*
PHONE ☐ *(215) 555-9423* AGE *50* WT *150*
Synthroid
tablets AMT *125 mcg*
SIG *tablet once a day*
FOR *Graves' Disease*
SIDE EFFECTS *No* REFILL
FOLLOW UP
No generics

FIGURE 6–6 Medical callback form

Procedures for Taking Messages Regarding an Illness

Ask:

1. Name of the patient
2. Name and relationship of the caller, if different from the patient
3. When the patient's symptoms first appeared
4. Whether the patient has had similar symptoms in the past
5. Whether the patient has a fever and, if so, the temperature

Many medical offices use a specially designed message form that provides space for both medical and general information. Some medical offices use a computer program that allows the medical assistant to key information on a message form shown on the computer screen as illustrated in Figure 6–7. If you listen carefully when you make business calls, you may be able to hear the sound of computer keys being struck as your message is taken. The message is then printed and delivered by hand to the recipient, or it may be sent to the recipient by electronic mail (see Chapter 8).

Handling Emergency Calls

Emergency calls represent potentially life-threatening situations and should be handled efficiently and quickly. The caller may be frightened and excited, which makes obtaining required information difficult. Review the following sample conversation between a medical assistant and an emergency patient. Also refer to the section called "Handling Emergencies" in Chapter 5 for a thorough review of emergency procedures.

Incoming Call — Emergency

Medical Assistant: Dr. Romaine's office. May I help you?
Caller: I need to talk to Dr. Romaine.
Medical Assistant: Dr. Romaine is not available at the moment. May I ask who is calling?
Caller: This is Larry Hamm.
Medical Assistant: Are you a patient of Dr. Romaine's?
Caller: Yes.
Medical Assistant: Would you like to make an appointment, Mr. Hamm?

```
Call to:   Dr. Margehon              Time:   9:15 A.M.

Call from: Joseph Petriccione        Date:   May 2, 20—
           Chamber of Commerce

Number:    (215) 555-7164

Needs to know how much time to schedule for your
presentation on medical malpractice.


Taken by:  Al Paige
```

FIGURE 6–7 Computer message screen

Caller:	No, I'd like to talk to Dr. Romaine.
Medical Assistant:	Is your call about a medical problem?
Caller:	Yes.
Medical Assistant:	If you will tell me your symptoms, I will check with the nurse who is available.
Caller:	I'm not feeling well. My left arm tingles, I'm sweating, and I'm having trouble breathing.
Medical Assistant:	When did this start?
Caller:	About an hour ago.
Medical Assistant:	Does your chest hurt?
Caller:	Not right this minute, but I had some really bad pains a few minutes ago. That's why I called.
Medical Assistant:	Is anyone with you, Mr. Hamm?
Caller:	No.
Medical Assistant:	I'll get Dr. Romaine. Stay on the line; she'll be right with you.

(Get the physician immediately. This patient may be experiencing a heart attack.)

Study the techniques listed in Figure 6–8 for more suggestions on using the telephone.

Telephone Techniques

1. **Put Yourself in the Caller's Place.** People who call a medical office are often sick or worried about a family member. When a caller sounds unfriendly, mentally put yourself in the person's place and treat the caller as you would like to be treated in a similar situation.

2. **Give Your Full Attention to the Caller.** When you are talking on the telephone, answer questions fully, even though you may be busy. Allow the caller to explain the reason for the call, and do not interrupt except to encourage information.

3. **Speak Clearly and Distinctly.** As you converse, speak directly into the mouthpiece. Talk clearly and distinctly. Never chew gum or eat while you talk because the noise is offensive and distracting to the listener.

4. **Use a Courteous Tone.** Say "Please" and "Thank you" as you would in a face-to-face conversation. Close the conversation on a pleasant note.

FIGURE 6–8 Telephone techniques

PLACING LOCAL AND LONG-DISTANCE CALLS

As a medical assistant, you will place many different types of local and long-distance calls. These may be to patients, consulting physicians, other medical facilities, and business associates. You may also make travel arrangements for the physician(s), order supplies of drugs and equipment, or request service providers. Wait until all patients have been greeted and registered before placing outgoing calls. Then make your business calls brief and to the point. Delay personal calls until lunch or a break. If your voice carries, do not place calls within earshot of people in the reception area.

Local Calls

To place a local call:

1. Dial the seven-digit telephone number. If your call must first go through a switchboard, dial 9 for an outside line. Then dial the seven-digit number at the sound of the tone.
2. Identify yourself and the medical office when the call is answered. If you are making the call for the physician, identify the physician.
3. Leave a message or explain that you will call again, if the person you are calling is unavailable.

Long-Distance Calls — AT&T and Alternative Services

The American Telephone and Telegraph Company, originally made up of several operating companies known as the Bell System, had very little competition for almost seventy years. However, in the late 1970s, the Federal Communications Commission opened the door for greater competition by breaking up the AT&T system and by allowing other companies to provide telephone service. Today MCI, Sprint, and many other alternative companies compete for long-distance service, resulting in reduced rates for consumers.

Long-distance users pay according to the type of call made and the amount of time spent on the line. As a medical assistant, you will be expected to know the differences among the varying services and their relative costs. Since service and rates differ among telephone companies and geographic locations, accurate national comparisons cannot be made. Contact the companies providing telephone service in your community for a complete listing of services and fees. By spending an hour comparison shopping, you may save your practice several hundred dollars each year in telephone charges.

Direct Distance Dialing

Direct Distance Dialing (**DDD**) refers to calls placed directly, without benefit of an operator. They offer a low-cost alternative to calls placed through an operator. Because telephone company personnel are not needed for DDD calls, the savings is passed along to the consumer in lower long-distance rates. Area codes for direct distance dialing to all parts of the country are located at the front of the white pages. If you are uncertain of an area code, look in the listing.

To place a DDD call within the same area code:

Dial 1 plus the number.

1-555-3875

(Note: In some parts of the country, dialing 1 is not necessary. Check your local directory.)

To place a DDD call to a different area code:

Dial 1 plus the area code plus the number.

1-614-555-7927

Operator-Assisted Calls

Operator assistance is provided for person-to-person calls, collect calls, calls charged to another number, some credit card calls, and station-to-station calls when requested by the caller.

To place an operator-assisted call within the same area code:

Dial 0 plus the number.

0-555-7927

To place an operator-assisted call to a different area code:

Dial 0 plus the area code plus the number.

0-614-555-7927

Advise the operator of the type of call you are making. If you reach an incorrect long-distance number, dial 0 and explain the problem to the operator. You will receive credit for the call.

Supervisors are available to assist telephone customers, even when information is sketchy. If you need to locate someone, dial 0 and make a person-to-person call, giving the operator any information you have, and ask for help. The operator will try to reach the designated person for you. For example, assume you need to reach your employer, who is attending a convention in another city. When you reach the convention area, you are told that the physicians are in one of three major meetings, all of which are accessible by telephone. The telephone operator will help you with this problem by calling each room to ask for the physician.

Station-to-Station and Person-to-Person Calls

A station-to-station call mean that the caller will talk to anyone who answers the telephone. A person-to-person call is made when the caller wishes to speak only to a specific person. Station-to-station charges begin as soon as the receiver is lifted, but person-to-person charges start only when the designated person answers the telephone. Station-to-station service calls cost less per minute than person-to-person service, but they may be more expensive if the recipient must be located or takes several minutes to answer the phone. Most people prefer to dial person-to-person calls directly without help from the operator as this illustration shows. The operator will ask who is being called after you direct dial.

(Dial 0 + Area Code + Number)

Medical Assistant: Operator, I'd like to talk with Mr. Dave Ciccone at Thresh and Company. This is Erika Silk calling from Dr. Bill Burrough's office in Philadelphia.

Operator: Thank you.

(Telephone rings and receptionist answers.)

Receptionist: Good morning, Thresh and Company.

Operator: I have a person-to-person call for Mr. Dave Ciccone.

Receptionist: May I ask who is calling?

Operator: Erika Silk with Dr. Bill Burrough's office in Philadelphia.

Receptionist: One moment, please. I'll ring Mr. Ciccone.

Collect Calls

Collect calls are sometimes known as "reversed calls" because the charge is reversed to the answering telephone. The person who answers must agree to pay for the call before the operator will make a connection. A collect call can be station-to-station or person-to-person.

You should not accept a collect call unless the caller's identity is clear and office policy permits acceptance. Some medical offices will accept collect calls from patients with an understanding that the cost will later be billed to the patient. Acceptable collect charges might include the following: (1) a call from your employer who is attending an out-of-state medical convention; (2) a call from the physician's spouse or children; and (3) a call from a patient undergoing continuing treatment for a medical condition. (Charges for this last call would be billed to the patient later.) Examples of unacceptable collect charges include calls from a medical supply company representative or a person whose name is unfamiliar. A typical collect telephone call is shown in the following dialogue:

Collect Station-to-Station Call

(Medical assistant answers)

Operator: I have a collect call for anyone from Mr. Lawrence Babbio. Will you accept?

Medical Assistant: Operator, I can't accept this call without additional information to identify Mr. Babbio.

Operator: Mr. Babbio, will you identify yourself further?

Caller: Yes, operator. I'm the brother of Dr. Kincaid's patient, Rebecca Watson. Rebecca is visiting me in California and has a medical problem that I need to discuss with the doctor.

Medical Assistant: Operator, I will accept the call.

(The medical assistant screens the call and refers it to the physician or takes a callback message.)

Conference Calls

Long-distance calls can be arranged to include several people in different locations speaking in conference at one time. Although conference calls are more expensive than single-line calls, a net savings may occur when conversations do not have to be repeated with several different people.

To place a conference call:

1. Dial 0 and give the operator the name, area code, and telephone number of each person who will participate in the conversation. Specify a time when the call should take place, for example, 2 PM Eastern Standard Time.
2. When all parties to the call are on the line, the operator contacts the originator of the call, and the conversation begins.

Sometimes when a patient is extremely ill, family members who live in different places may wish to discuss with the physician the details of the illness, the length of hospitalization, and the

patient's chances of recovery. The time of day is important to consider when arranging for this type of conference call. You will want to place the call at a time convenient for the family members, some of whom may live in different time zones.

Credit Card Calls

Credit cards are issued by the telephone company so customers can eliminate collect calls. Using a credit card is convenient and usually saves the caller time.

To make a credit card call:

1. Dial 0 plus the area code, if different from yours, plus the number.
2. Advise the operator that you are making a credit card call and give your credit card number. From many telephones, a long tone indicates to the caller to key the credit card number into the telephone keypad, eliminating the need for an operator.

Time Zones

As a medical assistant, you must understand time zones if you are to use long-distance service successfully. Because there is a three-hour time difference between the East and West coasts, a person who places a 9:00 AM call in New York City will awaken California residents at 6:00 AM and receive no answer in California offices. The time zone map in Figure 6–9 shows time zones in the continental United States and adjacent Canadian provinces. Use the map to determine the appropriate time to place a call. The city of origination determines whether day, evening, or night telephone rates apply.

Directory Assistance

An operator can assist with locating unknown numbers. However, because you may be charged for directory assistance, requests should be kept to a minimum. You should first check for the number in telephone directories. Your public library will carry telephone directories for major cities in the United States. The charge for directory assistance is explained in the front of the white pages.

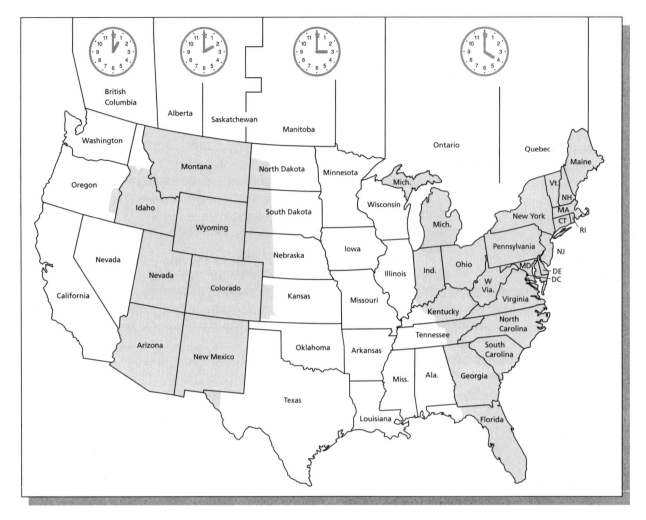

FIGURE 6–9 Time zone map

To call directory assistance locally or nationally:

Dial 411.

Telephone Log

As a medical assistant, you should keep a log of all long-distance telephone calls so that, if appropriate, the charges can be passed along to patients or charged to the practice's account. A long-distance telephone log should show the name of the caller, the person called, the date and time of the call, the city called, whether the call was station-to-station or person-to-person, the approximate length of the call, the name of the account to be charged, and the purposed of the call. Star all collect calls. An example of a telephone log is shown in Figure 6–10.

Monthly Telephone Charges

Charges for directory assistance and long-distance calls are shown on the monthly telephone statement along with charges for local service. Each month you should check the telephone bill closely to make sure that your practice was charged properly and that directory assistance is not being abused. Too many directory assistance charges might indicate that the staff is not checking the directory before asking for assistance.

Follow these procedures for checking the monthly telephone bill:

1. Match all charged items with the telephone log.
2. Charge individual patient accounts for long-distance calls pertaining to individual patients.

To	From	Date	Time	City	Type of Call	Length	Account to be Charged	Purpose
Rebecca Flamis	Vanessa Greene	5/2	9:15	New Rochelle	P-P	8 min.	Office	Supplies shipment
Vera Candes	Dr. Shellbaugh	5/2	11:45	Kansas City	S-S	20 min.	Howard Dietrich	Discuss her husband's condition
Suzanne Bourdes	Dr. Shellbaugh	5/2	12:15	Burlington	P-P	5 min.	Office	AMA talk
Century Drugs	Vanessa Greene	5/2	12:30	Kansas City	S-S	3 min.	Howard Dietrich	Mr. Rovele's prescription
George Motter	Sui Sing	5/2	1:00	Hesperia	P-P	7 min.	Sui Sing	Personal
*DL Dodson	Vanessa Greene	5/3	10:00	Marlington, WV	S-S	1 min.	DL Dodson	His vacation accident
DL Dodson	Dr. Shellbaugh	5/3	11:45	Marlington, WV	P-P	8 min.	DL Dodson	His accident
Maglia Valdez	Dr. Shellbaugh	5/3	12:00	Cape Girardeau	P-P	5 min.	Office	Review AMA talk

*Collect

FIGURE 6–10 Long-distance telephone log

3. Check all starred collect calls and charge to the appropriate account.
4. Cross through each call listing after the charge has been noted on the correct account.
5. Circle any questionable calls.
6. Calculate the total for calls to be charged to the practice and charge the proper practice account or make a note for the accountant.
7. Contact the local telephone business office about discrepancies between your records and the statement.

IN YOUR OPINION

1. How can you save your office money if you make a great many long-distance calls to suppliers and research institutions?
2. What do you think would be a reasonable policy on making and receiving personal calls while at the office?
3. How would you find the phone number of the author of an article in a medical journal? Name several ways.

Telephone Number File

You should keep frequently used telephone numbers in a handy file at your desk, in addition to any computerized telephone index you may have. Many medical assistants maintain their telephone numbers and addresses in Outlook Express or a similar program. Patients' numbers are usually located in an alphabetical card file or in their medical record. In addition, you should maintain a rotary card file for business-related numbers such as the cleaning service, the electric company, and suppliers. Use a separate card for each name. Emergency numbers such as police, fire department, rescue squad, the doctor's personal physician, and local hospitals should be typed on a blank card and taped to the telephone or desk. A rotary telephone number card is shown in Figure 6–11, a computer telephone file

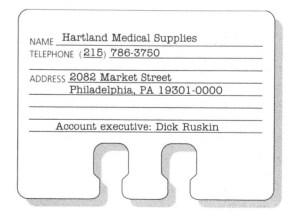

FIGURE 6–11 Rotary telephone number file

Address Book

Name	E-mail Address	Work Phone	Home Phone
Jesus Ramiz	jesusr@free.com	717-555-0123	717-555-0145
James Revere	Revere@nowmail.net	215-555-0156	215-555-0198
Esperanza Sanchez	espan@nowmail.net	215-555-0168	215-555-0185
Dr. Angelo Seda	aseda@primail.com	717-555-0165	717-555-0145
Mary Smith	m.smith@runmail.com	717-555-0134	717-555-0154

FIGURE 6–12 Computerized telephone file

Fire Department	498-1023
Police Department	498-1047
Dr. Natalie Baker (Dr. Joyce's physician)	624-5542
Harris Paramedic Service	624-9443
Center City Medical Service	624-1049
Cabrini Ambulance Company	498-6169
Memorial Hospital	498-6263

FIGURE 6–13 Emergency telephone number list

is shown in Figure 6–12, and an emergency telephone number list is shown in Figure 6–13.

USING THE TELEPHONE DIRECTORY

The telephone directory is a valuable but often unappreciated resource. Depending on the size of the geographic area served, one or more directories are required to contain all the information about telephone company customers. These are the five commonly used directories or parts of a directory:

1. The white pages list the names and telephone numbers for all telephone accounts for a specified calling area.

2. A special section of white pages lists business names and numbers.
3. The yellow pages list business and professional accounts for the same calling area covered by the white pages. Many of these listings also have special display ads that advertise the business.
4. The pink pages list business and professional accounts for a smaller geographic portion of the primary calling area.
5. The blue pages list special telephone numbers, including numbers for social service agencies; local, state, and federal government offices; and schools. The directories for each city vary, but typical telephone directories include some of the resource material discussed here.

Locating a Number

Because the names listed in a telephone directory are in alphabetical order, most numbers are easy to locate. However, certain names are confusing and more difficult to find. Although the guidelines for locating names in a telephone directory are similar to basic filing guidelines, they are not identical because most telephone directories are organized in the following ways:

1. Abbreviations are spelled out. To find "St. Joseph's Center," look for "Saint Joseph's Center."

2. Names with initials are listed before full first names. "Lawson, M." comes before "Lawson, Michael."

3. Names with prefixes are listed as one word. "duPont" follows "Duke"; "McDonald" follows "MacDonald."

4. Sometimes letters are used as names. When a name, usually a business name, is comprised of all capital letters, look in the beginning of the particular letter section. For example, "CC Medical Supplies" appears at the beginning of the "C" section, and "WBL TV" appears at the beginning of the "W" section.

5. Numbers are spelled out. Numbers used as names are spelled out and listed in alphabetical order. "19th Street Cafe" appears as "Nineteenth Street Cafe."

6. "The" follows the company name. "The Emerson Drug Store" appears as "Emerson Drug Store The."

7. Company names made up of two words are listed in alphabetical order by the first name. Hyphens (-), ampersands (&), and apostrophes (') are ignored. "Hewitt-Baker Medical Supplies" comes before "Hewitt & Banks Medical Laboratory." "Medical Professional Center" comes before "Medical-Prosthetic Devices." "Jacob's Pharmacy" appears as "Jacobs Pharmacy."

8. Some names can be spelled different ways. "Smith" may be spelled "Smyth" or "Smythe"; "Cohen" might be spelled "Coan," "Kohen," "Coahen," "Cohan," "Kohan," "Cohn," "Kohn," or "Kone." Suggestions for different spellings appear at the beginning of the most common last name listings.

9. Look for alternative listings. "Marshall Warner Associates" might appear under "Warner Marshall Associates."

10. Government listings are found in the blue pages in many cities. If your directory does not have a blue pages section, look for federal government agencies under "United States Government." Look for state agencies under the name of the state, city agencies under the name of the city, and municipal agencies under the name of the town.

USING ANSWERING SERVICES AND TELEPHONE ANSWERING DEVICES

Two methods are generally used to assure that calls to physicians or their associates are answered after hours and on weekends. As a medical assistant, you will be responsible for maintaining an answering system that meets the needs of the practice and the patients. Refer to the yellow pages in your community for the names of answering services and the names of companies that sell telephone answering devices (TADs).

Answering Services

Answering services are twenty-four hour services that, for a monthly fee, answer the medical office telephone number from a remote location. If a switching device is installed, the service can automatically answer the medical office telephone when it is unanswered. The service then locates the physician at an alternate number or on a paging device. If the answering service does not have the capability to switch on and off automatically, the medical assistant calls the service and advises the time to begin answering, the physician's location, and the time to stop answering. After returning to the office, the medical assistant checks with the service for messages. Because many answering services charge by the number of calls answered and the time spent tracking the physician, the service should be used only when necessary.

Answering Machines

Answering machines give a recorded message and a number where the physician can be reached. Because answering devices appear impersonal, some physicians do not use them. The medical assistant often records the greeting that patients hear. If this is your responsibility, follow these guidelines to reduce the negative effect of a machine greeting:

• Face a mirror and smile as you record.
• Use a warm tone of voice.

- Speak clearly and distinctly.
- Use informal, but professional, language
- Provide complete information about when the office staff will be available.
- Give details regarding how the physician can be located in case of an emergency.

Voice Mail

Telecommunications companies such as Verizon, Sprint, and Cingular offer **voice mail** service that eliminates the need for an answering machine. Voice mail provides the same type of impersonal greeting as an answering machine; however, by using a service that is handled directly by the phone company, one piece of additional office equipment is eliminated.

Cellular Phones and Beepers

Notice a physician's belt or pocket, and you may see both a **cellular phone** and a beeper attached. These devices maintain a physician's connection to the medical office at all times. Often the two devices are used in combination to eliminate the possibility of the phone ringing at an inappropriate time, for example, when the physician is with a patient at the hospital or in some other setting where taking a call would be distracting.

The medical assistant or other caller dials the beeper, which pulses to alert the physician of an incoming call. At a glance of the beeper's name and number screen, the physician can see who is calling and determine whether the call needs to be returned immediately. If the call is urgent, the physician asks to be excused and places the call on the cellular phone.

A medical assistant should use good judgment regarding when to interrupt the physician through a pager or cell phone. The general rule of thumb is to call only when a message is so important it cannot wait until the physician returns to the office.

Fax

Fax, or facsimile transmission, allows you to send a "picture" of a document over telephone lines to anyone who also has a fax machine. Data, charts, even sketches and drawings, can be sent in this way in a matter of seconds or minutes. A fax is especially useful when sending documents that are needed urgently.

Confidentiality issues are important to consider when using fax. Because most fax machines are not in secure locations and incoming fax messages may be read by anyone passing by, take care in using fax for transmitting confidential data.

Newer fax machines receive and print onto ordinary copy paper. Older fax machines use a thermal paper that usually comes in a roll. The paper is thin and shiny and images on this paper last only about a year. If a permanent record of incoming fax data is needed for legal purposes, the thermal message should be photocopied and the photocopy filed promptly. A fax is illustrated in Figure 6–14.

TELECOMMUNICATIONS FOR DIAGNOSIS AND TREATMENT

Medical telecommunication lines use data, video, and sound to assess, diagnose, and treat a patient in a remote location. Through telephone lines and computers, patients who might have died in the past before a physician could arrive to treat them now have some of the finest medical care available. Specific rewards of new sources of medical communication include these:
- Patients remotely located from medical care can now receive good primary care.
- The caregivers' range is extended, which makes them more productive.
- The resources available to caregivers are greatly increased.

FAX
Seriph Medical Associates

To: Marcus Hagard

From: Marimba Lopez

Date: October 27, 20–

Pages: 2, including cover sheet

Fax No.:   513-555-6956

Attached please find our purchase order No. 3278 for medical and surgical supplies. All items are subject to cancellation if delivered after the requested delivery dates.

Please let me know by Friday if any of the items require longer lead times.

FIGURE 6–14   Fax message

INTERNET ACTIVITY

Go to the Web site of American Connect at www.mediconnect.com or the Web site for Sickbay Health and Wellness at www.sickbay.com. Read the section *About Us* from one of the sites and describe the telecommunication services available. Complete and submit a request for information form from one of the companies and wait for the response.

STUDENT STUDY CHECKLIST

Workbook

1. Complete Chapter 6 activities in the workbook.

Administrative CD-ROM

1. Go to the Library on the CD-ROM and play the interactive games for Chapter 6.
2. Go to the Patient Reception area of the office and click on the telephone. Complete the exercises.
3. List five ways a telephone is essential in a medical office.

REFERENCES

Career Solutions Training Group. *The Quick Skills Series: Embracing Diversity.* Cincinnati, OH: South-Western, 2001.

Career Solutions Training Group. *The Quick Skills Series: Speaking and Presenting.* Cincinnati, OH: South-Western, 2000.

Career Solutions Training Group. *10-Hour Series: Videoconferencing.* Cincinnati, OH: South-Western, 2003.

Lindh, Wilberta Q., Marilyn S. Pooler, and Carol D. Tamparo. *Administrative Medical Assisting,* 2nd ed. Clifton Park, NY: Delmar Learning, 2002.

Super Pages. Philadelphia, PA: Verizon, 2002.

CHAPTER ACTIVITIES

PERFORMANCE-BASED ACTIVITIES

1. You have been asked to record the voice mail message for Riley and Bromberg Internal Medicine, P.C. that all patients and other callers will hear when they call the office after hours. Write the message you will record.

   _____

   _____

   _____

2. You receive an emergency phone call from a first-time mother of a 6-week-old infant whose temperature is 102°. The mother is very upset and keeps interrupting her conversation with you to attend the baby. You are having a hard time understanding the baby's problem and obviously need to lead the mother in providing you with the proper information. Write a list of questions you will ask the mother. Recommend how you will deal with the mother's anxiety.

   Questions to ask:

   _____

   _____

   _____

   Recommendations for dealing with the mother's anxiety:

   _____

   _____

   _____

3. Prepare a fax message using the format below. State that Dr. William Lennart will arrive in Dr. Marisol Chile's office at 10:00 AM on March 9 for a consultation regarding infant Jon Verex's brain surgery. Ask for confirmation by fax that Dr. Chile will be available.

   Doctor's Office
   Fax Note

   To: _____

   From: _____

   Date: _____

   Fax #: _____

   No. of pages: _____

4. Compile a packet of materials on cellular communication from your local telephone office. Develop a summary of services offered by the company.

EXPANDING YOUR THINKING

1. Role-play a screening of the following callers to determine their business.

    a. Sales person from a pharmaceutical firm

    b. Golf partner of the physician

    c. Fund raiser from the physician's alma mater

    d. Patient with excessive pain the day after outpatient surgery

    e. Mother whose child has a fever of 104.5°F

    f. Patient who does not understand instructions on medication

    g. Insurance company seeking records

2. Locate the following, and compile name, address, and phone number for each:

    a. A medical supply house in your state

    b. A medical school in your state or in an adjoining state

    c. A service that searches medical databases and can provide articles on requested topics

    d. A local uniform supply business

    e. A British dermatologist

    f. A manufacturer of medical instruments

    g. Three associates that serve the medical field

3. Assemble a list of emergency phone numbers that you think should be posted in the average home. Compile a similar list of emergency numbers for a medical practice.

Home

1. _____

2. _____

3. _____

4. _____

5. _____

6. _____

Medical Practice

1. _____

2. _____

3. _____

4. _____

5. _____

6. _____

CHAPTER 7

Scheduling Appointments

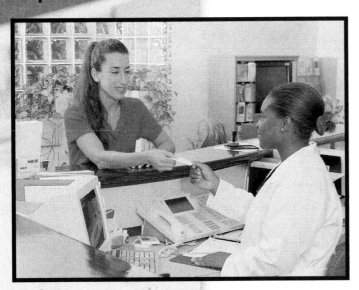

SAUSALITO, CALIFORNIA

I manage a medium-sized group practice. A few weeks ago we were short-handed and our most recently hired medical assistant, Zannah, had to schedule appointments for a couple of days. I had forgotten — we all had forgotten — that Zannah didn't have any hands-on scheduling experience. Because she had learned medical office scheduling in school, she thought she could handle it. We're still recovering from her well-intentioned oversights and mistakes. She feels embarrassed, and I feel that it's my responsibility.

We've had to reschedule some of her appointments to give doctors more time with each patient. Rescheduling annoys some patients. Every couple of days, when we haven't been able to reschedule, we get back-ups in the office because Zannah had underestimated the length of the examinations. The office will get over it, and so will Zannah. She's bright and caring, and once she's given a chance to learn, she's quick. As I say, her mistakes were my fault as a manager. Don't ever, even for a second, think scheduling is simple — until you've mastered it.

Rosemary Storey
Medical Office Manager

PERFORMANCE-BASED COMPETENCIES

After completing this chapter, you should be able to:
1. Evaluate different means of scheduling.
2. Schedule patient and nonpatient appointments.
3. Analyze the time required by different patients and procedures.

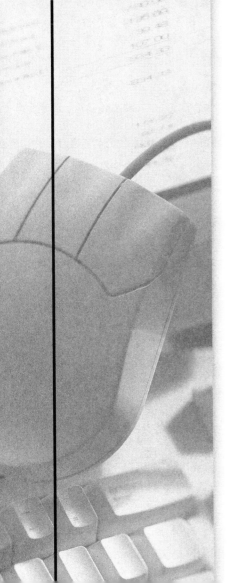

4. Choose among options for handling delays to the schedule.
5. Screen nonpatient appointments.
6. Prepare the daily master schedule.
7. Coordinate scheduling of patients at other medical facilities.
8. Measure the performance of the actual to planned schedule.

VOCABULARY

Allocation   Deciding how to divide available resources, such as time, among conflicting demands.

Appointment book   A daily record of each patient's name, telephone number, appointment time, and the reason for the medical visit.

Computer scheduling   Scheduling patient appointments with computer software.

Daily list of appointments   A list showing names of all patients who will be seen in one day.

Effective   Achieving the mission of the practice in serving patients, whether or not resources are used efficiently.

Efficient   Making good use of available resources.

No show   The term given to a patient who fails to keep an appointment.

Optimal   Making the best use of a resource.

Overbooking   Scheduling more patients than the physician can see in the time available.

Progress appointments   Follow-up appointments that monitor the progress of treatment.

Referral   Determination by a physician that a patient should see a specialist or subspecialist for a consultation.

Schedule   The daily calendar of times when patients will be seen.

Triage   Screening calls, usually associated with emergencies, to prioritize the schedule, putting worst cases first.

Wave scheduling   Clustering appointments by time block; flow is maintained by rotating patients among needed procedures.

Time is a scarce resource, like money, and scheduling is the tool for managing that resource. Whether appointments are scheduled by hand in a day book or with a computer using scheduling software, the entire staff depends on a smooth flow of patient traffic to maintain a workable schedule. Appointments must be made so they allow sufficient time for each patient's medical problem to be treated thoroughly, yet without long waits.

As a medical assistant, you will schedule appointments based on several factors such as the availability of time, the type of patient being treated, the type of medical problem, and the personal preferences of the medical staff. Trade-offs will always occur because days are too short, emergencies interrupt, and the doctors run late from making rounds or attending meetings. Learning to manage these schedule changes is part of learning how to manage the daily routine.

To make rational decisions about the allocation of time, you will screen and evaluate callers. If the call is truly urgent, you will have to find time for the patient to see the physician. For other problems, you will work with the patient to schedule a convenient appointment.

You will find human relations and organizational skills to be important qualities in balancing your schedule (Figure 7–1). As you monitor patient flow, you must strive to maintain both a calm and unhurried environment and an efficient system. Although these two characteristics may appear to be opposites, they actually complement one another.

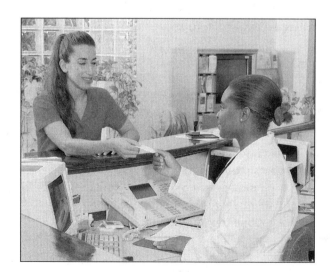

FIGURE 7–1   Scheduling appointments requires problem-solving skills.

SCHEDULING ACCORDING TO A SYSTEM

The type of practice, the physician's time management preferences, and the age of the patients contribute to the final decision regarding which of several scheduling systems a medical office will use. The key to any system is its structure and its flexibility. It must be able to accommodate emergencies, work-ins, cancellations, and no shows while also ensuring a smooth flow of patient traffic with minimal patient waiting time.

Streaming

You are probably most accustomed to stream scheduling where a steady stream of patients has been previously scheduled through the day, usually in fifteen-minute segments (Figure 7–2). Under this system, patients who need thirty minutes for an appointment are given two fifteen-minute segments, patients who need forty-five minutes are given three fifteen-minute appointments, and so on. Some physicians prefer to schedule longer appointments for specific times of the day, for example, early morning. It is helpful to establish time guidelines for specific types of appointment, such as thirty minutes for six-month checkups or one hour for new patients.

Double Booking

In a practice where several medical staff members are available to work with patients, two or more patients are given the same appointment time. For example, a patient for a six-month checkup might be seen at the same time as a patient being seen for sinusitis. As the staff completes the six-month patient's weigh-in and takes the person's vital signs, the physician examines the patient with sinusitis symptoms. This method can be very effective, but if not monitored carefully, it can result in long wait time for patients.

Clustering

In some medical offices, specific appointment times are set aside during the day or week for certain types of patients. For example, all patients requiring physician examinations might be scheduled for early morning or late afternoon, and all consultations might be scheduled during a designated time. This type of clustering works well in obstetrics and gynecology practices where all new mothers might be seen on a specified day of the week and all expectant mothers at another designated time. Early pregnancy patients might be seen after lunch so their morning sickness will have disappeared. When patients can be scheduled in clusters, the physician and staff usually increase their efficiency.

Wave

When a practice has access to several procedure rooms and a large staff, wave scheduling is a viable option. With the wave system, patients are scheduled in the first half of each hour. Work-ins and late arrivals are accommodated in the second half of each hour. Wave scheduling requires precision planning and can result in wasted time, patient delays for seeing the physician, and staffing conflicts.

Modified Wave

Established as an alternative to wave scheduling, the modified wave system allows two or three patients to be scheduled at the beginning of each hour, followed by single appointments every ten to twenty minutes thereafter. Often, major or time-consuming examinations, such as new patients, are scheduled at the beginning of the

---

Stream Schedule for Internal Medicine Practice	
New Patients	30 minutes
Patients for consultation	45 minutes
Patients requiring complete physical examinations	45 minutes
All other patients (minor illnesses, routine checkups, etc.)	15 minutes

FIGURE 7–2 Stream schedule for an internal medicine practice

hour, and minor examinations, such as suture removal, are scheduled twenty to thirty minutes after the hour. Walk-in and late appointments can be accommodated at the end of the hour. Good planning will determine the success of this method.

Open Hours

This method refers to first-come, first-served scheduling, and patients are seen throughout the day. Emergency rooms and clinics choose this method because they see a large number of patients who are unable to make appointments.

MAINTAINING THE APPOINTMENT SCHEDULE

Appointments for patients and other visitors are recorded in the appointment book or in a computer software system. With either arrangement, the appointment schedule serves as the daily planning guide by showing (1) the names of all patients to be seen each day, (2) the time of each patient's appointment, (3) the patient's telephone number, and (4) a brief reason for the visit. From this information, the doctors and other office personnel determine approximately how much time is needed for their portion of the patient's treatment and which medical instruments and supplies will be required for the examination.

Patient Appointments

Patient appointments are usually requested by the patient or a relative, by notes or messages from the physician or nurse, or by a referring physician. When a patient requests an appointment, ask for a specific description of the symptoms. If, in your judgment, the complaint is serious enough to justify an immediate examination, look through the day's schedule for the first vacant time period. If no openings exist, find a time when the patient can be "worked in." For example, an elderly patient suffering from chest pain might be in the preliminary stages of a heart attack and should be seen as soon as possible. In this case, you must make room in the schedule for an immediate appointment, even though

other patients will be delayed. If the patient's request is not urgent, such as for a routine physical exam, a recheck, or a minor ache or pain, search the appointment schedule for the first vacant time period. Give the patient one or two alternative times and then schedule the appointment according to the patient's wishes.

Verifying Details

Ask established patients if their addresses or telephone numbers have changed recently. If so, note any changes in their medical record. To increase efficiency, ask new patients to arrive at the office about fifteen minutes early so that they can complete forms needed to open accounts.

Do not schedule a day completely full. Last-minute adjustments will almost certainly occur, and you will be able to react to them more easily if you have built some flexibility into your plan. Cancelled patient appointments and other time vacancies allow late afternoon patients to come in for earlier appointments. When a cancellation occurs, review the schedule to determine which patients can be moved to the opening caused by the cancellation. Then call the patients until you locate a person who wishes to make a change. Always try to fill openings made available through cancellations so all patients can be served and the physician and staff can practice at top efficiency.

Acquiring Information

Some patients prefer to provide information about their symptoms to the doctor only, but part of your job will be to screen requests for appointments and make a rational determination of their urgency. This will be an opportunity to use your human relations skills to acquire the necessary information. Patients frequently decide to talk after a little encouragement. Determining a patient's condition involves asking several questions, including the following:

Procedures to Help Identify a Patient's Complaint

Ask these questions:

1. What are your symptoms?
2. Are your symptoms related to a previous illness?

3. Has the doctor treated you for this condition before?
4. How long have you been ill?
5. Is your problem urgent or routine?
6. Would you like a consultation with the doctor (if the patient refuses to talk about the illness or the reason for the visit)?

Most appointments are made by telephone, and you will not always recognize the name or the voice. When you do not recognize the patient's name, ask, "Are you a new or an established patient of our office?" You may also ask, "Have you seen Dr. Cooper previously?" Or "When were you last seen by anyone in this office?"

Recording the Appointment

You will record appointments either manually in a daily appointment book or electronically using computer software. With an appointment book, you will search for "holes" in the schedule by flipping through each page until you find an opening appropriate for the patient's symptoms. With a computerized system, you will enter information about the appointment, and the system will offer scheduling options that allow you to maintain an optimal plan.

The Appointment Book

A typical appointment book is divided into days of the week, with each day broken into fifteen-minute segments. You will block out as many fifteen-minute segments as necessary to provide time for each examination. For example, a new patient visit, which in most offices requires thirty minutes, would use two fifteen-minute segments as shown in Figure 7–3. To record an appointment, follow these procedures.

Procedures to Record an Appointment in the Appointment Book

1. List the patient's first and last names in pencil.
2. Draw a slash after the name; then list the patient's complaint or reason for the visit.
3. Draw another slash; then write the patient's telephone number.
4. Write "New" if the patient is visiting the physician for the first time.

5. Mark out additional time periods with an arrow if more than fifteen minutes are needed for the examination. By doing so, you will not schedule two patients for the same time.
6. Make sure your handwriting is legible.
7. Review the appointment book at the end of each day to be sure it is accurate for all patients seen that day. This step is important because the appointment book might be used as evidence in a court case.
8. Make a note of changes and interruptions to the schedule, and measure how well the staff was able to perform against the schedule. This will allow you to improve the effectiveness of future schedules.

Physicians must often be away from the office to make hospital rounds, perform surgery, or handle personal business, and these absences are also recorded in the appointment book. When the physician will be out of the office, draw an "X" in pencil through the appropriate time period and date; then write a brief explanation. This information is for staff knowledge only and should not be given to patients. The appointment book in Figure 7–3 shows Dr. Ferguson's planned absence at 5:00 PM on May 14.

Computer Scheduling

Appointment scheduling can be done by computer using a variety of scheduling software. When you need to allocate time for an appointment, the computer system searches through the database of current appointments for an open slot and schedules the appointment according to your instructions. In some systems, you must enter a code for the type of appointment required. For example, after you enter the code "CPE" to request an appointment for a complete physical examination, the computer searches for the first opening with the appropriate time length. If the patient agrees to the time, you enter the person's name, and the computer automatically schedules the appointment. You can also request a specific date and time, and the computer will search for time availability. If the time is unavailable, the program will request an alternate time. You can continue your search until the computer locates a time slot the patient prefers.

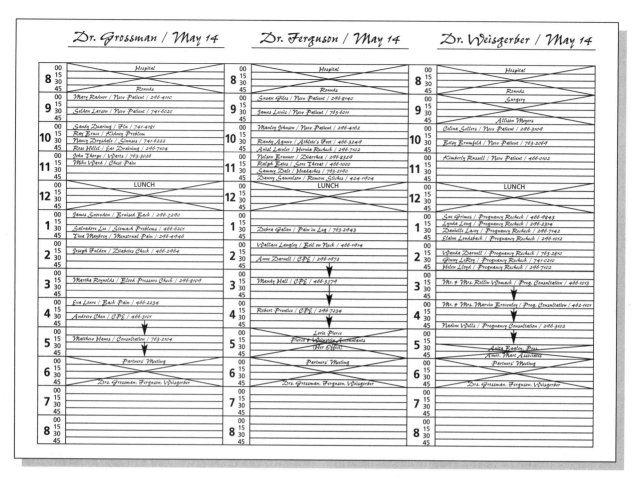

| Dr. Grossman / May 14 | Dr. Ferguson / May 14 | Dr. Weisgerber / May 14 |

Time	Dr. Grossman	Dr. Ferguson	Dr. Weisgerber
8:00–8:45	Hospital / Rounds	Hospital / Rounds	Hospital / Rounds / Surgery
9:00	Mary Radnor / New Patient / 296-4110	Susan Giles / New Patient / 296-8140	
9:30	Seldon Larson / New Patient / 741-6020	James Lewis / New Patient / 763-6011	Allison Meyers
10:00	Sandy Dearing / Flu / 741-4181	Manley Johnson / New Patient / 296-4162	Celina Sellers / New Patient / 296-3109
10:15	Ray Bruce / Kidney Problem		
10:30	Nancy Drysdale / Sinuses / 741-6222	Randy Agnew / Athlete's Foot / 466-3249	Betsy Brumfeld / New Patient / 763-2069
10:45	Rose Hillel / Ear Draining / 296-7104	Aniol Lawler / Hernia Recheck / 296-7102	
11:00	John Thorpe / Warts / 763-3026	Nelson Brunner / Diarrhea / 296-8329	Kimberly Russell / New Patient / 466-0102
11:15	Mike Ward / Chest Pain	Ralph Bates / Sore Throat / 466-1000	
11:30		Sammy Dale / Headaches / 763-2190	
11:45		Danny Samuelson / Remove Stiches / 424-1904	
12:00	LUNCH	LUNCH	LUNCH
1:00	James Snowdon / Bruised Back / 296-3290		Sue Grimes / Pregnancy Recheck / 466-9843
1:15			Lynda Long / Pregnancy Recheck / 296-2314
1:30	Salvadore Lee / Stomach Problems / 466-6201	Debra Galion / Pain in Leg / 763-2943	Danielle Lavey / Pregnancy Recheck / 296-7142
1:45	Tina Maybrey / Menstrual Pain / 296-4946		Elaine Londsback / Pregnancy Recheck / 296-1012
2:00		Wallace Langley / Boil on Neck / 466-1914	
2:15	Joseph Fuldon / Diabetes Check / 466-2964		Wanda Darnell / Pregnancy Recheck / 763-2810
2:30		Anne Darnell / CPE / 296-1972	Ginny LeRoy / Pregnancy Recheck / 741-0210
2:45			Helen Lloyd / Pregnancy Recheck / 296-7102
3:15	Martha Reynolds / Blood Pressure Check / 296-8109	Mandy Hall / CPE / 466-3379	Mr. & Mrs. Rollin Womack / Preg. Consultation / 466-1013
4:00	Eva Lenre / Back Pain / 466-2234		Mr. & Mrs. Marvin Brownley / Preg. Consultation / 462-1101
4:15	Andrew Chen / CPE / 466-3101	Robert Prentice / CPE / 296-7234	
4:45			Nadine Wells / Pregnancy Consultation / 296-3102
5:00	Matthew Hanes / Consultation / 763-2104	Lorie Pierce / Pierce & Weinstein Accountants (Her Office)	Anita Bagley, Pres. / Amer. Mart Associates
6:00	Partners' Meeting	Partners' Meeting	Partners' Meeting
6:45	Drs. Grossman, Ferguson, Weisgerber	Drs. Grossman, Ferguson, Weisgerber	Drs. Grossman, Ferguson, Weisgerber

FIGURE 7–3 Appointment book page from a group practice

Figure 7–4 shows a medical assistant using computerized scheduling software to arrange patient appointments.

Overbooking Patients

Overbooking or **double tracking** refers to scheduling more patients than the physician can see during a reasonable period of time. Overbooking is not recommended because it often delays the schedule and frustrates the patients, physician, and staff. You should avoid overbooking unless an emergency patient or a very sick patient must see the doctor immediately. Many physicians like to schedule a thirty-minute break once or twice a day to ease scheduling pressures. In Figure 7–3 Drs. Grossman and Weisgerber have set aside thirty unscheduled minutes at 11:30 AM to compensate for any delays in the morning. Dr. Ferguson has thirty minutes unscheduled at 1:00 PM, allowing the lunch hour to be pushed

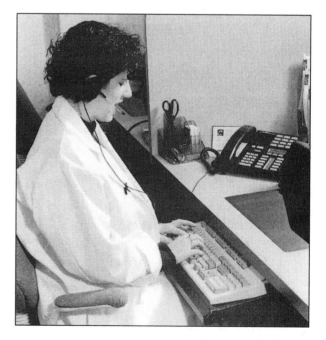

FIGURE 7–4 Appointment scheduling on the computer can save time.

back if necessary to accommodate patients. If physician assistants perform preliminary examinations, patients can be scheduled more closely.

Rescheduling and Canceling Appointments

A patient may sometimes need to reschedule an appointment for a later date, or may decide to cancel the appointment altogether. Because rescheduling and canceling appointments disrupt the schedule, patients should be encouraged to give early notice when they will not be able to keep an appointment. Follow these procedures to reschedule or cancel an appointment.

Procedures to Reschedule an Appointment in the Appointment Book

1. Erase the patient's name at the original appointment time to indicate that the slot is once again available for scheduling.
2. Give the patient one or two alternative dates and times; then ask which time is more convenient.
3. Transfer the patient's name and the reason for the visit to the new date and time.

Procedures to Cancel an Appointment in the Appointment Book

1. Erase the patient's name.
2. Record the cancellation in the patient's medical record. (If the same patient cancels several appointments, tactfully suggest that no further cancellations should be made. You may say, "Mr. Reynolds, will you check your calendar, please, before we schedule this appointment? You had to cancel your three previous appointments.")

Procedures to Reschedule or Cancel an Appointment by Computer

In most computer systems, rescheduling and cancellations are accomplished by deleting the patient's name from the appointed time slot and adding it at another time. The first slot then becomes available for other appointments. Because it is important to maintain a list of cancellations for legal purposes, refer to your software manual to determine whether your system provides a method of record keeping for canceled appointments. If not, maintain a separate list of all cancellations. Also, record the cancellation in the patient's medical record.

Handling Emergency Appointments

An emergency patient should be allowed to see the physician immediately, even though the emergency delays other patients.

Determining how soon a patient needs to see the doctor requires skill. This process of screening is called triage and is usually associated with emergencies. Appropriate questions need to be asked to identify the urgency of the problem:

- How long have the symptoms/problem been present?
- Is the patient bleeding?
- Is another type of discharge occurring?
- Is pain present? If so, how severe?
- Is another individual present to help the patient?

When emergencies occur, you should call all patients who are affected by the delay and reschedule their appointments for another time. Advise patients already in the office of the emergency and give them the option of waiting for the physician or rescheduling their appointments. When a waiting patient's complaint is serious, work the waiting patient into the schedule as soon as possible the same day. To avoid overcrowding the schedule, delay other appointments until a later date. Most people are understanding of the need for rescheduling because of an emergency. They will appreciate having a choice about waiting, returning, or rescheduling.

Coordinating Delays and Unexpected Appointments

The appointment schedule cannot be followed at all times even in the most efficient and organized medical office. Delays are caused by (1) examinations that take longer than expected, (2) patients who arrive late for their appointments, (3) tests that the doctor orders for patients, (4) important telephone calls that the physician must take between appointments, (5) patients who wish to talk to the physician following their examinations, and (6) other unforeseen reasons. When delays interrupt the appointment schedule, you must adjust the daily routine so the medical staff can return to the schedule. This can be done in several ways:

Procedures to Adjust the Daily Schedule

1. Alert the physician and medical staff that appointments are behind schedule.
2. Volunteer for some tasks that other office personnel ordinarily handle, for example, clearing examination rooms and preparing them for patients.
3. Determine whether later appointments can be rescheduled for another time. Check with the physician before taking this step.

When the physician will be delayed more than thirty minutes, inform patients waiting in the reception area. They can select magazines, engage in conversation with other patients, or run errands. You will avoid complaints by advising patients of the approximate length of the delay.

Rescheduling Missed Appointments

Some patients miss appointments without calling to cancel. When a patient misses an appointment, draw a line through the name in the appointment book and write "Missed" or "No show" beside the name. Refer to your computer software manual for instructions for noting a missed appointment in the computer system. Record the missed appointment in the patient's medical record and mail a card to the person as a reminder. Figure 7–5 illustrates an appointment book page showing a missed appointment. Figure 7–6 shows a reminder that is mailed to the patient.

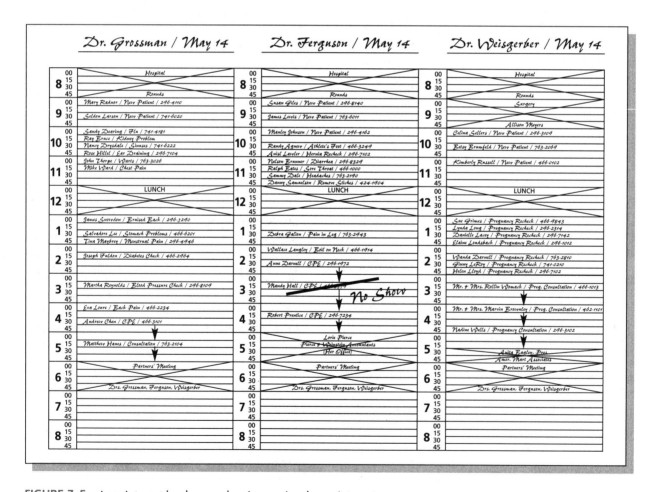

FIGURE 7–5 Appointment book page showing a missed appointment

DID YOU FORGET...

your appointment on _____May 16_____ at
_____9:45 am_____?

Please let us know when you would like to
reschedule your appointment.

Molly Bertrand, M.D.
89 Lancaster Highway
Philadelphia, PA 19301
(215) 555-0293

FIGURE 7–6   Missed appointment card

Some medical offices charge for missed appointments because the doctor wastes valuable time and they reduce the medical practice's income. You should review office policy carefully regarding this issue since ill will generated by a missed appointment charge may be too big a risk to take. When missed appointments are charged, print the notice on the bottom of monthly statements and in any other materials given to patients.

Nonpatient Appointments

People besides patients frequently request appointments with physicians. These may be sales representatives for pharmaceutical companies, medical equipment manufacturers, medical supply companies, or office supply companies; the doctor's accountant or attorney; representatives from civic or charitable organizations; or other doctors. You should ask your employer which visitors should be scheduled routinely. Do not schedule others unless you believe their business can be handled only by the physician. When you think the physician would like to see a person who is not a patient, schedule the appointment at a time that will not interrupt the daily routine, such as in the late afternoon.

You can handle many of the nonpatient appointments personally, or if not, you may refer them to other staff members. Because nonpatient callers can take up a great deal of time, only those who have important business or who can be helpful to the practice in some way should be

scheduled. Figure 7–5 shows a nonpatient appointment for Dr. Weisgerber at 5:30 PM on May 14.

Sales Representatives

Most physicians are interested in new pharmaceutical products and innovative or improved medical equipment and supplies. Your responsibility is to distinguish between the sales representatives whose products should be seen personally by the physician and the representatives whose products can be evaluated by you or someone else. An appointment with a sales representative should be scheduled for approximately fifteen minutes, unless the physician agrees to a longer appointment. Because most sales representatives believe their product is valuable, some may be intimidating in their efforts to convince you to schedule an appointment. Therefore, you must be firm in denying the appointment if you think it is unnecessary.

Most sales representatives are open and straightforward about their business; however, some may attempt to see the physician without disclosing the purpose of the call. For this reason, you must screen all visitors carefully. Ask questions that will extract the information you need. Then if a caller does not provide an adequate explanation, consider the business unimportant and do not schedule an appointment.

SITUATION ONE

Medical Assistant: May I help you?

Visitor: Dr. Weisgerber is expecting me.

Medical Assistant: Do you have an appointment?

Visitor: No, but she wants to see the results of the first clinical testing of our new product.

Medical Assistant: Our staff members review new products first and make recommendations. Would you like to make an appointment with the office manager?

Visitor: No, I'd prefer to see Dr. Weisgerber. If she's too busy today, I'll come back another day.

Medical Assistant: Dr. Weisgerber will not see you until your product is reviewed by other staff members.

Visitor:	This will only take a minute. I'll just wait and you can work me in between patients.
Medical Assistant:	I regret that I can't do that.
Visitor:	I know you're doing your job. But I think Dr. Weisgerber will be very upset if she learns that you wouldn't allow me to see her.
Medical Assistant:	As I said you may make an appointment with the office manager if you like. I'll advise her that you'd like to see her.
Visitor:	All right, I'll wait.

SITUATION TWO

Medical Assistant:	May I help you?
Visitor:	I'd like to see Dr. Ferguson
Medical Assistant:	Are you a patient?
Visitor:	No.
Medical Assistant:	Does this concern one of our patients?
Visitor:	No.
Medical Assistant:	May I ask the purpose of the appointment then?
Visitor:	It's personal.
Medical Assistant:	Are you a friend of Dr. Ferguson?
Visitor:	No, I just need to see him.
Medical Assistant:	You need to give me additional information before I can schedule an appointment. Would you give me your name and the name of your company, please?
Visitor:	Elinor Post, from Eastern Office Technology.
Medical Assistant:	Is this a sales call regarding one of your products?
Visitor:	Well, I want to show him the new computer software we've developed especially for medical offices.
Medical Assistant:	Perhaps I could review your software. If you will leave me a brochure and any special information you think I should have, I'll be glad to study it.
Visitor:	Do you make the purchasing decisions?
Medical Assistant:	I review all office products and make recommendations to Dr. Ferguson.

Visitor:	Since this represents a major purchase, I think I should talk to the doctor.
Medical Assistant:	He is not available without an appointment.
Visitor:	I'll come back next week.

(Note: If this visitor returns, she should not be given an appointment with the physician.)

Representatives from Charitable Organizations

Physicians often are asked to contribute their time or money to charities. Although most physicians are supportive of charitable organizations and participate in their activities when possible, they do not have time to speak to each representative. Therefore, you should ask the representative for complete details about the organization, the nature of the request, and the date and time of any events in which the doctor might participate. Leave a note for the doctor to review and ask the representative to call you back for the doctor's decision regarding participation or a donation. If the physician wants to participate and wishes to talk to the representative, you can arrange an appointment later. If the physician makes a donation, you can forward a check to the organization.

The Physician's Business Associates

The physician's accountant, stockbroker, or other business associates may occasionally ask for an appointment. Check with the physician in advance to determine which of these people should routinely be given an appointment. If you have a question about a person requesting an appointment, do not schedule it until after you have talked to the physician.

Occasionally other physicians may wish to meet with your employer. As a professional courtesy, escort them to a private office immediately and advise your employer of their presence. Do not ask a visiting physician to wait with patients in the reception area.

IN YOUR OPINION

1. What are the characteristics of good and poor scheduling?
2. How do you know a schedule is a good schedule?
3. What are the factors you must balance in maintaining a schedule?

PREPARING A DAILY LIST OF APPOINTMENTS

The daily list of appointments is prepared at the end of each business day for the next day or in the morning before patients begin arriving. The list shows the names of all patients who will be seen, the time of their appointments, and the reason for the visit. The list is typed neatly on plain paper with the doctor's name and the date centered near the top of the page. A copy is made for each person who works with patients, including the physician, nurses, medical assistants, and others.

Each staff member places a check mark (✔) beside the patient's name after seeing or treating the person. The medical assistant checks off the name after preparing the patient's medical record for the nurse, the nurse or medical assistant checks off the name after routine tests have been administered, and the physician checks off the name following examination and treatment. Figure 7–7 shows a computerized daily list that was automatically prepared by computer software.

```
05/18/--              APPOINTMENTS WORKSHEET REPORT BY DOCTOR      Page 3
                            Annette Grossman, M.D.
                        Dates 05/18/--  —  05/18/--

  Time        Patient              Length     Reason             Exam Rm
================================================================================
  05/18/--    Thursday
--------------------------------------------------------------------------------
   8:30
   8:45
   9:00
   9:15
   9:30
   9:45
  10:00
  10:15
  10:30     Weiss, Bruce            1        1 -General Check-up        1
  10:45
  11:00
  11:15
  11:30     Mignotti, Jason         2        5 -General Examination     1
  11:45     Lusaki, Jennifer        -        5 -General Examination     2
  11:45     Gillerman, Lesley       2        5 -General Examination     3
  12:00     Sanchez, Maritsa        -        5 -General Examination     1
  12:15
  12:30
  12:45
   1:00     Carleton, Charles       1        1 -General Check-up        1
   1:15
   1:30
   1:45
   2:00     Lafflit, Tarela         1        1 -General Check-up        1
   2:15
   2:30
   2:45
   3:00
   3:15
   3:45
   4:00
   4:15
   4:30
   4:45
   5:00
```

FIGURE 7–7 Computerized daily list of appointments

SCHEDULING PATIENTS FOR OTHER MEDICAL UNITS

Physicians refer their patients to hospitals for outpatient care, inpatient care, and surgery; to laboratories for tests; to other physicians for consultations; to nursing homes and rehabilitation centers for long-term care; and to other medical facilities that treat special problems. You, as a medical assistant, will be responsible for coordinating the patient's arrangements, whether this means simply providing the patient with the name, telephone number, and address of another physician or making complete arrangements, including calling for the appointment and scheduling the tests (Figure 7–8).

Scheduling Patients for the Hospital

One of your duties will be to make arrangements for patients who must be admitted to the hospital. Based on the physician's instructions, you will call the hospital admitting clerk and provide the following information:

- Patient's name, address, and telephone number
- Admitting physician's name
- Date of admission
- Admitting diagnosis
- Consulting physicians' names

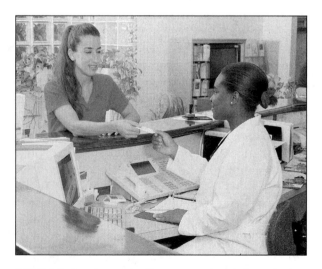

FIGURE 7–8 The medical assistant may need to schedule patients for outside facilities or for referral to other physicians.

After making hospital arrangements, you must call the patient to give him the admission date and check-in time. Any special instructions, such as no food or drink after a certain hour, must also be communicated at this time. As a courtesy, you should always ask if the patient has any questions about the hospitalization.

Scheduling Patients for Surgery

When surgery is to be performed, the time for the surgery is arranged with the surgery scheduling clerk, who must be given the following information:

- Patient's name and address
- Nature of the surgery
- Surgeon's name
- Assisting surgeon's name
- Names of other assisting physicians, such as the anesthesiologist or the pediatrician, in the case of a child's surgery
- Names of other operating room personnel

After arrangements are complete, call the patient with full information about the surgery. Provide any special instructions, for example, how many hours before surgery the patient can eat. Tell the patient the name of the surgeon and all assisting physicians; then try to answer any questions. If the patient has questions you cannot answer, ask the physician to call. Schedule the surgery in the practice's appointment book or computer as shown in Figure 7–9 so that the staff will know the physician will be unavailable during this time period.

Scheduling Patients for Outside Facilities

Patients frequently require medical service that must be performed outside the physician's office, either by another physician, a laboratory, or a specialty medical service. These patients may be asked to schedule their own appointments, or you may be asked to schedule the appointment for them. If you make the arrangements, call while the patient is in the office. Provide the scheduling clerk with the patient's name, the physician's name, the diagnosis, any necessary details regarding the service to be performed,

Dr. Joseph Felske
Surgery Schedule, July 14, 20–

7:00 AM	Carolyn Sinclair/D & C/Dr. Ingram assisting
7:15 AM	
7:30 AM	
7:45 AM	Suzanne Pittsfield/Hysterectomy/ Dr. Romalo assisting
8:00 AM	
8:15 AM	
8:30 AM	
8:45 AM	
9:00 AM	Edward Greer/Maltoma/Dr. Ingram assisting
9:15 AM	
9:30 AM	
9:45 AM	
10:00 AM	
10:30 AM	
10:45 AM	
11:00 AM	Charlene Reeves/Lumpectomy/ Dr. Sparkman assisting

FIGURE 7–9   Appointment book showing surgery schedule

Hilary Groche is scheduled for an appointment with Dr. _Concord_ at _2_ AM/**PM** on _June 19, 20–_ .

Elaine Shrager, M.D.

FIGURE 7–10   Referral card

Prepare an information card for the patient who is being referred. Include (1) the name of the referring physician, (2) the address and telephone number of the consulting physician, and (3) the date and time of the appointment. A preprinted form or a blank 3" × 5" card may be used for this purpose. A referral card is shown in Figure 7–10.

FOLLOW-UP APPOINTMENTS

Monitoring an existing health condition and preventive medicine are accomplished through follow-up appointments. These can be: (1) progress appointments designed to check on and control an existing condition or (2) periodic routine appointments that allow the physician to evaluate a patient's health. Both types of follow-up appointments are important for the overall care of patients, and you must assist patients in arranging follow-up appointments that will encourage good health practices. Follow-up appointments can be tracked easily by computer. You will enter a command to store the patient's name for a follow-up appointment in the future, usually for a specific month. Later, when you recall all follow-up appointments needed that month, you will be given the patient's name. The computer can also print a follow-up reminder card.

Progress Appointments

Many patients see their physician for follow-up appointments to monitor the progress of their treatment. Ask the patient to make arrangements before leaving the office at the time of the current visit. Then prepare a card showing the date

and the previous treatment. When arrangements are complete, give the patient a card showing the date, time, and place of the appointment.

Scheduling Patients for Referral

Primary care physicians sometimes refer patients to consulting physicians for additional tests and examinations or for a second opinion. You may be asked to make the appointment or to give the name and telephone number of the consulting physician to the patient. Keep a handy list of names, addresses, and telephone numbers of all physicians to whom patients are routinely referred.

Give the following information to the medical assistant at the consulting physician's office:

- Patient's name
- Preliminary diagnosis
- Previous treatment
- Service to be provided
- Referring physician's name

```
_____Sven Nordquist_____ is scheduled for an
appointment with Dr. _____Patrice_____ on
_____July 30_____ at _____3:00_____ AM/PM.

                        Gerard L. W. Miller, M.D.
                        89 Windwood Lane
                        Nashville, TN 37215
                        615-555-0293
```

FIGURE 7–11   Progress appointment follow-up

and time of the next appointment and give it to the patient. A progress follow-up card is shown in Figure 7–11.

Routine Periodic Appointments

Patients who see their physicians for routine appointments on a regular schedule, for example, every six months or once a year, may prefer to wait until a time close to the required date to make arrangements. You should maintain a tickler file containing the name and approximate follow-up date for each patient. A few weeks before the follow-up is due, mail a reminder notice to the patient.

Some offices use a different system. You may ask patients to address a preprinted reminder card before leaving the office at the current visit. A few weeks before the appointment is due, stamp and mail the card, thus giving the patient adequate time to schedule a follow-up. Medical offices that are computerized may instruct the computer to print reminder notices on a regular schedule. For example, once-a-month reminders can be printed for all patients who need to schedule an appointment within the next month or two. A reminder card is shown in Figure 7–12.

IN YOUR OPINION

1. Explain this statement, "A schedule is a good servant, but a poor master."
2. What would cause the following practices to need flexibility in scheduling: (1) pediatrics, (2) orthopedic surgery, (3) obstetrics, and (4) dermatology?
3. How can good scheduling improve patient satisfaction? The financial performance of the practice?

Front of card

```
IT'S TIME for your _____ month checkup.

Please call the office for an appointment.

                        Jennifer Tinnari, M.D.
                        89 Dick Lane
                        Trevose, PA 19301
                        215-555-0293
```

Back of card

FIGURE 7–12   Reminder card

INTERNET ACTIVITY

Go to the *Schedule View* Web site at http://www.scheduleview.com and download the Trial Edition of this scheduling software. Analyze the software, then prepare a short memo to your fictitious physician employer giving your opinion of the value of the software for the practice.

STUDENT STUDY CHECKLIST

Workbook

1. Complete Chapter 7 exercises in the workbook.
2. Complete Chapter 7 simulations in the workbook that access the CD-ROM in the back of the book.

Administrative Skills CD-ROM

1. Go to the Library on the CD-ROM and play the interactive games for Chapter 7.
2. Go to the Patient Reception area of the office and click on the computer. Take the tour and complete the exercises.
3. List the four scheduling systems, identifying what you like and dislike about each.

REFERENCES

Fordney, Marilyn T., and Joan J. Follis. *Administrative Medical Assisting*, 4th ed. Clifton Park, NY: Delmar Learning, 1998.

Humphrey, Doris. *Pediatric Associates, P.C.—The Medical Secretary.* Cincinnati, OH: South-Western, 1997.

Lindh, Wilburta Q., Marilyn S. Pooler, Carol D. Tamparo. *Administrative Medical Assisting*, 2nd ed. Clifton Park, NY: Delmar Learning, 2002.

CHAPTER ACTIVITIES

PERFORMANCE-BASED ACTIVITIES

1. Assume you are to begin work in a few weeks for a pediatric practice. Recommend what you believe is the best type of scheduling system and explain the reasons for your choice.

   Type of system recommended: _____

   Reason for this choice: _____

   _____

   _____

   _____

   _____

2. Develop a plan for the following schedule interruption: A blizzard has caused the physician and much of the office staff to be late. Several patients negotiated the bad roads and are waiting.

   _____

   _____

   _____

   _____

3. Create practice guidelines for building flexibility into a schedule.

   _____

   _____

   _____

   _____

4. Using information from this chapter, design and key or desktop publish a form that can be used to acquire information from patients before they are scheduled for hospital admission.

EXPANDING YOUR THINKING

1. Log on to Google or another search engine and enter the key words Medical Scheduling Software. Review the Web site for three software products and write a brief summary of the basic features that can be found in each package.

2. Your practice consists of three physicians. One is a single mother and the other two are a married couple with children. The practice is open six days a week. Each physician wishes to work five days a week. Construct two different schedules for a one-month period, and assess the advantages of each.

3. Linda Hebert has a condition the physician is unable to diagnose and is being referred to Dr. Raisa Van Doren for consultation. Your employer asks you to make the arrangements. List the steps you will follow and include any conversations you will have.

Referral Procedure

Information Needed	*Person to Contact*
1.	
2.	
3.	
4.	
5.	
6.	

PART III

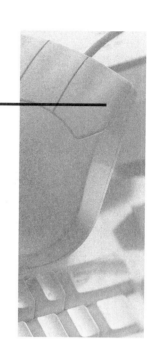

Computers and Information Processing in the Medical Office

Computers, originally used in the medical field by hospitals for billing and administration also play an important role in private medical practices. Computers are used for most administrative tasks, such as billing and collection, check writing, payroll management, accounts management, personnel records, drug and supply inventory, recall notices, and financial and tax applications. In addition, computers give physicians access to the most current medical research and opinion from around the world through medical databases and bulletin boards.

A computerized medical office usually is more productive, efficient, and organized. Computers simplify tasks that are difficult, repetitive, and time-consuming. That leads to improved employee morale and patients receive speedier service with fewer mistakes. As a medical assistant, you will be expected to know about computing in general and medical computing in particular. You will create, maintain, store, retrieve, and route data and documents of many types. In addition to conventional U.S. Mail, you will use various forms of expedited mail, such as Federal Express, United Parcel Service Priority Mail, and even couriers. Intelligent selection among these choices will result in high-quality, cost-effective service.

CHAPTER 8

Computerizing the Medical Office

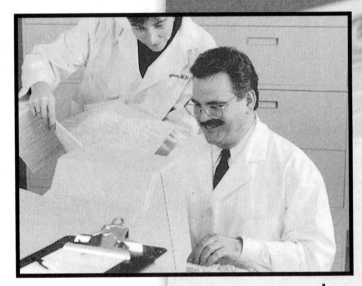

FLAGSTAFF, ARIZONA

When our doctors moved this practice to a different building four years ago, they installed a new computer system and purchased medical office management software. Because I had prior computer experience, I was designated the lead person to interact with the computer company for in-service training. The doctors assigned me to choose and set up programs that would help the staff become more efficient.

We now use computers for everything from word processing and mail merge to desktop publishing and presentation programs. The system includes a patient scheduling application that has done wonders for reducing patient wait. The database of patient files allows us to compare average length of visit per physician, sorted by patient complaint, age, and gender. Additionally, we're able to see whether one physician goes through inventory faster than others.

Recently, a software upgrade has given us new opportunities. Now, I can set up a program that compares the prescription practices of our doctors — analyzing which of them typically prescribes which drug for a given ailment. We're beginning to analyze just about everything.

Bonnie Byrd
Medical Assistant

PERFORMANCE-BASED COMPTENCIES

After completing this chapter, you should be able to:
1. Identify software applications and how they can be used in a medical office.
2. Discuss how to set up an inventory.
3. Analyze critical components of computer maintenance agreements.

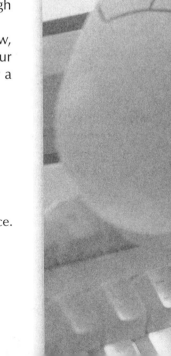

Computers have revolutionized medical offices in the last few years primarily because of two factors: (1) spectacular advances in computer clinical applications and (2) a drop in the price of computer processing power. The introduction into the practice of the whole-body scanner, computerized analysis of test results, and computerized laboratory equipment allows physicians to perform procedures in the office that previously were performed only at hospitals.

Today's computers that sit on a desk and cost less than $1,000 have the processing power of the room-size computers of the 1960s. Lower prices for high-powered systems make computing affordable for even the smallest practice, and most practitioners use computers to handle routine office applications.

HIGH TECH MEDICAL OFFICES

Among career experts, "every job is a high-tech job." The implications for you as a medical assistant are far-reaching. You are about to enter the medical assisting field at a time when caregivers are trying to become more efficient, while also being more cautious. According to the June 17, 2002 *Investor's Business Daily*, a 1999 Institute of Medicine report alerted the medical community that many deaths from medical errors might have been prevented with better record keeping. This encouraged physicians to invest in computer systems that can organize paperwork and store large amounts of patient data.

Alan Kells, director of investor relations for Cerner Corporation, a company that helps medical facilities track patient records by computer, was quoted in *Investor's Business Daily*, "When physicians use a pen, as opposed to computerized patient entries, the patient care is based on memory. When the pen is taken away and a computer with built-in logic is put in front of them, the computer can say, 'Wrong prescription. The patient's kidneys will fail, given their lab results.'"

Medical malpractice lawsuits, managed health care plans, convenience, and more enlightened patients have driven the surge toward high technology in medical offices. Figure 8–1 lists some of the many ways that medical offices rely on computers.

Any person who works in a medical office should be knowledgeable about computers and

Accounting

Accounts payable
Annual statements to patients
Cash report
Cash register
Check writing
Cross-posting in multiphysician practices
Daily log
Deposit slip
General ledger
Income and expense statement
Payroll
Profit and loss statements
Retirement plan accounting
W-2 forms
1099 forms

Billing, collecting, and insurance

Accounts receivable
Aging accounts receivable
Billing forms
Collection letters
Electronic form submission
Insurance claim form processing
Patient billing

Clinical

Access to national data banks
CME (continuing medical education) programs
Diagnosis and treatment
Drug interaction and allergy checks
Laboratory results system
Patient education
Prescription writing and tracking
Protocols, diagnosis, and treatment
Remote diagnosis and treatment
Retrieving medical research

Desktop publishing

Brochures
Business cards
Forms
Patient instructions
Stationery

Medical records

Case management
Clinical terminology
Electronic transcription services
Electronic transmission and retrieval

Practice management

E-mail
Employee vacation and sick-time records
Hospital lists and charges
Inventories and drug supplies
Ordering drugs and supplies
Patient profiles by age, diagnosis, etc.
Practice profiles by diagnosis, procedure, service
Production reports by physicians
Referrals

Research

Clinical information
Professional journals
Office administration
Health care trends
All medical and nonmedical subjects

Scheduling

Appointment scheduling
Follow-up scheduling
Patient recall lists
Patient reminders

Travel planning

Flight schedules
Fares and fees
Hotel and car reservations

Word processing

Articles
Consultation reports
Correspondence
Labels and addressing
Memos
Thank you letters
Welcome-to-practice letters

FIGURE 8–1 What computers can do in a medical office

proficient with all software applications. As a medical assistant, you may be the most knowledgeable person about computers in the office, because your training will be recent. This chapter will help define the medical assistant's overall responsibilities for computing and the broad issues involved in computerizing a medical office.

The Computer System

People often refer to installing a computer "system," leaving the impression that they are about to do something that will take up a large amount of space. Actually, the term computer system simply refers to all the various equipment or programs needed to turn a manual task into an electronic task, for example, producing and storing electronic documents with word processing software, instead of handwriting or typing documents and storing them in a file cabinet. Computers do not eliminate the need for manual tasks, but they simplify daily chores and reduce the amount of time required to perform the work.

A computer system consists of hardware and software. You are probably familiar with the key elements of a computer system, but for a quick review the components are briefly discussed below.

Hardware

The equipment or machines in a computer system are known collectively as hardware and include the following common components:

- Keyboard, the keys used to enter data
- Central processing unit (CPU), the electronic circuitry that translates the software instructions
- Monitor, the screen
- Modem, a device that converts a sending computer's message into telephone signals that can be received by other computers with a modem
- Mouse, the pointing device that controls the cursor
- Printer, the device that provides words and images on paper
- Data storage devices, including internal and external devices that can read and write on floppy disks, zip disks, and compact disks.

A typical computer system is made up of several pieces of hardware.

Software

The programs that give instructions to the computer are known collectively as software. The most frequently used programs in medical offices perform the following functions:

1. Give instructions to prepare documents or medical records (word processing)
2. Complete financial functions (spreadsheet)
3. Develop lists of patients, vendors, employees, associations, or others (database)
4. Prepare charts, graphs, or pictures (graphics)
5. Desktop publishing (create brochures and similar items)
6. Create presentations for meetings of conferences (presentation software)

Some medical office programs are integrated, or bundled, into one program called practice management software that performs all the functions named above. A medical office may use these integrated programs or combine a practice management program with other common business software such as Microsoft Windows.

MEDICAL SOFTWARE APPLICATIONS

Medical offices can purchase or lease practice management software ready-made or customized. In addition, a wide variety of general use computer software programs are available. General programs do not offer the special features of programs developed specifically for medical computing, and their use is diminishing while the use of specialized medical software is increasing. A practice will likely choose a system with scheduling and billing capabilities developed especially for medical offices.

One of your responsibilities as a medical assistant will be to review equipment and software contracts. Use the guidelines given in Figure 8–2 to review contracts of all types.

No one piece of software can handle all computing functions, and the specific needs and

1. Specify all terms and conditions of the contract. Write as part of the contract any verbal agreements between the physician and the vendor or between you and the vendor related to the system's performance.
2. Is the price standard or is it a negotiable item? Does it include the printer, hard disk, monitor, modem, mouse, central processing unit, and keyboard?
3. Make sure the maintenance support agreements and guarantees are detailed to identify how the equipment and software will perform.
4. Have the physician's accountant or attorney review the contract. Will the vendor assume liability when the computer is down?
5. Does the practice's current insurance coverage include financial losses when extended maintenance for the system is required?

FIGURE 8–2   Guidelines for reviewing contracts

priorities of each medical office must be analyzed to determine how software can be most useful. Ready-made software packages, customized software packages, or a combination of the two may provide the proper alternative.

Medical offices use software programs to process data. For example, when a patient visits a physician, a software program calculates the charges, subtracts payments and adjustments, adds the previous balance, and produces a current balance. As a medical assistant, if you key a number incorrectly, the computer will produce an incorrect result. The term "GIGO," or "Garbage In, Garbage Out," is applied to computer mistakes caused by human error. Perhaps you have received an incorrect bill for services at some time. When you questioned the mistake, you may have been told "the computer made a mistake." Most of the time, the computer only processed a mistake made by a human.

Word Processing

The major advantages of word processing are: (1) ease of making changes and (2) the ability to cut and paste from various documents to create a new document. Many programs can integrate graphics and data into the text. Word processing is one of the most frequently used medical software applications.

Spreadsheet

Applications that involve rows and columns of numbers requiring calculation usually use spreadsheet software, although word processing software can also create tables. Financial reporting, tax, and money management programs are spreadsheets that have been customized for a specific purpose. Popular spreadsheets allow users to enter their own formulas. For example, instructions in the expense spreadsheet in Figure 8–3 tell the computer to add both down and across, so that day and expense category totals can be seen. Medical billing software is based on spreadsheet applications.

Database

Computers are excellent at sorting and arranging records in databases. Applications that involve many records, such as patient files and inventory records, are good candidates for database software. Each piece of data in the record, such as the patient's name, address, age, and sex, is stored separately.

Databases are valuable because they can sort by characteristics. For example, how many patients are six years old and younger? How many are female? How many are six feet or taller? Lists can be produced and printed in alphabetic or numeric order using any characteristic in the database, including number of visits, number of prescriptions issued, or average length of appointment. Only data entered can be extracted, so database applications require good planning. Medical scheduling software is developed around database guidelines.

The medical assistant should meet with the medical staff to identify the types of reports needed before creating databases. Collecting and storing

	Ground Trans	Meals	Lodging	Mileage	Parking/ Tips	Other	Totals
Monday		23.41		10.08		25.6	$59.09
Tuesday	65.14	26.24	52.19				$143.57
Wednesday	43.80	20.44	87.75				$151.99
Thursday	43.96	16.40	80.64	10.08	26.00	1.40	$178.48
Friday							$0.00
Totals	$152.90	$86.49	$220.58	$20.16	$26.00	$27.00	$533.13

FIGURE 8–3   Expense spreadsheet

data that is "nice to know" rather than "needed to know" should be avoided. The medical assistant should review all reports periodically to make sure they are being used by the staff. A good way to audit this is to continue to run a report without distributing it to see if anyone complains. High-volume, repetitive transactions are the most cost effective to complete by computer. Figure 8–4 shows a partial database of patients.

Graphics

Graphs and charts are excellent for presenting information that can be interpreted at a glance. Integrated software converts spreadsheet or database data into charts and graphs such as those shown in Figures 8–5a, b, and c.

When graphing a chart choose the type of chart that pictures the information most effectively. For example, monthly financial data can be graphed to show how income changes over time. Intelligent use of graphics can save the medical staff valuable time when they read reports.

Desktop Publishing

Using desktop publishing software and a computer, a medical assistant can produce professional-looking documents such as flyers, brochures, reports, newsletters, and pamphlets. Years ago, the preparation of these documents involved many participants including a copywriter, an editor, a designer, a typesetter, and a paste-up artist. Today, the tasks can be performed by one person.

Name	Age	Gender	Race
Ramon Lucas	15	M	African-American
Serena Baldwin	10	F	Caucasian
Dale Leman	11	F	Native American
Carlos Lucerez	12	M	Latino
Phillipe St. Lucio	14	F	Caucasian
Patty Parker	12	F	Caucasian

FIGURE 8–4   Partial database of patients

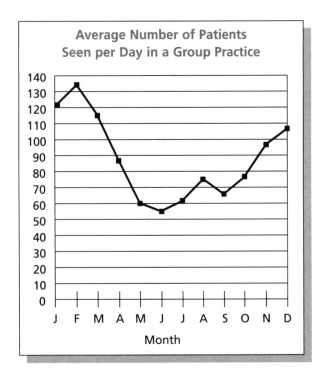

FIGURE 8–5A Line graph

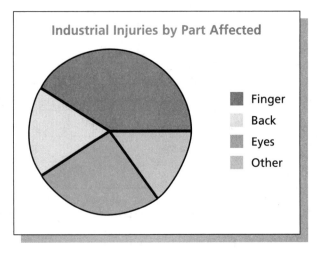

FIGURE 8–5B Pie chart

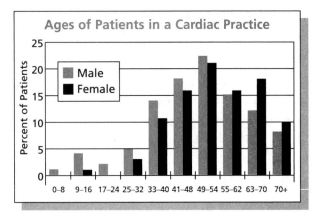

FIGURE 8–5C Bar chart

Attractive letterhead stationery and business cards can be created easily and inexpensively with desktop publishing software. By using a scanner — a machine that "reads" photographs or other images — to merge photographs with words, a medical assistant can include pictures of the medical office or its patients in a brochure. This textbook, including the cover, was created with desktop publishing software.

Presentations

Presentation programs are another form of graphics. Using presentation software, a computer, and a projector for on-screen electronic presentations allows the physician or medical assistant to bring together and present a variety of special effects and features. For example, the spreadsheet in Figure 8–3, the partial database of patients in Figure 8–4, and the graphs in Figures 8–5a, 8–5b, and 8–5c could be merged into a presentation program for showing during a meeting.

A physician might ask the medical assistant to prepare an electronic presentation combining words and illustrations of diseased lungs for a meeting on pulmonary problems or a slide pre-sentation using graphs and words to show the cost of medical malpractice insurance with different companies. Presentation graphics programs are excellent for creating on-screen materials.

DEVELOPING PRACTICE LISTS AND REPORTS

One of your responsibilities as a medical assistant will be to develop weekly or monthly lists and reports. The software manuals accompanying your system will illustrate many types of reports pre-programmed into the software. You can use these to create similar reports or you may wish to customize report formats specific to your practice. Figure 8–6 shows a database of drugs and codes used in one practice.

```
                              DRUG CODE LIST                          03/17/-
                                                                      Page 1
=============================================================================
Identification No.         Drug Code      Name
=============================================================================
         54)               ADRIA          ADRIAMYCIN
         15)               ALBUT          ALBUTEROL
         24)               ALDOMET        ALPHA METHYL DGPA
         35)               ELAVIL         AMITRIPTYLINE
         18)               AMP            AMPICILLIN
         12)               ASA            ASPIRIN
          6)               ATEN           ATEOLOL (TENORMIN)
         61)               BRONK          BROKOSOL
         66)               CAPTO          CAPTOPRIL
         55)               CARD           CARDIAZEM
         63)               LIBRIUM        CHLORDIAZEPOXIDE
         25)               CATPRESS       CLONIDINE (CATAPRES)
         17)               TRANX          CLORAZEPATE
         62)               LOTRIM         CLOTRIMAZOLE
         51)               PREMAR         CONUGATED ESTROGENS
         31)               CORG           CORGARD
         50)               COUM           COUMADIN
         26)               B12            CYANOCOBALAMIN
          9)               DEPOSE         DEPO-ESTRADIOL
         69)               DESIMPR        DESIMPRAMINE
         68)               DESIP          DESIPRAMINE
         46)               DIAB           DIABINESE (CHLORPRO)
         11)               DIG            DIGOXIN
         47)               PERSANT        DIAPYRIDAMOLE
         21)               DYAZ           DYAZIDE
         53)               ESDERM         ESTRADERM
         36)               LIDEX          FLUOCINONIDE
         49)               LASIX          FUROSEMIDE
          4)               FASIX          FUROSEMIDE
         64)               GLUC           FLUCOTROL
         43)               HYDER          HYDERGINE
          7)               HCTZ           HYDROCHLOROTHIAZIDE
         27)               NUPRIN         IBUPROFEN
         37)               IMIP           IMIPRAMINE
         22)               ISORDL         ISOSORBIDE DI (NO3)
         59)               ALUPENT        METAPROTERENOL
         28)               MINI           MINI-PRESS
         52)               NAP            NAPROSYN
         10)               NAPROS         NAPROXEN
          1)               NTG            NITROGLYCERIN SL
          3)               NPH            NPH INSULIN U-100
         20)               TALWIN         PENTAZOCINE
         41)               PERIAC         PERIACTIN
         45)               PERS           PERSANTIN
          8)               KCL            POTASSIUM CHLORIDE
         33)               MINPRES        PRAZOSIN
         60)               PRED           PREDNISONE
         30)               PREM           PREMARIN
         23)               PROCAN         PROCAINAMIDE
         56)               INDERAL        PROPRANOL
```

FIGURE 8–6 Partial database of drug and drug codes used in one practice

The following guide suggests several lists and reports that are generally helpful in a medical practice. Most of these are easily created by using information stored in the computer's database. This list is not intended to be comprehensive, but it should serve as a guide to the types of reports that are available.

Useful Computerized Lists and Reports

Patient-Related Information

- Patient names, addresses, telephone numbers, and patient numbers, if used
- Frequently used insurance company names and addresses
- Frequently used provider names, addresses, and telephone numbers, including hospitals, laboratories, and consulting physicians
- Emergency medical services in the area
- ICD codes and descriptions not listed on the superbill but frequently used
- CPT codes and descriptions not listed on the superbill but frequently used
- Codes for drugs commonly used by the practice (see Figure 8–6)
- Zip codes of nearby towns and cities

Practiced Management Information

- Staff names, addresses, telephone numbers, and social security numbers
- Vacation and holiday schedules
- Payroll information, including FICA and other taxes paid by each employee and the practice
- Transaction report for each physician by day, week, month, or year
- Productivity report by procedure; for example, the number of ECGs performed in one week
- List of all clinical and office equipment and dates of purchase or contract renewal, if leased
- Calendar of warranty requirements and maintenance dates of all equipment

INVENTORIES

A well-managed supply of office and clinical equipment and supplies enables a medical practice to deliver good service efficiently. The objective of an inventory system is to have the needed item available on time without excess stock. Items must be of the quality needed at the best price available.

Equipment Inventories

Once a year the medical assistant should review the inventory list of all equipment to make sure it is current. Clinical and office equipment may be listed together or separately. If all items are included in one list, the inventory may be easier to maintain; however, some medical assistants prefer to separate the inventory according to clinical or office functions or disposable or nondisposable. Some offices also include paintings, rugs, and other office furnishings. This decision should be made in coordination with the practice's financial advisors, as they may wish to categorize equipment for tax purposes.

After the first equipment inventory is created and keyed into the database, it is a simple matter to add or delete items. For example, when any item is purchased, sold, traded, or replaced, the appropriate information should be immediately keyed into the inventory database. In the partial inventory list shown in Figure 8–7, notice that a computer at the reception desk was upgraded on December 15, 2003. The disposition of the old computer is shown, as well as information about the new computer. The software can be instructed to print a current inventory at any time.

Clinical Supplies

Keeping a separate list of clinical and office supplies is a good idea. Depending on the type of

Office Equipment Inventory				
Item	Serial Number	Purchase Date	Location	Disposition
Dell computer	196-40268789	6/24/2002	Reception	Gave to Martin Elementary School
Dell computer	195-98293857	12/15/2003	Reception	
Panasonic copier	AB-L0142	9/18/2002	Billing	Trade in
Panasonic copier	RL-P334	4/14/2003	Reception	

FIGURE 8–7   Partial inventory of equipment

practice, the clinical supplies will vary from a very few to a large quantity. For example, in a psychiatric practice, the number of supplies is usually small, consisting primarily of medications. However, a pediatric practice requires bandages, tapes, medications, adhesive bandages, suture supplies, scissors, needles, and a wide variety of other items. A complete inventory must include a count of each of these (Figure 8–8).

Office Supplies

Paper, pens, scratch pads, superbills, staples, paper clips, printer paper and cartridges, and other office supplies are listed by number of boxes, reams, or packages in the inventory. An up-to-date stock of both clinical and office supplies is basic to a successful practice, and it will be your responsibility as a medical assistant to

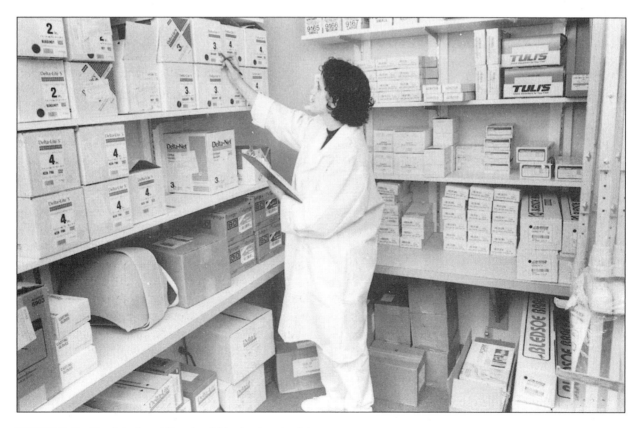

FIGURE 8–8   The list of supplies should be kept up to date.

have supplies available when needed. There are two goals that may seem contradictory in managing an inventory: "do not run out and do not have excess." Some tips for managing inventories are listed below:

1. Know what you have. If you do not know what you have, you will not know what to buy and may maintain expensive duplication. Think of supplies as money sitting on the shelf.
2. Keep track of how fast you use supplies. When you run out or something, check to see the last time you purchased it. Buy in quantities appropriate to your rate of usage. Do not tie up extra money in inventories.
3. Categorize your inventory according to the chart in Figure 8–9.
4. Some office and medical suppliers may be willing to hold inventories for you to get your business. They will bill you only when you "call out" or order supplies. This can save your employer thousands of dollars in supplies and office space. The supplier may even agree to come in weekly to review supplies and replenish them to your desired level. This saves the practice administrative costs.
5. Label shelves where supplies are kept, and group supplies of a similar type. On a monthly basis, review the most frequently used supplies to make sure the actual supply matches your computer record. If it does not match, review your procedure for updating receipts and issues of supplies at the time when they occur.

Purchasing

Purchasing is an important function that can save your practice considerable money. The purchasing objective is to buy the right quality of supplies for the right price. The right price is not always the cheapest initial cost but should take into consideration the total cost of using the item over its period of use. A piece of equipment that rarely breaks down, for example, may easily justify a higher initial cost than a cheaper alternative.

Purchasing software is available. This type of software shows inventory balances, prints orders,

Inventory Categories

Type of item	Inventory objective
Inexpensive, often used, like tongue depressors	Buy in bulk, never run out
Dated supplies	Review for expiration date, discard properly, do not store excess
Items similar to one another, such as gauze pads of different sizes	Eliminate duplication where possible and buy only needed sizes
Expensive, often used	Monitor often and buy carefully
Expensive, rarely used	Locate a source that can rapidly supply this item
Items that have not been used for six months or more	Review for possible disposal; storage costs money and prevents you from keeping a tidy supply area
Items that have a long "lead time"	Order far enough ahead of time to avoid last-minute crises and expensive delivery charges
Items that can be substituted for out-of-stock items, for example, a larger gauze pad could be used if the smaller size is out of stock.	Develop a list of substitutes

FIGURE 8–9 Categories for an office inventory

tracks items on order, shows inventory transactions such as issues and receipts, and tracks prices paid. An office that uses a modem may be able to order supplies directly if the supply house provides this service.

MISCELLANEOUS COMPUTER TIPS

The following suggestions will help with office computerization.

Mechanical Failures

Do not be concerned about whether a computer will ever malfunction. Sooner or later it will. The essential question is how rapidly can you get it repaired. All hardware should be covered by a maintenance agreement that guarantees service within a few hours. It is important for the medical assistant to make sure that the turn-around time is short. This is a matter on which you should insist.

When a medical office is fully automated, the computer's down time can destroy the practice's schedule and organization. Consider, for example, the office that stores all patient accounts and medical records in a computer. If the computer is down, no financial transactions can be completed, and medical histories cannot be reviewed unless a paper file exists.

Maintenance agreements are invaluable. Computer equipment should be covered by a contract, preferably by the same vendor who sold it. Otherwise, each vendor may say someone else is responsible for maintenance and repair.

Larger practices may contract with firms that provide back-up systems, including memory, that enable the practice to continue operating, even when they experience computer failure. The computer system for the practice is networked to the disaster service so that data is backed up in a remote location.

Bypassing Frustration

Computers do not always do what the user wants. Software generally causes more problems than hardware because each program has its own quirks. The best way to bypass frustration is to refer to the software manual. For example, when unable to print, find the section on printing in the manual and read the troubleshooting tips. To eliminate the frustration of lost data, back up your files on a daily or weekly basis.

Do Not Panic: Call the 800 Number

Many software vendors provide a toll-free 800 number for the moments when all best efforts fail, even though all the manual's instructions have been conscientiously followed. The 800 number should be used any time assistance is needed because a technical support representative who will understand your problem is sitting by a telephone waiting for such calls. As a caller, you must, however, be able to specify exactly what happened before, during, and after a procedure. Generalities are not good enough. For example, someone who cannot print from a particular program might say, "When I depressed CODE and PRINT, the screen locked. Just before that I had saved my document to a new disk." The representative will offer suggestions until the trouble has been cleared up. It is also a good idea to be sitting at the computer terminal and to have the machine on during the call.

IN YOUR OPINION

1. What transactions in a medical office might not justify the time and money to computerize?
2. Name medical supplies for which quality is more important than initial cost.
3. The computer says you have sutures, but there are none on the shelf. What could have caused the discrepancy?

INTERNET ACTIVITY

Go to the WebMD Web site http://www.medical-manager.com and take the tour called *A Day in the Life*. It includes one day in a typical practice using medical software. Describe any usage you did not know about before.

STUDENT STUDY CHECKLIST

Workbook

1. Complete Chapter 8 activities in the workbook.
2. Complete Chapter 8 simulations in the workbook that access the CD-ROM in the back of the book.

Administrative CD-ROM

1. Go to the Library on the CD-ROM and play the interactive games for Chapter 8.
2. Visit three areas of the medical office on the CD-ROM. Describe what applications computers perform in each area.

REFERENCES

Howell, Donna. "More Doctors Prescribe Software," *Investor's Business Daily*, June 17, 2002.

Pusins, Dolores Wells and Ann-Peele Ambrose. *Computer Concepts.* Cambridge, MA: Thomson Learning/Course Technology, 2001.

WebMD Web site, Medical Manager Health Systems Products, 2002.

CHAPTER ACTIVITIES

PERFORMANCE-BASED ACTIVITIES

1. Compare two maintenance agreements for office or lab equipment. Using the format below, analyze the features of each to determine which is a better contract. Summarize the pros and cons of each contract.

   *Type of equipment*_____ *Purpose* _____

   Contract Features

   Contract 1   *Contract 2*

   1. _____

   2. _____

   3. _____

   4. _____

   5. _____

   Summary of advantages

   1. _____

   2. _____

   3. _____

   Summary of disadvantages

   1. _____

   2. _____

   3. _____

2. Assume you work for a medical practice that is actively involved in a number of activities. The practice is moving to a new, larger location and patients will be invited to an open house. Over the next month, you will be asked to perform the following tasks. Identify the software application you will use to complete the task and explain why the application was chosen.

   April 4   Prepare a list of the names, addresses, and zip codes of all patients seen in the last two years, so they can be invited to the open house.

   Software application: _____

   Reason chosen: _____

   _____

   April 6   Prepare an invitation to the open house.

   Software application: _____

   Reason chosen: _____

   _____

April 10   Create an attractive brochure that provides information about the practice, including the new hours, the address, the names of the doctors, and pictures of the staff at work.

Software application: _____

Reason chosen: _____

_____

April 11   Write a letter explaining the move, one that can be inserted in the envelope with the invitation and brochure.

Software application: _____

Reason chosen: _____

_____

April 15   Prepare and print the rough draft speech Dr. Wamder's wrote for the open house.

Software application: _____

Reason chosen: _____

_____

April 16   Prepare slides and visuals for Dr. Wamder to use electronically as part of his presentation.

Software application: _____

Reason chosen: _____

_____

3. Develop a list of guidelines that will help you maintain an accurate inventory count.

4. Decide whether word processing, spreadsheet, graphics, or database software is the best application to accomplish each task named below. Justify your answer.

Task	Software Applications	Reason for Application
Indexing medical journals	Database	Alphabetizes and sorts a lengthy list
Determining rate of usage of disposable supplies	Spreadsheet keeps up with quantity used and time frame	
Creating holiday card list		
Calculating mortgage payments		
Maintaining patient records		
Logging vehicle mileage		
Writing memos		
Preparing income statements		
Presenting a research paper		
Compiling credit card expenditures		
Creating correspondence		
Maintaining payroll records		

EXPANDING YOUR THINKING

1. List several ways computers can help each of the following:
   a. The physician
   b. The medical assistant
   c. The nurse
   d. The laboratory assistant

2. Develop a list of questions to ask a prospective maintenance company that wishes to service your computer system.

3. Assume you are speaking with a medical assistant applicant who wishes to work for your group practice. What questions about using computer software would you want the medical assistant to answer? Role-play the interview with a classmate who will assume the role of the applicant.

CHAPTER 9

Medical Documents and Word Processing

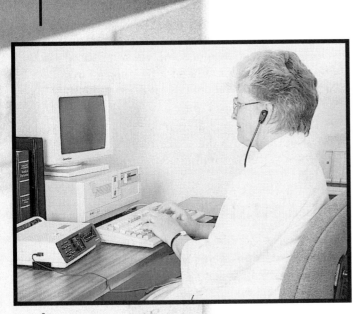

HARTFORD, CONNECTICUT

Something that sets our practice apart from many others is the crisp, precise, and professional way we conduct our business. Don't get me wrong; we're warm and caring too, but we work hard at doing things right. That includes our correspondence and other word processing output. Everyone in the practice uses the same format for letters and reports, and all are computerized and standardized to that style.

This sounds fussy, and I guess it is, but there's a purpose. We want to present a professional image. That includes the way we present ourselves in our written communications — margins, spelling, grammar, tone, and style. Appearances are not deceiving.

Fortunately, our computer software allows us to program document setup for letters, reports, files, articles, and presentations. Beyond that, spell checking is a lifesaver, as is the grammar alert. It's nice to have all those memory chips supporting our quest for perfection.

Even so, we still take time to proofread new output, sometimes even reading it aloud to each other — just to make sure that we didn't key something the computer couldn't catch — for instance accidentally keying "their" when we should have keyed "there." Reading aloud pinpoints technically correct but poorly written sentences. We have a reputation among our patients and in the medical community for being one of the best practices in the area. Our attention to image and detail is part of the reason.

Sebastian Angelino
Medical Assistant

After completing this chapter, you should be able to:

1. Create written communication appropriate to the reader's ability to understand.
2. Demonstrate comprehension of guidelines for medical correspondence by developing form letters and medical documents.
3. Adapt available word processing technology to medical applications.
4. Apply proofreading techniques to rough draft and finished copy.
5. Use proper methods in transcribing by machine.

VOCABULARY

Block   Letter format in which all lines begin at the left margin.

Formatting   Placement of the parts of a letter or medical document.

Gender bias   Subtle form of verbal sex discrimination.

Gender neutral   Language that is not biased toward either sex.

Modified block   Format in which the date and closing lines begin at center.

Proofread   To examine a document for errors.

Redundancy   Unnecessary repetition of words.

Stored letter parts   Standard paragraphs that are stored in the computer's memory.

Thesaurus   Reference book or word processing feature containing synonyms and antonyms.

Tone   Sound of letters; what is said and how the writer chooses to say it.

Transcription   To write from one source to another.

"You" viewpoint   Focusing the language of a written document on the best interests of the reader.

As a medical assistant, you may compose some of the general correspondence and reports for your practice. Letters concerning business matters, such as leases or equipment repair, and reports about office management or a comparative study of computer systems, are items that physicians usually do not write themselves. They leave these and similar writing responsibilities to the medical assistant. As a result, the medical assistant must be prepared to create documents that represent the practice. This involves an understanding of writing principles and objectives.

For some people, writing well is an ability developed during their formative years but everyone can improve their ability to produce clear documents and letters. The ability to write well increases your value as a medical assistant.

Your professional writing will probably include: (1) correspondence for your personal signature, (2) correspondence for the physician's signature, (3) informal notes to other staff members, (4) standard fill-in forms or cards to be mailed, and (5) occasional practice or research reports. If you are also the office manager, your writing responsibilities will be even greater.

LETTER WRITING

Because many people, including physicians, write poorly, demonstrating your ability to write clear and informative letters provides a distinct professional advantage. Some people resist writing letters because they believe letter writing requires an innate creativity. Actually, becoming a good writer only requires practice. If your writing skills are limited, register for a class that provides the guidance you will need to improve.

Professional-looking and-sounding letters project a positive image for the medical office. They require time, energy, skill, and a good knowledge of grammar usage, punctuation, and spelling. Because letters often serve as legal documentation, they must be well written and accurate.

Medical assistants often are responsible for composing and formatting routine or non-clinical letters to patients, such as referrals, instructions, or hospital scheduling information. They also write to suppliers, insurance companies, and organizations. Other written communications that a medical assistant may write include:

- Memos
- E-mails and fax correspondence
- Meeting reports
- Practice brochures

Developing Tone

Musicians tune their instruments before every concert so the sound will be pleasing to listeners. Good orchestra leaders know that an out-of-tune instrument can spoil the effect of a lovely composition. In the same way, the tone or sound of letters should be pleasing to the readers. What is said and how the writer chooses to say it determines a letter's tone. Appropriate tone in a letter is conversational, informal, and business-like but it should not be too familiar, chatty, or pretentious.

"You" Viewpoint

A letter is written for the benefit of the reader. Therefore, the reader's wants, needs, feelings, and emotions come before the writer's wants, needs, feelings, and emotions. For example, a letter requesting payment for an overdue account should focus on the reader's desire to maintain a good credit rating, not on the practice's desire to collect money. Commonly called the **"you" viewpoint** or the "you" attitude, this concept of letter writing might be described as "putting yourself in the reader's place." The "you" viewpoint is accomplished through a positive, pleasant tone that focuses on the reader. It does not mean that the word "you" is overused.

The opposite of the "you" viewpoint is the "I" (or "we") viewpoint, a letter based on the writer's needs. "I" letters sound selfish and turn the reader off from the message. Read the following examples of the two viewpoints.

"You" Viewpoint

Dear Mr. Shuba:

Good health is the key to a good life, and you obviously had that thought in mind when you asked us to remind you of your annual physical examination. It is once again time for your annual checkup.

If you will call the office at your convenience, we will schedule an appointment for a day that won't interfere with your work. The telephone number is 555-3867.

"I" Viewpoint

Dear Mr. Shuba:

Our calendar shows that it is time for your annual physical examination, and I would like to schedule an appointment that fits Dr. Carerra's schedule within the next month. Please call me so I can determine what appointment time is best for us.

Use Positive Words Instead of Negative

Positive words add pleasure to letter reading and should be used abundantly. Negative words are worthwhile only if they add meaning or make an important point. by reconstructing sentences, positive words can usually be substituted for most negative words. In addition to "no," "not," "never," and other generally recognized negatives, the connotations of some words also set a negative tone. Figure 9–1 lists some negative words and phrases.

Saying "No" in a "Yes" Way

Letters should speak of what can be done instead of what cannot be done. Letters whose purpose is essentially negative, even credit rejection letters, can be written to say "no" in a "yes" way. The following two letters were written by a medical assistant for the physician's signature. Compare the ways in which the negative letter was rewritten to say "no" in a positive way.

Negative Treatment

Dear Ms. Phillieo:

I am sorry to say that your failure to keep your last two appointments forces me to withdraw from treating your medical condition. It is useless for me to continue to make recommendations, since my efforts are in vain.

Negative Words and Phrases

dumb	inconsistent
unsuccessful	reject
useless	in vain
impossible	mistake
failed	oversight
inadvertent	mess
fiasco	limit
sorry	withdraw
stupid	beg your pardon
correct me if I'm wrong	disagree

FIGURE 9–1 Negative words and phrases

Positive Treatment

Dear Ms. Phillieo:

Your good health is important to me, so I was naturally concerned when you missed your last two appointments. Routine appointments to evaluate your condition are important for your continuing successful recovery.

Unless we can arrange a suitable schedule of checkups, I will be unable to continue as your physician. Will you please call me so we can discuss the future direction of your treatment.

Correct Word Choice

Using the right word at the right time is a gift for some letter writers. However, even the person who is not naturally gifted in writing can develop skill in choosing the right words. A few liberally applied guidelines, as well as a thesaurus for strengthening vocabulary and a dictionary for correct spelling, will ensure correct word choice (Figure 9–2).

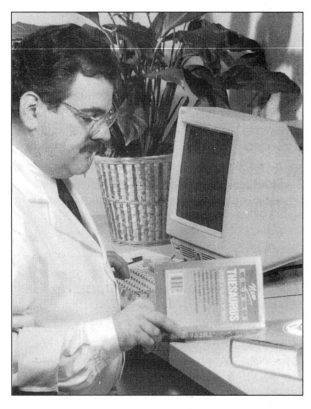

FIGURE 9–2 Use reference books to check vocabulary and spelling.

Communicating at the Reader's Level

To understand the importance of writing to a specific audience, consider these questions:

- Should a teacher write a first grader a note using twelfth-grade words?
- Should an engineer use engineering terms in a memorandum to a botanist?
- Should a medical assistant use technical medical terminology when writing to a patient?

The answer to all of these questions is "no." Unfortunately, some writers fail to consider the reader's background. Because of this, they write letters that fail to deliver their messages because the language is too technical or too sophisticated for the reader to understand. Direct the message to the educational level, maturity, and experience of the reader. For example, a letter to a consulting physician to arrange an appointment may use medical terminology. Patients, however, may not understand medical terminology, and letters sprinkled with medical terms confuse and frustrate them. A comparison of technical terminology and ordinary words is shown in Figure 9–3. It is appropriate to use the terminology on the left in a letter to a medically trained person. A letter to a nonmedical person should use the common language substitutes.

Gender Bias

Occupations that once were dominated by men or dominated by women are now gender neutral because of federal legislation to eliminate bias in employment. It is difficult to change habits of thought and speech, so gender-restrictive terms continue to be a part of language. Although the number of female physicians has grown in recent years and male nurses are becoming more common, some people still visualize "doctors" as men and "nurses" as women (Figure 9–4). Always strive to eliminate gender bias in writing. Sometimes this is as simple as being aware of the subtle biases that exist in the subconscious. Thinking in nongender terms will make writing much easier. By substituting a word, reworking a sentence, or changing a pronoun from singular to plural, gender bias can usually be eliminated from writing. Review the lists in Figure 9–5 to learn some acceptable substitutes for sexist words or phrases.

Technical Terminology	Common Language Substitute
myocardial infarction	heart attack
hypertension	high blood pressure
diabetes mellitus	diabetes
carcinoma	cancer
arteriosclerotic heart disease	hardening of the arteries
deglutition	swallowing
erythrocyte	red blood cell
h.s.	at bedtime
hyperglycemia	excessive sugar in the blood
inspiration	breathing
trauma	injury

FIGURE 9–3   Comparison of medical and nonmedical terminology

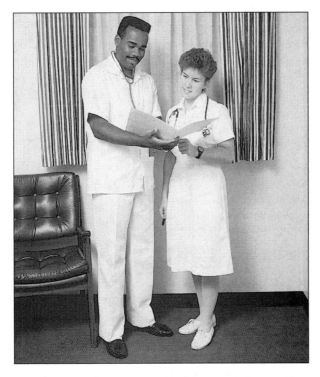

FIGURE 9–4   Occupations that were once dominated by one sex, such as nursing, are now gender neutral. Be aware of gender biases you may have.

Gender-Biased Language	Substitute for Gender Bias
female nurse	nurse
male orderly	medical attendant
stewardess	flight attendant
foreman	supervisor
cleaning ladies	cleaning crew, janitorial staff
physician wore his lab coat	physician wore a lab coat
nurse called her husband	nurse called a spouse
medical assistant spoke her mind	medical assistant commented
reviewed his paperwork	reviewed the paperwork

FIGURE 9–5   Substitutes for gender-biased language

Use Active Instead of Passive Voice

Active verbs make writing more direct and easier to read. The difference between an enticing and a boring piece of communication may rest in the choice of verbs. Review the examples of sentences with active verbs or passive verbs in Figure 9–6.

Use Short Sentences and Paragraphs

Short sentences and paragraphs are more readable than long sentences and paragraphs. A sentence should state the point directly and concisely. Twenty words is considered the maximum limit for a good sentence. Eliminate unnecessary words and phrases that do not contribute to the sentence and combine short sentences that sound choppy and monotonous.

Comparison of Active and Passive Verbs

Active Voice	Passive Voice
The medical assistant filed the patient's records.	The patient's records were filed by the medical assistant.
An emergency physician saves lives daily.	Lives are saved daily by an emergency physician.
The mother brought her baby in for a checkup.	The baby was brought in by the mother for a checkup.
The young children disrupted the entire staff.	The entire staff was disrupted by the young children.

FIGURE 9–6   Active and passive voice

Short Choppy Sentences:

Dr. Ashley examined the patient. The patient complained of headaches to the doctor. The doctor prescribed medication. The patient took the medication and felt better.

Long Sentence:

The patient complained to Dr. Ashley about headaches; then Dr. Ashley examined the patient and prescribed medication, which the patient took before feeling better.

Well-Constructed Sentence:

Dr. Ashley examined the patient who complained of headaches. After taking the medication the doctor prescribed, the patient felt better.

FIGURE 9–7   Comparison of sentence structure

Constructing sentences that are clear, yet not wordy or choppy is a challenge. Study the sample sentences in Figure 9–7.

A paragraph should cover only one point and contain from two to five sentences. Readers lose interest when a paragraph is too long.

Eliminate Redundant Words

The saying "I didn't have time to write a short letter, so I wrote a long one" means that a writer finds it takes less time to be wordy than concise. Being concise takes time because it requires thought. Never use two words when one will do. Using excessive words makes reading tedious and causes the reader to lose interest.

Redundancy means the unnecessary repetition of words. Redundant use of language shows up too often in business correspondence. Does that mean the writer is lazy? Or does the writer not understand how redundancy affects the communication process? After each letter, memo, or report, analyze the paragraphs to check for redundancy. Eliminate or rephrase any part that bogs down the message. Figure 9–8 lists some common redundant expressions. In each case, the phrase can be replaced with one word.

Redundant Expression	Replacement
repeat again	repeat
forever after	forever
reverse order	reverse
close up	close
very latest	latest
now and forever	always
first and foremost	first
each and every	each
absolutely free	free
invisible to the eye	invisible
physician's patient	patient
patient's illness	illness

FIGURE 9–8   Redundant expressions and substitutions

DEVELOPING YOUR COMMUNICATIONS

Consider a request to compose letters, reports, memorandums, and other materials as a compliment. Only a person with advanced grammar, punctuation, spelling, human relations, and organizational skills is given this assignment. A medical assistant asked to compose a communication should start by developing a plan. One system that works well is the simplified five-step plan which significantly reduces the time required for composing. The plan is given in Figure 9–9.

WRITING FOR THE PHYSICIAN'S SIGNATURE

Composing a letter to be signed by another person poses a challenge because the writer must duplicate the signer's writing style. As a medical assistant, you will routinely key the physician's dictated communications and thus gain a feel for the person's style of writing. You can also review other documents written by the physician to learn the particular style used. When you are asked to write a letter, search the files for a letter on the same subject that the physician previously dictated or wrote. Substitute current details in the appropriate spots and update the letter with names, times, and specific details. The first two or three times you compose a document for the physician, submit a rough draft for approval or revision. After keying the changes, print the final document in correct format for the physician's signature.

Your responsibility for report writing as a medical assistant probably will be limited. The amount of report writing you do will depend on the degree to which you become involved in the physician's outside activities. Some physicians who engage in research, public speaking, writing articles, and related activities may ask a medical assistant to research the Internet, periodicals, newspapers, and books for specific information necessary for these activities. Someone who is both a medical assistant and an office manager may be called on to develop a report on office procedures, office equipment, or personnel matters. The basic rules that apply to writing letters are also useful for writing reports, although special rules exist for developing and preparing a report.

COMPOSING AT THE COMPUTER

Word processing software offers the opportunity to compose at the computer, thus saving an enormous amount of time. The screen can be considered a clean sheet of paper on which to write thoughts. As you develop your e-mails, letters, reports, or other documents, read them for tone and word choice. When you find redundancies, gender bias, overuse or inappropriate use of the passive voice, or overly short or overly long sentences, edit your documents on the screen. Then, print a draft copy for final review and correction. Finally, edit the document on the screen and make final changes before printing the finished copy. Although composing at the computer may be a bit awkward at first, you will soon wonder how you ever found the time to hand write rough drafts in the past.

Electronic Mail

Electronic mail, or e-mail, fulfills a very important function in today's medical office. Using e-mail properly shortens the response between when a question is asked or a concern is voiced and the answer or solution is available. The writing principles for an e-mail are the same as for a letter or other written medical information.

Most e-mail messages are written in a simple, straightforward paragraph format. When it is possible to use bullets or other formatting techniques, do so to enhance the readability of your message. Several important guidelines should be followed when writing and sending an e-mail.

- Never write anything you would not want to be seen in a letter. Any inappropriate remark will surely get into unintended hands. Computers can be confiscated by the authorities and their files used as evidence in legal proceedings.

Step One: Define the Problem and the Audience.   Classify the purpose of the communication: informational, request, collection, thank you, or other. Determine the nature and background of the communication and the reader's view of the situation: Has previous correspondence been exchanged? Will the reader be receptive to the document?

Identify the reader by considering education, economic status, marital status (if appropriate), experience, age, attitude, biases, and other factors you consider relevant.

Step Two: Create an Outline.   Prepare a brief outline with a one-word identifier that describes the content of each paragraph. The following outline is suggested for a letter advising patients that a new physician has joined the practice.

First paragraph:	Announcement
Second paragraph:	Background
Third paragraph:	Good will

Step Three: Brainstorm Ideas.   Jot down thoughts that can be included in each paragraph. Do not worry about the order in which you write them at this stage. The identifiers listed above suggest that the first paragraph of the letter will announce the new physician's name and starting date. The second paragraph describes the physician's medical background. The last paragraph builds good will by explaining how patients will benefit from an additional physician. A brief list of ideas might look like this one:

First paragraph:	Dr. Rogers joining practice June 26
	Available on full-time basis August 15
Second paragraph:	Specialty, Family Practice
	Johns Hopkins University
	Internship, Albert Einstein Medical Center
Third paragraph:	Waiting time reduced for patients
	Taking new patients
	Auxiliary staff increased

Step Four: Put Ideas into Order.   Review all the ideas written in Step Three. Choose the best and list them in the order in which they should be presented in the letter.

First paragraph:	Dr. Rogers joining practice
	Available on limited basis beginning June 26
	Full-time after August 15
Second paragraph:	Graduated from Johns Hopkins University School of Medicine
	Specialty, Family Practice Internship, Albert Einstein Medical Center
Third paragraph:	Waiting time reduced for established patients
	Taking new patients
	Auxiliary staff increased

Step Five: Write the Paragraphs.   The letter is now ready to be written. Construct concise, complete sentences in the order shown in Step Four. Add transitional words as necessary to create a smooth writing style.

FIGURE 9–9   Five-step plan for composing

- Keep the e-mail message brief. Write just a few lines or only one or two short paragraphs.
- Proofread all e-mail correspondence carefully. Print a copy and ask a coworker to read any e-mail that holds important or potentially controversial information.
- Make sure all grammatical and typographical errors are corrected. Just because e-mail is informal does not mean that standards should be low for the content.
- Remember that e-mail is not private. Some people forget that e-mail is as easily reproducible as a letter and can be forwarded to many people quickly. Recognize that your employer or supervisor can check your e-mail.
- Handle conflict in person, if possible, rather than by e-mail. Written messages can be more readily misunderstood, and they live on after the matter has been settled.
- Try to keep your system of sending e-mail copies simple and sensible. Do not send copies of messages to others unless required.
- File e-mails in appropriate cyber folders as received. Otherwise, they will multiply faster than you ever expected.

IN YOUR OPINION

1. Do you think that e-mails have replaced letters as a form of written communication?
2. Can you think of gender-neutral alternatives for these words; Man hours, office girl, workmen, mankind, lab girl, manpower?
3. What steps can you take to make sure you are writing at the reader's level?

SOURCES OF INPUT

The correspondence, memos, and medical reports that medical assistants create and edit on the computer come from a variety of sources, both inside and outside the medical office. Whatever the source, you as a medical assistant will be responsible for organizing and producing the information in the documents so that it is attractive and clear. Here are some of the more common forms of information you will key, edit, proof, and file:

- The physician's dictation
- The physician's notes
- Patient information sheets
- Case histories and other medical reports
- Memos and letters
- Speeches

Rough Draft Input

Handwritten source documents are popular because they can be created at almost any time and in any place. Input from rough draft documents has both advantages and disadvantages.

Advantages
- Documents can be created quickly without concern for appearance.
- Many people think best when they use a pencil to add, delete, and cross out.
- Medical terminology is usually spelled correctly and accents and dialects are added which makes the document easier to key.

Pitfalls
- Physicians are notorious for their hard-to-read handwriting.
- Rough draft materials often have been cut and re-taped, making them difficult to follow.
- Copy may be sprinkled throughout with correction fluid that is written over.
- Several different type styles may appear in the same document.
- Different word processing drafts may exist causing confusion over which is most current.

Tips for Managing Rough Drafts
- Read the entire document to be sure you understand it.
- Recopy poor handwriting.
- Trace inserted material to its proper location in the document, drawing arrows as needed.
- Add missing information, such as an address or title.
- Correct spelling and grammar and add punctuation as needed.
- Use proofreading marks to clarify editing.
- Circle special notes in red.
- Add formatting comments or other information that will aid in keying the document.

- Make sure you always work with the most recent draft.
- Destroy previous revisions.

Study the proofreader's marks shown in Figure 9–10 and review the rough draft typed case history in Figure 9–11 to determine the reason for the proofreader's marks.

Word processing is especially helpful for a previously keyed rough draft letter that must be edited.

Dictation and Transcription

The threat of medical malpractice lawsuits has forced physicians to document thoroughly all medications, instructions, procedures, treatments, and services for each patient. Many physicians use machine dictation for their correspondence and medical reports. Machine transcription also has its advantages and disadvantages.

Voice-Activated Dictation: Brave New World

Physicians commonly dictate into a machine for transcription at another time. With computer based voice activated dictation, the physician records several hundred words in the voice activated system. The system learns to recognize the physician's pronunciation. The system rapidly creates a draft document, which is proofread for errors. Voice activated systems have a good degree of accuracy at recognizing spoken words and they make the dictation process much faster.

The medical assistant is freed from the laborious process of transcription and takes on the higher level skill of editing.

Machine Dictation

Some physicians return to their offices to dictate reports and doctor's notes on a desktop dictating unit after treating each patient. Other physicians dictate on a portable dictating machine in the examining room in the patient's presence. This method helps to reduce malpractice claims because (1) the physician dictates the report before any important portion of the visit is forgotten, and (2) the patient knows that a report covering the visit is on file. If there is a discrepancy between the patient's and the physician's understanding of the procedure or treatment, the patient has an opportunity to ask questions after hearing the dictation.

Advantages
- The medical assistant can perform other functions while the physician dictates.
- The material can be transcribed later.

Pitfalls
- Dictation from physicians with foreign accents and regional dialects may be difficult to understand.
- The transcriber must use medical dictionaries and other reference books to locate spellings and meanings that fit the context of medical documents. (Some software packages have a spell checker.)

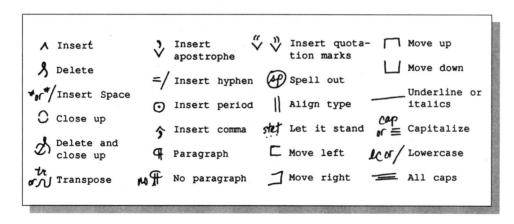

FIGURE 9–10 Proofreader's marks

PATIENT CASE HISTORY

MADELINE HAST, M.D.

NAME ____Robert ᴬMcElroy_____

DATE _____August 16, 20—_____

PATIENT NUMBER _____894_____

CHIEF COMPLAINT: This twelve-year-old ~~patient~~ *female* came to my office with ~~his~~ *her*
mother. ~~His~~ *Her* symptoms ~~are~~ *were* headaches, sore throat, and *a cough.*
She had been ʌcoughing for four days. Fever ~~had~~ been present for two
days. A week ago ʌ*s*he ~~spent~~ the night with a friend who
has ʌ*since* been diagnosed for strep ʌthroat.

EXAMINATION: Examination shows a generally healthy ʌ*female* child who is
developed and nourished well. ~~She~~ weighs ~~64~~ *84* pounds and
5'0"   is ~~4~~ feet ~~8~~ inches tall. Her temperature is 101.4
degrees. ~~B~~.p. is 100/60.
⟨*Sp.*⟩

Throat, glands and tympanic membranes are clear. Ears
and neck are within limits. Eyes are clear. Rales are
within normal limits present in the lower chest on respiration. Abdomen is
ʌ~~okay~~. The patient is lethargic.

LAB TESTS: None.

DIAGNOSOS: Lower pneumonia.

TREATMENT: *cc.* *twice a day*
Erthromycin, 100 ~~cc.~~ 1 teaspoon ~~bid~~ with food
Phenergan VC with codeine, 1 ~~t.bid.~~ *teaspoon twice a day*
Recheck in one week.

REMARKS: *t*
This patient appears very umcomfor~~a~~ble.

FAMILY HISTORY: ~~PATIENT IS THE OLDEST~~ of four children. All are in
good general health. The parents are also in good general
health. The maternal grandmother ~~has~~ *suffers from* high blood pressure.

PERSONAL HISTORY: Patient is active. She is fifth grade cheerleader and
also dances. She is successful academically.

_____
Madeline Hast, M.D.

FIGURE 9–11 Proofreading sample

- Medical transcription is more difficult than general transcription.

Some hints for successful transcription are listed below:

Machine and Transcription Tips

- Use the operator's manual extensively until you learn the machine (Figure 9–12).
- Rely on the electronic indicator panel of your unit for document length.
- Always review the special instructions and comments first.
- Follow the rule, "Listen to an earful, then type."
- Do not listen too long before you begin to key.
- Play back any material you do not understand; previously dictated material may clarify what comes next.
- Punctuate as you go.
- If the dictator does not use punctuation, listen for breaks that indicate punctuation.
- When you are unsure of punctuation, refer to a punctuation manual after completing the document.
- Leave a blank space for medical words you cannot comprehend.
- Remember, a medical malpractice lawsuit can be decided on the evidence in a medical report.
- Make a list of all notes to ask the doctor at one time rather than repeatedly interrupting.

Importance of Medical Terminology

Chapter 1 reviews common medical terminology. If you do not already own a medical dictionary such as *Taber's Cyclopedic Medical Dictionary* or *Dorland's Illustrated Medical Dictionary*, purchase a copy before you begin your first job (or early in your schooling). Even if transcription is not one of your responsibilities, you will use these dictionaries often. Figure 9–13 provides a brief description of medical terminology.

IN YOUR OPINION

1. How could a medical transcriptionist overcome the tedium of routine and consistent keying?
2. Medical transcriptionists often mention poor dictation practices by the originator of a source document as a major problem. What do you think dictators can do to aid transcriptionists? How can transcriptionists facilitate this?
3. Which do you think would be easier — transcription from rough draft or by machine? Explain why.

Medical Terminology

1. Many medical words sound alike but have different meanings, for example, hyperthyroidism and hypothyroidism, or do not sound alike but have the same meaning.
2. Abbreviations are often used. Some should be spelled out, but others should not. Refer to a medical dictionary when in doubt.
3. Latin or Greek beginnings and endings are used to form many medical words. Learn the most commonly used prefixes and suffixes.
4. Many medical words come from Latin or Greek root words. Learn the common roots.
5. Diagnoses and treatments have certain aspects in common. Compare the two when a question exists about a word.

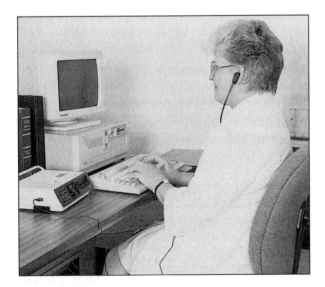

FIGURE 9–12 Dictation-transcription continues to be an important function in medical offices.

FIGURE 9–13 Medical terminology

WORD PROCESSING SOFTWARE

Using word processing software and a letter quality or laser printer, creates attractive correspondence and medical reports. The basic word processing features are display, editing, storage, and printing. With these capabilities, the user can create new documents — or store standard documents such as form letters, insurance forms, and recall notices — and retrieve them as needed.

Today's software packages have many advanced features that make it easy to create professional documents and letter-perfect correspondence. Listed below are some of these time-saving features and how they can be helpful in a medical office:

- A customized medical dictionary containing specific medical terms and physicians' names and used with the spell checker saves valuable time.
- Inserting graphics, charts, and diagrams directly into a document keeps all information together and results in a professional-looking document.
- Word processing "equation editors" enable the use of symbols and other special characters when typing equations and other formulas in a document.
- Using a database of patients or physicians and merging it with a form letter results in an automated office correspondence procedure.

Functions of Word Processing Software

Life is much easier for a transcriptionist who has access to an easy-to-use general purpose word processing software package. Most features are standard in the best known programs, but all of them work a little differently, depending on the specific program. Create and Edit are two primary word processing functions.

Creating Text

The software will ask for a document file name and identify the document by that name each time it is recalled for editing, formatting, or printing. The document can be revised and stored under the original name. If both the original version and the revised version will be used, an alternate name can be given to the second version.

Editing Text

Characters, words, sentences, or paragraphs can be added, deleted, changed, or moved within a draft or previously stored document. Some commonly used editing commands are shown in Figure 9–14.

OUTPUT

Output refers to the finished product after text is keyed and processed. Output takes many forms, including letters, memos, research articles, insurance forms, completed superbills and ledger cards, medical reports, graphs, charts, computer-output microforms, graphics, and other documents. The user is responsible for formatting the output, although some information will be printed on specially designed forms such as insurance claim forms. However, most of the medical assistant's word processing time is spent formatting correspondence and medical documents. Standard formatting guidelines that can be used on any type of keyboard in addition to illustrations of typical formats are shown in the following section.

Formatting Word Processing Correspondence

The term formatting refers to placement of the parts of a letter or medical document. Any formatted communication should be attractive and easy to read. Because letters and internal memorandums account for a large portion of the physician's correspondence, the medical staff should establish standard formats for greatest efficiency. Simple formats are best, especially with electronic equipment. This is because the greatest efficiency comes when a minimum number of keystrokes is required and when standard parts of a document are stored and retrieved as needed. Several procedures for creating an attractive document are appropriate, whether you use a typewriter or word processor to create your documents.

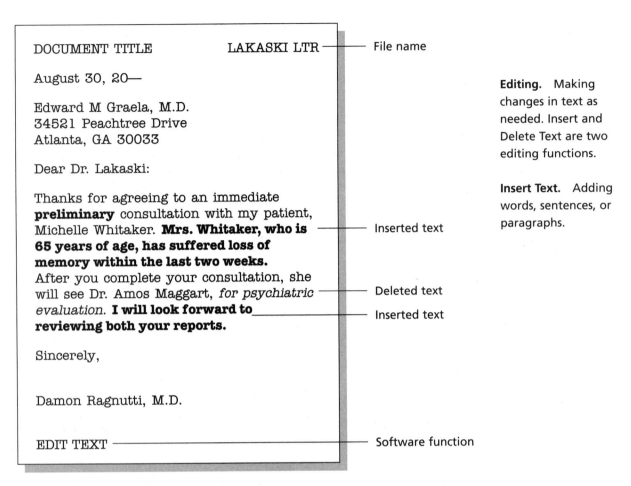

DOCUMENT TITLE   LAKASKI LTR —————— File name

August 30, 20—

Edward M Graela, M.D.
34521 Peachtree Drive
Atlanta, GA 30033

Dear Dr. Lakaski:

Thanks for agreeing to an immediate **preliminary** consultation with my patient, Michelle Whitaker. **Mrs. Whitaker, who is** ————— Inserted text
65 years of age, has suffered loss of
memory within the last two weeks.
After you complete your consultation, she will see Dr. Amos Maggart, *for psychiatric* ————— Deleted text
evaluation. **I will look forward to** ————— Inserted text
reviewing both your reports.

Sincerely,

Damon Ragnutti, M.D.

EDIT TEXT ————————————————— Software function

Editing. Making changes in text as needed. Insert and Delete Text are two editing functions.

Insert Text. Adding words, sentences, or paragraphs.

FIGURE 9–14 Edited document showing inserted text in bold and deleted text in italic.

Procedures for Formatting Documents

Several specific formatting suggestions follow. Refer to your software manual for short cuts offered by the software.

1. Place your document on the page, as you would place a picture within a frame.
2. Leave plenty of white space in the frame.
3. Center the document on the page.
4. Make sure top, bottom, and side margins are neither too narrow nor too wide. Use the word count feature in your software's spell check to determine the number of words in your document. The number of words will determine how wide or narrow the margin should be.

Block and Modified Block Letter Formats, Open and Mixed Punctuation

The two most common letter formats are block, in which all lines begin at the left margin, and modified block, in which the date and closing lines begin at the center. In both styles, paragraphs may be indented or they may begin at the left margin.

Open and mixed punctuation refers to the punctuation after the salutation and the complimentary close of a letter. When no punctuation appears after these parts, punctuation is said to be "open." When a colon follows the salutation and a comma follows the complimentary close, punctuation is referred to as "mixed."

Figure 9–15 illustrates a block style letter with no paragraph indents and open punctuation. Figure 9–16 illustrates a modified block letter with no paragraph indents and mixed punctuation. Figure 9–17 illustrates a modified block letter with open punctuation and paragraph indents. Block is recommended for letters, especially when electronic equipment is used, because it increases efficiency by reducing keystrokes.

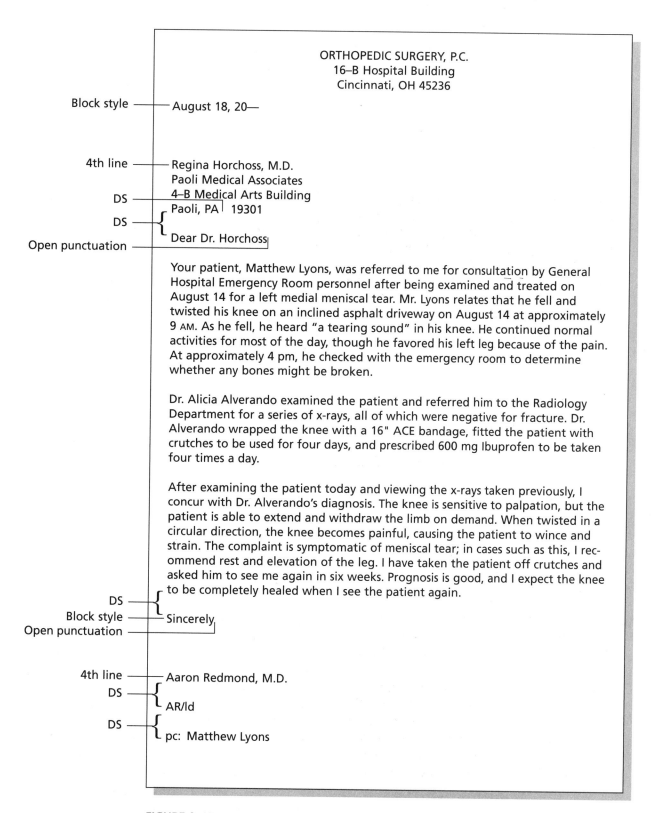

Block style — August 18, 20—

ORTHOPEDIC SURGERY, P.C.
16–B Hospital Building
Cincinnati, OH 45236

4th line — Regina Horchoss, M.D.
Paoli Medical Associates
DS — 4–B Medical Arts Building
Paoli, PA 19301

DS —
Open punctuation — Dear Dr. Horchoss

Your patient, Matthew Lyons, was referred to me for consultation by General Hospital Emergency Room personnel after being examined and treated on August 14 for a left medial meniscal tear. Mr. Lyons relates that he fell and twisted his knee on an inclined asphalt driveway on August 14 at approximately 9 AM. As he fell, he heard "a tearing sound" in his knee. He continued normal activities for most of the day, though he favored his left leg because of the pain. At approximately 4 pm, he checked with the emergency room to determine whether any bones might be broken.

Dr. Alicia Alverando examined the patient and referred him to the Radiology Department for a series of x-rays, all of which were negative for fracture. Dr. Alverando wrapped the knee with a 16" ACE bandage, fitted the patient with crutches to be used for four days, and prescribed 600 mg Ibuprofen to be taken four times a day.

After examining the patient today and viewing the x-rays taken previously, I concur with Dr. Alverando's diagnosis. The knee is sensitive to palpation, but the patient is able to extend and withdraw the limb on demand. When twisted in a circular direction, the knee becomes painful, causing the patient to wince and strain. The complaint is symptomatic of meniscal tear; in cases such as this, I recommend rest and elevation of the leg. I have taken the patient off crutches and asked him to see me again in six weeks. Prognosis is good, and I expect the knee to be completely healed when I see the patient again.

DS —
Block style — Sincerely
Open punctuation —

4th line — Aaron Redmond, M.D.
DS — AR/ld

DS — pc: Matthew Lyons

FIGURE 9–15   Block style with open punctuation

ORTHOPEDIC SURGERY, P.C.
16–B Hospital Building
Cincinnati, OH 45236

Modified block style — August 18, 20—

Regina Horchoss, M.D.
Paoli Medical Associates
4–B Medical Arts Building
Paoli, PA 19301

Dear Dr. Horchoss: — Closed punctuation

Your patient, Matthew Lyons, was referred to me for consultation by General Hospital Emergency Room personnel after being examined and treated on August 14 for a left medial meniscal tear. Mr. Lyons relates that he fell and twisted his knee on an inclined asphalt driveway on August 14 at approximately 9 AM. As he fell, he heard "a tearing sound" in his knee. He continued normal activities for most of the day, though he favored his left leg because of the pain. At approximately 4 PM, he checked with the emergency room to determine whether any bones might be broken.

Dr. Alicia Alverando examined the patient and referred him to the Radiology Department for a series of x-rays, all of which were negative for fracture. Dr. Alverando wrapped the knee with a 16" ACE bandage, fitted the patient with crutches to be used for four days, and prescribed 600 mg Ibuprofen to be taken four times a day.

After examining the patient today and viewing the x-rays taken previously, I concur with Dr. Alverando's diagnosis. The knee is sensitive to palpation, but the patient is able to extend and withdraw the limb on demand. When twisted in a circular direction, the knee becomes painful, causing the patient to wince and strain. The complaint is symptomatic of meniscal tear; in cases such as this, I recommend rest and elevation of the leg. I have taken the patient off crutches and asked him to see me again in six weeks. Prognosis is good, and I expect the knee to be completely healed when I see the patient again.

Modified block style — Sincerely,
Closed punctuation

Aaron Redmond, M.D.

FIGURE 9–16 Modified block letter with no indents and mixed punctuation

ORTHOPEDIC SURGERY, P.C.
16–B Hospital Building
Cincinnati, OH 45236

August 18, 20—

Regina Horchoss, M.D.
Paoli Medical Associates
4–B Medical Arts Building
Paoli, PA   19301

Dear Dr. Horchoss

    Your patient, Matthew Lyons, was referred to me for consultation by General Hospital Emergency Room personnel after being examined and treated on August 14 for a left medial meniscal tear. Mr. Lyons relates that he fell and twisted his knee on an inclined asphalt driveway on August 14 at approximately 9 AM. As he fell, he heard "a tearing sound" in his knee. He continued normal activities for most of the day, though he favored his left leg because of the pain. At approximately 4 PM, he checked with the emergency room to determine whether any bones might be broken.

    Dr. Alicia Alverando examined the patient and referred him to the Radiology Department for a series of x-rays, all of which were negative for fracture. Dr. Alverando wrapped the knee with a 16" ACE bandage, fitted the patient with crutches to be used for four days, and prescribed 600 mg Ibuprofen to be taken four times a day.

    After examining the patient today and viewing the x-rays taken previously, I concur with Dr. Alverando's diagnosis. The knee is sensitive to palpation, but the patient is able to extend and withdraw the limb on demand. When twisted in a circular direction, the knee becomes painful, causing the patient to wince and strain. The complaint is symptomatic of meniscal tear; in cases such as this, I recommend rest and elevation of the leg. I have taken the patient off crutches and asked him to see me again in six weeks. Prognosis is good, and I expect the knee to be completely healed when I see the patient again.

Sincerely

Aaron Redmond, M.D.

Labels at left:
- Modified block style
- Open punctuation
- Indented paragraphs (5 spaces)

FIGURE 9–17   Modified block letter with open punctuation and paragraph indents

```
Mr. Adam Janus                        2                        May 5, 20—
```

FIGURE 9–18   Second-page heading when copy is long

```
Mr. Adam Janus
Page 2
May 5, 20—
```

FIGURE 9–19   Second-page heading when copy is short

Second-Page Headings

Second-page headings may be formatted in two ways, depending on the length of the second-page copy. When the copy is long, the heading should be formatted as one horizontal line. If the page needs to appear fuller because the copy is short, the heading should be formatted vertically. In either case, the name of the person to whom the letter is sent comes first, followed by the page number and the date. Both types are illustrated in Figures 9–18 and 9–19.

Stored Letter Parts

Electronic equipment allows parts of documents, such as the date or closing, to be standardized and saved for quick retrieval and output. Figure 9–20 shows a date, salutation, and closing lines that might be stored in a word processor. At the beginning of each day, the numerals in the date can be changed to reflect the current date.

Merged Paragraphs

No discussion of word processing is complete without mentioning a special type of letter created from **merged paragraphs**. This refers to standard paragraphs that are stored in the computer's memory and combined later to form letters or other documents. For example, a medical assistant may be asked to key and save several different paragraphs that can be used in credit

August 18, 20—	(Stored Date)
Dear :	(Stored Salutation. The addressee's name is keyed before the colon. The body of the letter begins two lines below the salutation.)
Sincerely yours,	(Stored Closing Lines. Closing lines are retrieved with two lines added after the body of the letter.)
Aaron Redmond, M.D.	
ms	(Stored Reference Initials. Other lines for carbon copy, photocopy notation, or enclosure are added as needed.)

FIGURE 9–20   Stored letter parts

letters. The paragraphs will differ depending on the delinquency of the patient accounts. By storing several paragraphs on the subject and selecting for each document only those needed, the medical assistant needs to key very little additional information. WordPerfect and other software packages have this capability. A great deal of time can be saved when the medical assistant combines pre-stored paragraphs. Examples of merged paragraphs and a complete letter are shown in Figures 9–21 and 9–22.

In Figure 9–22, paragraphs 1, 4, 7, and 8 are retrieved from memory and then combined and formatted into a form letter. Only the patient's name and address need to be keyed.

Memorandums

The size of a medical facility determines the number and frequency of memorandums. In a small facility with only one physician and one or two employees, much communication is oral. However, as a practice grows, memorandums become more necessary. Memo headings follow a standard format that can be stored. A standard memorandum format, containing a To, From, Date, and Subject line, is shown in Figure 9–23.

Formatting Medical Reports

In a private practice, case history/physical examinations and consulting physician reports are

(1) Dear

(2) Your account is past due by 30 days, and we would appreciate your immediate payment. If you have overlooked your account, will you please send a check immediately.

(3) Your account is past due by 60 days, and we have not heard from you. If there is a problem with our account or if you need to discuss your financial situation, please call the matter to our attention.

(4) Your account is past due for more than 90 days and we cannot understand why you have delayed payment. After repeated notices and a request that you call us to explain your problem, we have not heard from you.

(5) You may call me at 555-8954 if there is a problem with your account. We look forward to receiving your payment.

(6) Contact me at 555-8954 if we can explain any portion of your statement that you do not understand. If we do not hear from you, we will expect payment within one month.

(7) We must turn your account over to a collection agency if we do not hear from you within two weeks. Please contact us at 555-8954 before that time in order to set up a payment plan.

(8) Sincerely,

Raymond R. Jackson, M.D.

FIGURE 9–21   Merged paragraphs

Dear

Your account is past due for more than 90 days and we cannot understand why you have delayed payment. After repeated notices and a request that you call us to explain your problem, we have not heard from you.

We must turn your account over to a collection agency if we do not hear from you within two weeks. Please contact us at 555-8954 before that time in order to set up a payment plan.

Sincerely,

Raymond R. Jackson, M.D.

FIGURE 9–22 Letter created from merged paragraphs

To: The Staff

From: Aaron Redmond, M.D.

Date: August 18, 20—

Subject: New Partner

Dr. Marcia Webster will join our practice as a partner on September 24. She is a graduate of Johns Hopkins University School of Medicine with a specialty in Neurology. Dr. Webster completed her internship at the Hospital of the University of Pennsylvania and her residency at Vanderbilt Hospital in Nashville, Tennessee. For the last four years, she has been stationed in Japan where she served in the U.S. Army.

Please join me in welcoming Dr. Webster to our staff. She will depend on you to help her make the adjustment to a new city and a new practice.

FIGURE 9–23 Memo heading aligned at colon indent

the most common medical documents produced. In a hospital, admission summaries, discharge summaries, and laboratory reports account for a large part of output. All of these documents follow a standard format, although it may vary slightly from one practice to another or from one hospital to another.

By storing the appropriate format and using it for each document, output time can be reduced dramatically. Figures 9–24 through 9–27 show typical formats for a case history and physical, consulting physician's report, laboratory report, and hospital discharge summary. Information for a hospital admission contains much of the same information found in the case history and physical. The desktop publishing features of Word-Perfect and Windows can be used to create a professional-looking report.

Patient Case History

Patient No. _____

Name ____Nathaniel Watson_____

Date of Visit ____August 24, 20–____

Address ____8204 Mayland Drive_____
____Richmond, VA 23233_____

Chief Complaint: This 28-year-old white male complains of headaches that began the day he came out of a halo/jacket after being treated for a fracture of C-6 following a fall from the top of a 20-foot ladder. Patient stepped off the ladder accidentally on April 4, 20–, while painting the gutters of his house. During the fall, he tore a ligament of the liver and jerked his neck so hard that he broke it.

Patient was admitted to General Hospital on April 4 where he underwent emergency surgery for the torn liver ligament and was placed in a halo/jacket. He remained neurologically intact during the six weeks of halo and came out of the halo six weeks ago. He had no headaches during the time he was in the halo, developed them the day he came out of halo, and has suffered with headache pain ever since. He experiences some mild numbness in his arms and occasionally mild neck pain.

Examination: Neurological examination reveals an alert, cooperative, slightly overweight male with two darkened points over each frontal region where his tongs had been placed.

No spasm in the neck. Range of motion is: 60°, right lateral flexion; 60°, left lateral flexion; 30°, flexion; 30°, extension; 80°, right rotation; 80°, left rotation.

Sensory system is entirely intact, and there is no atrophy or fasciculation of the motor system. Reflexes are entirely intact; head shows no tenderness over the superficial aspect of the greater occipital nerves. Cranial nerves are intact; pupils were equal and reacted well to light.

Lab Tests: Skull x-rays reveal no osteomyelitis at the tong sites. Cervical spine x-rays reveal a minimal compression fracture of C-7 and a bridge formation between C-6 and C-7. The spine is well aligned, and lumbosacral spine x-rays are within normal limits.

Diagnosis: Status post C-7 compression fracture, now fusing spontaneously to C-6. Neurologically intact. Headaches appear to be a muscular contraction form of headache.

Treatment: Treatment will be supportive with liberal use of aspirin recommended. If headaches persist or if patient develops radicular symptoms, he is to see me again for evaluation.

Remarks: Patient feels he cannot go back to work on either a full-time or part-time basis. I recommend that he take off one more week and return to work on a part-time basis thereafter.

Family History: Patient is married and the father of four children, ages 1–7, all of whom are in good general health. Father is a paraplegic resulting from an automobile accident, mother is diabetic. The patient has one sister and one brother, both in good general health.

Personal History: Patient has had no previous accidents or illnesses. He leads an active life and is involved with his children's activities. Since his accident, he has curtailed many of his activities and seems hesitant to resume them for fear of further damaging his neck.

Katherine R. Santiago, M.D.

FIGURE 9–24 Case history and physical report

Jackson R. Westfallen, M.D., P.A.
22 Elmwood Drive
Riverside, RI 02915

CONSULTING PHYSICIAN'S REPORT

Neurological Re-evaluation for
NATHANIEL WATSON
February 23, 20—

This patient was referred to me by Katherine R. Santiago, M.D., of Wayne, Pennsylvania, after the patient relocated to my area. I am to recommend a primary care physician and continue to follow the patient on a consulting basis as needed. Dr. Santiago treated the patient for three years following an accident in which he stepped off the top of a 20-foot ladder, breaking his neck and tearing a ligament of the liver. The patient has been taking Sygesic and Parafon Forte regularly. He is taking Elavil on a p.r.n. basis. He had an ENT evaluation in Philadelphia for an ear problem, but he did not learn anything further about his condition. He has a balance problem at night and in the dark. He has neck pain extending into the left shoulder and across the right arm. He works sporadically as a general contractor.

Examination:

Patient is alert and oriented without impairment of mental function.

Gait and Station: There is no ataxia. Tandem walking is well performed. Romberg sign is not present.

Cerebellar-coordination: There is no tremor, abnormal movement, dysmetria or dysdiadochokinesis. Finger to nose to finger and heel to shin testing are well performed.

Motor System: Strength, tone, and muscle mass are intact in all muscle groups tested. There is no evidence of focal atrophy or fasciculations.

Sensation: Examination reveals a diminished sensation to a pin in the left upper extremity over the shoulder. Touch, position, and vibration are intact. Cortical sensation is normal.

Cranial nerves are unchanged from the prior evaluation.

Deep Tendon Reflexes:	BJ	TJ	BR	PJ	AJ	PL
Right:	++	++	++	++	++	flexor
Left:	++	++	++	++	++	flexor

Miscellaneous:

Dorsal lumbar range of mobility is full.

Cervical range of motion is limited to:

Flexion	50 degrees
Extension	35 degrees
Right lateral rotation	30 degrees
Left lateral rotation	30 degrees
Right lateral flexion	20 degrees
Left lateral flexion	15–20 degrees

Impression:
1. Status post cervical fracture.
2. Chronic irritation of the left axillary nerve.
3. Recurrent headaches.
4. Hearing loss, bilateral.

The patient is advised to continue medical management under the primary care of Dr. John S. Camp.

Jackson R. Westfallen, M.D., P.A.

rs

FIGURE 9–25 Consulting physician's report

DEPARTMENT OF NEUROLOGY   Report of ___Electromyogram___

PATIENT'S NAME:	Nathaniel Watson
EMG#:	S507
AGE:	29
DATE:	December 16, 20–
REFERRED BY:	Katherine R. Santiago, M.D.

NERVE CONDUCTION: Motor and sensory nerve conduction studies were performed in the left upper limb and were within normal limits.

ELECTROMYOGRAPHY: EMG of the muscles of the left upper extremity and the cervical paraspinals was performed. There were no fibrillations, positive waves or fasciculations. The motor unit potentials were of normal amplitude and duration. The interference patterns were normal.

IMPRESSION: 1) Normal nerve conduction studies in the left upper extremity.

2) No evidence of denervation was found in the muscles sampled.

_____
Ashar Ramed, M.D.

FIGURE 9–26   Laboratory report

Formatting Business Reports

Word processing is also used for a variety of business reports or manuscripts the physician writes. This activity requires attention to detail and proofreading skill. The attractiveness and accuracy of the report reflect on the medical assistant's ability to organize and manage a project without supervision. Most reports today are edited several times before the final document is distributed. The original should be printed on bond paper with photocopies for general distribution. Desktop published reports can look just like those printed at a professional shop.

Reports must be organized completely before the first word is keyed. Otherwise, the final document will be a hodgepodge of pages that lack a polished appearance. Follow the procedures below as you organize and key reports.

Job Instructions

A job instruction sheet is invaluable for report planners. Every conceivable question that may arise during the report process should be listed and answered. When more than one person keys a report, the job instruction sheet is essential because, without such a guide, each page or section might be formatted differently at the whim of each person keying the document. Figure 9–28 lists some of the basic instructions that apply to every kind of report. The instructions provided apply to a left-bound manuscript only. Add other questions and instructions as they apply to each specific job.

Margin Guide

Word processing software often counts lines as material is keyed. When using equipment without line counters, prepare a margin guide to extend ½ inch beyond the right margin, so you will be able to count lines as you key.

GENERAL HOSPITAL

COLUMBUS, OH 44211

DISCHARGE SUMMARY

PATIENT:	NATHANIEL WATSON
ADMISSION DATE:	April 4, 20–
DISCHARGE DATE:	APRIL 16, 20–
ADMISSION DIAGNOSIS:	Multiple trauma
DISCHARGE DIAGNOSIS:	C-7 Compression fracture Torn ligament of liver
OPERATIONS/PROCEDURES:	Exploratory laparotomy Ligation of falciform ligament
INFECTIONS:	None
CONDITION ON DISCHARGE:	Improving

BRIEF HISTORY AND PHYSICAL: This patient was admitted to the General Surgery Service on April 4, 20–, and the attending physician was Dr. Francisco Endrile. Patient was transferred to the Orthopedic Unit on April 10, 20–, where the attending physician was Dr. Marguerite Thaxson. This discharge summary will cover the patient's orthopedic care from April 10 to April 16.

The patient is a 28-year-old white male, status post fall from a ladder, 20 feet, sustaining multiple trauma, including neck and shoulder pain. He was admitted to the General Surgery Service where he had an exploratory laparotomy and ligation of the falciform ligament on April 4, 20–. He also sustained a minimally compressed fracture of C-7 and underwent a workup for this injury. He always stayed neurovascularly intact.

PERTINENT LAB AND X-RAY DATA: Tomograms were taken that showed significant combination of the body of C-7, but the posterior elements were intact, and the pieces reduced quite well in extension.

HOSPITAL COURSE: Patient was placed in a halo vest jacket and has remained neurovascularly intact. X-rays in the halo vest show the reduction to be adequate with no subluxation.

DISCHARGE MEDICATIONS AND INSTRUCTIONS: Tylenol with Codeine p.r.n.

DISPOSITION: Home, to be seen in the Spine Clinic in one week.

PROGNOSIS: Good.

_____

Katherine R. Santiago, M.D.

FIGURE 9–27   Discharge summary

1. **Type of paper** — 16 pound bond or less for the rough draft, letterhead quality for the final version.

2. **Size of paper** — 8½" × 11" unless otherwise instructed.

3. **Number of copies** — original plus one copy, original for author, and copy for medical assistant to file.

4. **Machine to be used** — typewriter, word processor, desktop publisher — word processor, electronic typewriter with memory, or desktop publisher if available.

5. **Color to be used** — black; color ribbons add excitement and readability to illustrations, figures, and graphs.

6. **Top and bottom margins for first page** — two-inch top margin; one-inch bottom margin.

7. **Top and bottom margins for all other pages** — one-inch top margin; one-inch bottom margin.

8. **Spacing requirements, single or double** — double, unless otherwise instructed.

9. **Paragraph indentions** — 5, 10, 15, or 20 spaces.

10. **Placement of headings and subheadings**

Title of Report, Chapter Title, and Chapter Number	All capitals and centered at top margin. Quadruple space to main heading.
Main Heading	Centered horizontally. Capitals for first letter of major words. Double space to first keyed line.
Subheading One	Flush with left margin. Underlined. Capitals for first letter of major words. Double space to first keyed line.
Subheading Two	Keyed at paragraph indention. Underlined. Capitals for first letter of major words. Double space to first keyed line.

11. **Pagination plan** — page number typed at right margin ½ inch from top of page.

12. **Footnote placement** — superior numbers typed at point of reference; footnotes at end of manuscript.

13. **Placement of illustrations, figures, and graphs** — to be easily read and visually attractive.

14. **Instructions for proofreading** — proof first for accuracy, reading numbers aloud to a second person; proof second for format and inconsistencies in style.

15. **Instructions for collating** — by machine if possible, otherwise collate from bottom up. Combine insets, joggles until perfectly aligned.

16. **Instructions for binding** — permanent binding with eyelets of spiral frame preferable, conservative color.

17. **Instructions for distribution** — based on instructions of author; if mailed, back the pages with sturdy cardboard.

18. **Time frame** — depends on length; schedule two days for ten pages — first day to key and proof, second day to edit at keyboard, keyboard, collate, bind, and distribute.

19. **Names and schedule of individuals who will key** — determined by practice policy.

20. **Reference books needed** — general dictionary, medical dictionary, *Physicians' Desk Reference* if drug names used widely, thesaurus if editorial decisions to be made, and report style manual.

FIGURE 9–28   Job instruction sheet for report formatting

Title Page

Each report should have a simple, attractive title page. Word processor or desktop publishing programs provide a number of creative type variations for the title page.

Type the title in all capital letters and center it approximately two inches from the top of the page. Center other information vertically and horizontally with the first letter of each word capitalized. WordPerfect and other word processing software offer short cuts in preparing the title page, as well as the table of contents and footnotes discussed below.

Table of Contents

Prepare a table of contents showing main divisions, chapters, and page numbers. Place the title of the division (for example, "Chapter") in all capitals in the left margin and the page numbers at the right margin. Divide division names and page numbers with leaders (. . .). Most word processing programs have a feature that automatically generates a table of contents based on the headings designated in a document — a great time-saver!

Footnotes

The use of electronic equipment has changed techniques of footnoting. Conventional footnotes are numbered in sequence on each page with the reference given at the bottom of the same page. However, it is becoming increasingly popular for all footnotes to be numbered sequentially but referenced only at the end of a manuscript. Refer to a report-writing style manual for the correct method of keying different types of footnotes.

Bibliography

The bibliography is the last item in a report; it contains references for all material cited in the body or used in the research. Bibliographical references are similar in form to footnotes, but the keying pattern is not identical. Refer to a report-writing style manual for the correct method of keying bibliographical entries.

Proofreading

No document is complete until it is proofread carefully. Creating a document and using sophis-

ticated software functions are preliminary to proofreading, and a poor proofreader cannot claim to be successful at word processing. Proofreading is not fun, and it is often dismissed or underrated by people who are too impatient to do the job carefully. Proofreading in a medical office is especially important because medical decisions are often based on information found in medical reports.

Documents that go out of the office represent the practice. If mistakes in grammar, punctuation, spelling, format, or content are present, they reflect negatively on the staff. One physician says it this way, "One good proofreader is worth two good typists in my office, and I want to hire people who can find the mistakes I overlook. After all, I'm not supposed to be the proofreader!"

Review these procedures for improving proofreading:

1. Read the document first for content mistakes. Patients' lives may depend on a correct report.
2. Read the document backwards the second time. This will force attention away from the content and allow you to concentrate on spelling, grammar, and punctuation.
3. Read silently with your lips. You may worry about how you look doing this, but that's a small price to pay for a perfect document.
4. Read the finished copy aloud to a partner against the rough draft. There is nothing wrong with admitting that you cannot always find all the mistakes in every document. Reading with a partner is especially valuable when statistical material is involved. Numbers are especially easy to transpose but difficult to find when one proofreads alone.
5. Exchange documents with another medical assistant. "You proofread my documents, and I'll proofread yours" is a workable technique when more than one person keys nonconfidential information.

Spell checking is built into most word processing programs. The spell checker stops at each word that it does not recognize and prompts you to allow it to make corrections. Typically, several suggested spellings are listed on the screen.

Although spell checker software is helpful for people with a poor spelling background, it is not the perfect solution for documents that include unusual words, foreign words, or abbreviations. Nor can a spell checker distinguish between homonyms (words that sound the same but have different meanings), such as "to," "two," and "too," or "flour" and "flower," or "weather" and "whether." For example, while a common spell checker would include the words "eyes," "ears," "nose," and "throat," it would not recognize the abbreviation "EENT." Special dictionaries or glossary space is available in most programs for adding words that occur frequently in individual offices. Each office adds the words it chooses, and they become a permanent part of the program. Medical spell checker software is available to accompany most programs and is recommended for people who use medical terminology. Punctuation checkers and grammar checkers have been introduced but are not yet as common as spell checkers. Word usage checkers are not yet available, but this software is expected.

IN YOUR OPINION

1. Can you think of some factors not mentioned in the text that make it difficult to read a finished document?
2. Why is the ability to write well a career advantage?
3. What methods have you found useful in proofreading?

INTERNET ACTIVITIES

Access the search engine Google.com and enter the phrase Business Correspondence Overview in the search box. When the reference list appears, read the article titled Style in Business Correspondence or read any other article on business writing, then list five new things you learned. How will your documents improve if you use these recommendations when you write?

STUDENT STUDY CHECKLIST

Workbook

1. Complete Chapter 9 exercises in the workbook
2. Complete Chapter 9 simulations in the workbook.

Administrative Skills CD-ROM

1. Go to the Library on the CD-ROM and play the interactive games for Chapter 9.
2. Go to the CD-ROM and click on several areas of the office. For which areas do you think a medical assistant might need to write letters.

REFERENCES

Career Solutions Training Group. *The Quick Skills Series: Writing in the Workplace*. Cincinnati, OH: South-Western, 2000.

Career Solutions Training Group. *Hands-On-Academics*. Paoli, PA: Career Solutions Training Group, 2002.

Humphrey, Doris. *Pediatric Associates, P.C.* Cincinnati, OH: South-Western, 1997.

McMurrey, David A. *Power Tools for Technical Communication*: Thomson Learning/Heinle, 2002.

Lindh, Wilburta Q., Marilyn S. Pooler, and Carol D. Tamparo. *Administrative Medical Assisting*, 2nd ed. Clifton Park, NY: Delmar Learning, 2002.

CHAPTER ACTIVITIES

PERFORMANCE-BASED ACTIVITIES

1. Your pediatric practice is celebrating its fifth birthday. Write a letter inviting Monique Santora, age 6, to the office birthday party. Write a second invitation letter to Monique's father. Key and print your letters in an appropriate format and include the letterhead information as shown below.

Pediatric Associates
17 Ranchero Drive, Boulder, CO 80302

---

2. One member of the office staff has been absent without excuse three times in the last month. Write a note warning of possible consequences of this behavior. Keep your note positive in tone. Key and print in an appropriate format, using the form below.

Cedarcrest Oncology Clinic

TO:

FROM:

DATE:

SUBJECT:

3. Exchange drafts of the letters in Nos. 1 and 2 with a classmate. Proofread each other's letters and mark with the correct proofreader's marks. Turn in the corrected draft with your finished letters.

4. Key the following information in acceptable case history form, using the format below.

Patient's Name, Juan Gomez
1233-B Nathan Court
Wayne, Pa 19087–0000
Date of Visit: 6/18/–

Chief Complaint: This seven-year-old Hispanic male was brought to my office by his grandfather. About 9:45 AM today the patient was sliding down a slide and cut his right foot on a brick at the base of the slide. Examination: Patient is alert but in pain. There is an approximate 2.5 cm laceration of the right foot, post/lateral aspect, with full ROM of toes and ankle. Skin is pink, warm, and dry. His temperature is 100°F, pulse 104, respiration 16. Lab Tests: None. Diagnosis: 1 in. × ¼ in. laceration of right foot.

Treatment: Betadine Surgical Scrub. Normal saline irrigation. 1% Lidocaine. Five No. 5.0 nylon sutures. Dry sterile dressing, 3 in. Kling bandage. Remarks: None. Family History: Patient is an only child. The father suffers from emphysema. The mother is in apparent good health. There is a family history of early heart disease and hypertension. Personal History: Patient is an active second grade student with a wide variety of outdoor interests. He plays soccer, football, T-ball, and softball. His development is normal.

DATE OF VISIT:

PATIENT'S ADDRESS:

CHIEF COMPLAINT:

EXAMINATION:

LAB TESTS:

DIAGNOSIS:

TREATMENT:

REMARKS:

FAMILY HISTORY:

PERSONAL HISTORY:

5. Key and print two case histories (from the instructor's manual) according to the format in No. 4.

6. Using the five-step letter writing plan given in this chapter, develop a plan and write a letter to Dr. R.S. Mason. Dr. Mason will be joining your practice as a partner on May 31. Your employer wishes to know what day Dr. Mason will arrive in town and whether his family will accompany him. Ask whether you should make hotel and transportation reservations, and if so, for how many days.

   Step 1. Define the problem and the audience

   Step 2. Create an outline

   Step 3. Brainstorm ideas

   Step 4. Put ideas in order

   Step 5. Write the letter

7. Compose an e-mail message to relay the following information. Include other points you think are important. Use your own wording.

   Mr. Ansel Harris asked you to e-mail him at his office regarding the day and time his surgery for prostate cancer is scheduled.

EXPANDING YOUR THINKING

1. Using a dictionary or thesaurus, list at least five other choices for each of the following over-used words. You may also use the thesaurus found in your software program.

   interesting _____

   important _____

   nice _____

2. Analyze the following letter written by for Dr. Emir Romelem, a neurologist. He is writing a follow-up letter to a patient who asked for a written explanation of her illness and some insight into how it can affect her in the future. Dr. Romelem knows his skills are in the practice of neurology, not in letter writing, and he has asked you to read and improve all his letters before they go out to patients. Describe what you believe are the good and bad points of the letter. Make recommendations for improvement.

   Ms. Lolinda Remes
   2302 Saughlin Lane
   Anderson, SC 29621

   Dear Ms. Remes:

   Your diagnosis came back as Multiple Sclerosis. Women between the ages of 20 and 40 get this disease the most, but that doesn't mean men can't get it too. It's baffling. We're still trying to find out what causes Multiple Sclerosis.

   You described your symptoms as numbness, tingling, and burning sensations on your skin. Other things can happen, too, from feeling your body is out of balance to losing your eyesight. Maybe this won't happen to you, though, since most people with MS live a full, active life and continue with all their previous activities. Some people have to go into wheelchairs.

   There is no cure for MS. The most common treatment is intravenous steroid infusions, administered over a period of several days. The good news is that the treatments make you feel better, but the bad news is that you'll have side effects such as water retention, weight gain, insomnia, and some other things. You'll have to make up your mind whether the symptoms or the side effects or worse. Either way, we can't get rid of the MS yet, though some breakthroughs are expected in the next ten years.

   You need to make another appointment with me, so I can see you in the next three weeks. If this isn't enough information before then, I have some brochures on MS that you can read. Some of them are very helpful.

   Sincerely,

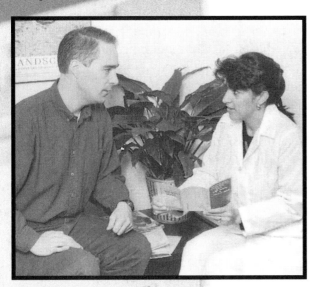

CHAPTER 10

Professional Activities, Travel Arrangements, and Postal and Delivery Services

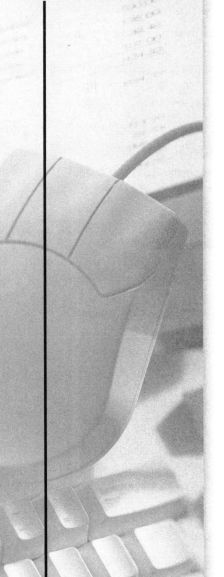

CASPER, WYOMING

Travel planning is something I enjoy doing, for myself and for the members of this small group practice. I've done enough traveling to take pleasure in putting together an itinerary that provides for nonstop flights where possible, and for flights with the shortest layovers or easiest transfers when direct flights are not available. The advent of online searching for the best fares and the best flights has added a new dimension to travel planning, making the search for the most cost-effective flights a lot easier. We depend on a local travel agent, one of our patients, to put the finished trip together for us.

Dr. Miller was invited to present a paper at a four-day conference in Paris. When I looked at the conference schedule, I realized that even if he presented his paper and attended every seminar he had expressed an interest in, he'd still have plenty of time to enjoy Paris. So I searched the Internet and identified half a dozen highly recommended Paris restaurants and gave him copies of the restaurant reviews and directions on how to get to the restaurant from his hotel.

I also had to do a preliminary literature search for him on the Internet to help him assemble materials for his paper. Fortunately, I spend a lot of my personal time at home using Internet search engines, so I was able to find material easily and quickly.

Carol Tremmel
Medical Assistant

After completing this chapter, you should be able to:

1. Complete Internet searches using keywords.
2. Manage the physician's travel schedule.
3. Make online travel reservations.
4. Use postage and delivery services effectively.
5. Instruct patients with special needs.
6. Teach patients methods of health promotion and disease prevention.
7. Orient and train coworkers.

VOCABULARY

Association   Organization that advocates special interests through information or lobbying.

Business class   Flight class that offers more amenities than coach, but fewer than first.

Direct flight   Flight that connects two cities without a plane change.

Domestic mail services   Mail services performed by the United States Postal Service.

Internet search   Locating information through the Internet.

Itinerary   Schedule of travel, including departure and arrival times, flight numbers, lodging, and telephone numbers.

Keywords   Words that identify the information you want to locate through the Internet.

Literature search   Review of published sources at the library or by computer to find articles on a specified topic.

Non-stop   Flight that connects two cities without making intermediate stops.

Objective   The intent of the process.

Orient   To provide an informational overview.

THE MEDICAL ASSISTANT'S PROFESSIONAL ACTIVITIES

Medical assistants enhance their value to a practice when their skills are broad. Some of your most important activities will include research, instructing patients, training staff, making travel arrangements, and developing a good mail management system.

As in many fields, physicians have access to a great deal of information. Although obtaining information is not a problem, getting exactly the information needed and nothing more can be a challenge. Because physicians engage in many professional activities, as a medical assistant you will often track down information for a talk, a report for a meeting, or an article for publication.

Physicians have many opportunities to take active leadership roles in their communities. A few of their activities are listed below:

- Marketing and public relations
- Civic affairs and public speaking
- Publication of research and other articles
- Training at professional forums
- Professional linkages with foundations, federal agencies, and research centers
- Recruitment and retention activities for health professionals
- Health policy monitoring and development
- Clinical trials with developers of health care products, such as pharmaceutical companies
- Advisory functions and technical assistance
- Disseminating resource information

Most of these activities involve information gathering and analysis. As a medical assistant, you may be asked to help the physician get started on one of these projects by conducting a preliminary literature search and screening.

Online Research

Internet research, or online research, is the fastest and easiest method of locating information on a specific subject. The Internet contains a wealth of information on just about every subject imaginable. In fact, the biggest challenge can be locating just what you need when so many facts are available. Great patience is required, or you can be overwhelmed.

When would you use the Internet? Here are a few examples:

1. The practice is considering hiring an office design expert to prepare sketches for the new waiting room. You would like to see what design services the furniture and equipment suppliers offer before committing to a consultant.
2. A new study on cystic fibrosis has been published in a medical journal and the physician asks you to summarize the study.

3. The physician will be traveling to a conference in Zurich, Switzerland and plans to take her family along for a vacation. She needs to know the flight schedules, and she would also like to find out what sightseeing her family can do while she is attending meetings.

4. At an upcoming meeting of the local AMA chapter, the physician will speak about new laws for compliance. He asks you to obtain the most recent guidelines.

5. Your employer, a radiologist, has been sued for malpractice because he misread an x-ray that showed a cancerous cyst in the throwing arm of a famous football quarterback. He wants all the information you can find on the particular type of cyst.

Using Search Engines

A search engine is a software program that locates information stored in thousands of Web sites written by individuals, associations, corporations, librarians, and others. There are numerous search engines, and each works a little differently, though the basic concept is the same.

Search engines allow the medical assistant to search for special words that an author might use in discussing the subject being researched, for example, "anorexia" or "eating disorders" might be used as **keywords** for researching a talk about teen health problems. If keywords are too general, such as "psychology" or "respiratory," too many references will be given. A more specific word should be substituted.

After a keyword is entered in the search engine, the computer goes on a hunt through all the Web pages in its database to try to find the word. A list of articles, reports, opinions, summaries, and other documents using the word will appear. Two examples of a keyword search are shown below:

Topic	Keywords
Medical insurance coding	ICD-9, CPT-5, medical insurance coding, diagnosis coding, procedure coding, International Classification of Diseases, Current Procedural Terminology, HCPCS, Health Care Procedure Coding System

continues

continued

Topic	Keywords
Office management	Office management, office administration, supervision, management, management styles, teams, staffing, office

Phrase Searching

Sometimes words need to appear next to each other when you are searching, for example, "medical insurance coding." In this case, enter quotation marks before and after the phrase. The search engine will locate only these words and only in the order you specify. If you are searching for more than one phrase, you can separate multiple phrases with a comma, for example, "medical insurance coding", "Current Procedural Terminology". Several popular search engines are shown in Figure 10–1.

If the practice's computers do not have Internet access, any large library allows the Internet search. The library may do the search, or the medical assistant may be required to do the research. The library may or may not charge a fee.

Professional organizations are among the best sources for specialized data. Figure 10–2 is a partial list of professional organizations where information can be obtained. These are only a few of the thousands of associations worldwide representing medical groups. Some of these associations may even provide speaker support kits with slides, graphs, and CDs to accompany a presentation. Federal agencies also produce research and publications. Contact them for additional information:

Health Care Finance Administration

Popular Search Engines

Alta Vista	www.altavista.com
Ask Jeeves	www.askjeeves.com
Google	www.google.com
Yahoo!	www.yahoo.com

FIGURE 10–1 Popular search engines

American Academy of Pediatrics

American Managed Care and Review Association

American Medical Association

American Medical Student Association

American Public Health Association

Association of American Dental Schools

Association for Health Services Research

Healthy Mothers, Healthy Babies Coalition

National Organization for Fetal Alcohol Syndrome

Nurse Practitioners in Reproductive Health

Society for Adolescent Medicine

FIGURE 10–2   Partial list of professional organizations

Public Health Office
    Office of Health Promotion and Disease Prevention
    Office of Minority Health
    National Vaccine Program
    Health Resources and Services Administration
        Bureau of Primary Health Care
        Bureau of Health Professions
        Bureau of Maternal and Child Health
    Centers for Disease Control and Prevention

The list goes on and on! You can see why it is a challenge to find the one piece of information needed.

After you conduct preliminary research and receive materials from periodicals, agencies, associations, and the Internet, you should organize your information according to the following steps:

1. Remove duplicate information
2. Organize information by topic
3. Put information in logical order
4. Highlight and mark materials so that the physician can quickly and easily review them when developing a speech or article

Doing research is an art and a science. Your proficiency in developing good sources of data and transforming that data into usable information will enhance your value to any medical practice.

IN YOUR OPINION

1. How could you organize materials on the subject of smoking-related diseases for a presentation to a high school group? What props would improve the presentation?
2. Think of a specialty that interests you. What types of research might a physician need the medical assistant to conduct?
3. Name several keywords to use in an Internet search on premature babies.

Training Coworkers

A big difference exists between knowing how to do something and being able to train someone else to do it. When a new employee joins the practice, whether it is a physician, receptionist, billing clerk, medical assistant, or other, you will need to explain some aspects of the work or how the office operates. To be an effective trainer, you need to follow a few important guidelines:

1. Explain the purpose or objective of the process or function being learned.

> "Our goal in answering the phones is to give callers prompt, courteous, service so they receive a good impression of our professionalism."

Compare this instruction that does not include an explanation.

> "Answer the phone by saying, 'Dr. Rugger's office.'"

2. Explain how this process or function fits into the office's system.

> "After we log the checks, we forward them to Carole. She photocopies the checks, deposits the checks in the bank, and returns the photocopies to us so that we can attach them to the patient file. That way, if there is a question about payment, we can refer to the patient file."

Compare that explanation with this one.

> When we get checks, we write the number in this book and then put them in this basket."

3. Break the training process down into steps, or functions and document each step. Processes or functions with many steps, a great deal of backtracking, and several exceptions are difficult and will be hard to learn. Often, trainees are blamed for mistakes when it is the process that is at fault. In the following example, a trainee would have a hard time remembering all the details.

> "We keep all patient files except for Dr. Mammet's in a central storage area. Dr. Mammet likes to keep his patient files in his office. Also, all our Medicaid patients' records are separated and filed in this blue filing cabinet, except for the patients who are not U.S. citizens. Those records go in here. Dr. Revere is doing a study of sexually transmitted diseases, so all the files of patients with those diagnoses go to her first before filing."

If a procedure is not written down, the medical assistant and trainee should document the steps. This will make subsequent training easier and more consistent.

4. Remember that people learn in different ways. Most people learn best with a combination of show and tell and lots of practice. Successful trainers use this technique along with support and encouragement.
5. Listen carefully to the person's questions. Feedback in the form of questions is important because you will not know what the trainee fails to grasp unless she follows up with questions.
6. Develop different ways of explaining the same thing; repeating the original explanation will not improve the person's understanding. Do not be afraid to say, "I don't know, but I'll find out." Explain *why* a trainee must do something, not just *how*. People are more likely to make correct decisions if they understand the intent of the process.

Patient Instruction

Patient instruction is an extremely valuable and rewarding activity. Often a doctor's office is the place where people discover major changes are about to occur in their lives and learn how to manage them. A mother learning how to parent a newborn, a patient with heart disease trying to diet and exercise properly, a child with diabetes learning to inject insulin, a teenager adjusting to adolescence, and a widowed spouse suffering from loneliness can benefit from information about their circumstances.

Giving clear, concise patient instructions and at the patient's level of understanding can make the difference between good and excellent service.

Figure 10–3 provides insight into how patients learn best.

Providing Patient Literature

Pamphlets and brochures that explain illnesses and treatments are invaluable. Because desktop publishing software is affordable and easy to use, every practice should develop a variety of attractive, informative brochures and make them available on a convenient rack or display stand. The literature distributed or made available in the waiting room may include general topics such as nutrition, but it should also include information on the major health issues for the patients of the practice. A psychiatrist's office might offer brochures on depression, obsessive-compulsive disorders, anxiety, and stress. An obstetrician might display pamphlets on breastfeeding, sex during and after pregnancy, back pain, and changing nutritional needs.

In most cases, it will not be necessary for a medical assistant to develop these materials. For

- Most people learn best at the time they need to know, as when they are hospitalized.

- Patients who understand a medical procedure will be more cooperative.

- Explanation of prescribed treatment encourages compliance with directions.

- Patients cannot be expected to understand and remember the reasons for health problems and details of treatment procedures after one explanation, especially in situations of high emotional impact.

- Patients may be reluctant to ask questions of the physician, especially if the doctor appears to be rushed.

- Health education material is more likely to be used if it is easily available.

FIGURE 10–3   Facts about how patients learn

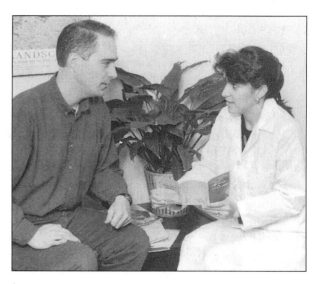

FIGURE 10–4   Explain to patients clearly, then ask for questions.

information related to medical conditions, materials from professional associations appropriate to your practice may be useful. You will find a great deal of information available at nominal cost. You will also locate an abundance of material about most health conditions on the Internet. *A word of caution:* Some Internet material is written by inexperienced or misinformed individuals. Check sources carefully before using any Internet material and ask the physician to approve all brochures before they are made available to patients.

The best method for explaining information to patients follows the simple format described below (Figure 10–4).

1. Sit with the patient in a private area free of distractions.
2. Explain the contents of a pamphlet in a clear tone of voice.
3. Be patient.
4. Pause frequently to see if the patient has a question or seems distracted or confused.
5. Be attentive to questions and concerns.
6. Give the patient a copy of the pamphlet.
7. Encourage patients to call you if they have questions.

Keep a follow-up list of patients who received instructions and call them a few days after their visits. This will not only impress them with the quality of your service, but may forestall problems and the need for another visit. A "tickler" file may be used for this purpose.

MANAGING TRAVEL

Physicians do not travel as often as business executives; however, they attend medical conventions, take vacations, and make other selected trips. As a medical assistant, you may be asked to make reservations for these trips by telephone through a private travel agency, directly with the airline, hotel, rental car agency, or over the Internet. The following discussion provides reference information about options you should consider when creating a travel plan for the physician.

Travel Agencies

A travel agent (1) researches the physician's destination and provides brochures about the area to be visited, (2) arranges for air and ground transportation, (3) develops highway routes for automobile travel, (4) creates an itinerary, (5) arranges for lodging in one or several locations, and (6) makes local entertainment and sightseeing suggestions. After a travel agent delivers tickets, check the tickets against the itinerary carefully. A good travel agent will maintain a list of the physician's seating preferences for air travel, a credit card number, and frequent flyer numbers. If a travel agent makes errors or fails to provide you with consistent, complete information about travel choices, investigate other travel suppliers.

Airline Travel

All major airlines have toll-free 800 numbers. If you know that only one or two carriers provide service on the route needed, you may wish to contact the airline yourself instead of working with a travel agent.

The two simplest ways to reduce the cost of air travel are to book ahead two weeks or more and to plan a Saturday overnight stay. The difference in cost can be several hundred dollars.

Several classes of service are available to airline passengers; first, business, and coach are the most common choices. The features of each of these classes are explained below.

- First class: Offers wider seats, more leg room, better food, and complimentary alcoholic beverages. There is no charge for movies if they are offered.

- Business class: Not offered by every airline or on every flight; most common for international or lengthy flights. Offers wider seats and more leg room than coach.

- Coach class: Up to 50 percent of the cost of first class. Can be uncomfortably crowded when the flight is full. Snacks only. Experienced travelers usually specify an aisle seat so that they can stand or move more easily, though some enjoy looking out a window.

Many physicians request the medical office assistant to make Internet airline reservations. The Internet affords a quick way to look at all flight options, show all connecting flights between the departure and destination cities, and see the ticket price immediately. The physician's choices for seating, food, and special accommodations can be requested, and automobile rental and hotel reservations can be made directly at the airline's Web site. A printout of all the flight alternatives can be given to the physician to review at a convenient time. Figure 10–5 shows the flight options from St. Louis, Missouri, to Austin, Texas.

Discount reservations companies compete to offer the lowest possible airline fares. Several hundred dollars often can be saved by using a discounting company. Be aware that some tickets are cheaper because they involve multiple connecting flights or changes of planes. The money saved may not be worth the physician's time loss and aggravation. Several discount reservations services and their Web site addresses are shown in Figure 10–6. Because Web site addresses change from time to time, you may use an alternate method if the site you choose from the figure is no longer available. Instead, type the keyword for the site, for example, Yahoo or Orbitz, into a search engine and wait for the reference to appear.

Tickets purchased through the Internet are called e-tickets. After the purchaser provides a credit card number and SENDS an okay to purchase, the airline E-mails a confirmation. This confirmation and a U.S. government-issued picture ID must be presented at the departure gate, or the passenger will not be allowed to board the airplane.

Ship

Physicians take cruises for both personal and business reasons. Continuing education requirements for license renewal can often be met through a work/pleasure cruise that offers a medical seminar or conference as part of the travel package. Often, these special trips are advertised to physicians through a sponsoring university, and the medical assistant's responsibility for scheduling is minimal. A medical assistant responsible for arranging such a trip may use a travel agent or the Internet.

278.50 Adult x 1 | **Depart** 9:31 pm Sun., Oct. 13   St. Louis (STL)
$278.50 Total (USD) | Arrive 11:39 pm Sun., Oct. 13   Austin (AUS)
Stops: 0 Travel Time: 2 hr 8 min

BUY

Return 1:40 pm Sun., Oct. 20   Austin (AUS)
Arrive 3:43 pm Sun., Oct. 20   St. Louis (STL)
Save
Stops: 0 Travel Time: 2 hr 3 min

278.50 Adult x 1 | **Depart** 9:31 pm Sun., Oct. 13   St. Louis (STL)
$278.50 Total (USD) | Arrive 11:39 pm Sun., Oct. 13   Austin (AUS)
Stops: 0 Travel Time: 2 hr 8 min

BUY

Return 10:54 am Sun., Oct. 20   Austin (AUS)
Arrive 12:59 pm Sun., Oct. 20   St. Louis (STL)
Save
Stops: 0 Travel Time: 2 hr 5 min

278.50 Adult x 1 | **Depart** 9:31 pm Sun., Oct. 13   St. Louis (STL)
$278.50 Total (USD) | Arrive 11:39 pm Sun., Oct. 13   Austin (AUS)
Stops: 0 Travel Time: 2 hr 8 min

BUY

Return 6:07 pm Sun., Oct. 20   Austin (AUS)
Arrive 8:12 pm Sun., Oct. 20   St. Louis (STL)
Save
Stops: 0 Travel Time: 2 hr 5 min

278.50 Adult x 1 | **Depart** 9:31 pm Sun., Oct. 13   St. Louis (STL)
$278.50 Total (USD) | Arrive 11:39 pm Sun., Oct. 13   Austin (AUS)
Stops: 0 Travel Time: 2 hr 8 min

BUY

Return 7:30 am Sun., Oct. 20   Austin (AUS)
Arrive 9:35 am Sun., Oct. 20   St. Louis (STL)
Save
Stops: 0 Travel Time: 2 hr 5 min

278.50 Adult x 1 | **Depart** 6:32 pm Sun., Oct. 13   St. Louis (STL)
$278.50 Total (USD) | Arrive 8:43 pm Sun., Oct. 13   Austin (AUS)

FIGURE 10–5 Flight options from St. Louis, MO, to Austin, TX

www.budgettravel.com
www.cheaptickets.com
www.orbitz.com
www.site59.com
www.travelocity.com

FIGURE 10–6 Discount reservation services

Train

Train travel is more attractive in some parts of the country than others. For example, physicians living in the Northeast often make short train commutes among Washington, New York, and their home cities to relieve the frustration of traffic congestion. Reservations can be made by phone or the Internet.

Automobile

A physician may wish to rent a car for in-town travel after flying to a destination. Automobiles for use anywhere in the world can be rented through a local rental-car franchise, such as Hertz or Avis, through a travel agent, or over the Internet. Auto rental companies all have 800 numbers. Usually, you can access car rental companies over the Internet with the http://www. address plus the company's name and .com (dot-com), for example, http://www.hertz.com will take you to Hertz car rentals. Or, go to a search engine and type in the keywords "Car Rental" plus the state or city where the rental will take place.

Be sure to ask about special weekend rates, upgrades, and other "deals." Membership in the rental company's preferred customer club will ensure the traveler quick service on arrival and departure. When the physician prefers to use an automobile for taking a long trip, you can access a route guide and highway map through http://www.mapquest.com. The physician may also subscribe to the American Automobile Association (AAA), a nationwide network that provides assistance to travelers. AAA will provide route guides, as well.

Lodging

Medical conferences are usually held in hotels with appropriate accommodations, and the sponsoring organization contracts for a large number of rooms to be used by conference participants. The advertisement for the convention frequently includes a room reservation form which the medical assistant completes and mails. A required deposit for one night's lodging can be made by check or credit card.

Lodging for trips unrelated to conferences can be arranged through a travel agent, the hotel or motel to be used, the local franchise of a hotel or motel chain, or by Internet. A written confirmation of all room reservations should be requested and included with the physician's itinerary. Major hotel chains have 800 numbers for reservations at locations worldwide.

Several types of information are required before a reservation for lodging can be made. These requirements are listed below.

- **Type of Room** — One room or a suite.
- **Type of Accommodations** — Twin beds, standard bed, or king-sized bed.
- **Date and Time of Arrival** — Arrivals after 6 PM require a deposit in advance for one night's lodging. This guarantee can be charged by telephone to the physician's credit card. Guarantees are not refundable.
- **Length of Time Room Is Needed** — One night, two nights, or longer.

Travel Funds

Costs associated with a physician's trip are closely monitored for income tax purposes. A travel advance request that allows funds to be drawn from the practice's business account can be completed before the trip, or the physician may used personal funds during the trip. The physician should complete a travel expense form for reimbursement from the practice account on return.

When funds are advanced, the medical assistant completes a travel advance form, and the bookkeeper or accountant prepares a check. The medical assistant may cash the check and give the money to the physician with the itinerary.

After the physician returns and provides the receipts, the medical assistant records all expenses including those for meals, lodging, transportation, tips, cash, and miscellaneous items on a travel expense form and turns it over to the accountant with all receipts. The extra paperwork is necessary to account properly for all funds at income tax time. A travel advance form is shown in Figure 10–7, and a travel expense form is shown in Figure 10–8.

International Travel

Several items must be considered when a physician takes a foreign trip. A travel agency should always arrange for international travel, because agents are experienced in planning such trips and often know shortcuts or can offer specific advice about entering individual countries.

Passport

The physician must acquire or renew a passport before entering any foreign country, except for Canada, Bermuda, the West Indies, Mexico, and a few others. In these countries, proof of U.S. citizenship is required.

To obtain a passport, an individual needs a completed application (which may be obtained from the post office), proof of U.S. citizenship, proof of identification with a personal signature, two photographs taken within the last six months by a passport photographer, and the passport fee. The Department of State requires as proof of citizenship a birth certificate with a raised seal; photocopies are not acceptable. It is a good idea to call ahead of time to verify acceptable documentation. A previously expired passport and

naturalization papers are other acceptable forms of proof of citizenship. Applications for a passport can be obtained from a travel agency; processing takes about two weeks, but renewals can be prepared in twenty-four to forty-eight hours.

Some foreign countries grant visa permission for individuals to enter. Usually, the visa appears as a stamped notation on the passport and designates the country to be entered and the amount of time approved. A travel agent can advise which countries require a visa.

Vaccinations

A travel agent or the Department of Health can provide information regarding vaccinations needed for visiting specific countries or recommended health precautions. Vaccinations are rarely required anymore, but typhoid vaccination, gamma globulin, current tetanus, or malaria suppressant may be recommended.

Preparing an Itinerary

The medical assistant should prepare a complete, concise itinerary before each trip. The travel agent will do this if an agency is used. The physician's spouse and business associates should receive extra copies, and the medical assistant should keep a copy in case the physician must be contacted during the trip. The itinerary shows travel times and destinations, meeting times, and lodging where the doctor will stay. Telephone and fax numbers and any appointments should also be included as a part of the trip.

The medical assistant should type the itinerary in neat, readable form, fold and insert it in a packet with the physician's airline ticket. All confirmations and notes about the trip should be stapled to the itinerary. An itinerary is shown in Figure 10–9.

TRAVELER'S NAME _____ DATE _____

NAME OF PRACTICE _____

PURPOSE OF TRAVEL _____

DEPARTURE TRAVEL TO _____ DATE ____

RETURN TRAVEL FROM _____ DATE ____

AMOUNT OF ADVANCE _____

SIGNATURE _____

FIGURE 10–7   Travel advance form

IN YOUR OPINION

1. What are the most important reasons for physicians to travel?
2. What are some travel pitfalls that can be avoided by careful planning?
3. Which of the physician's travel preferences should you know to make planning easier and more effective?

Travel Expense Statement

NAME _____Anderson Marcus Adam, M.D._____ SOC. SEC. NO. _____238-54-1345_____

NAME _____Physician_____ TRAVEL DATES FROM __April 1__ TO ___3, 2002___

PURPOSE OF TRIP _____AIDS Conference_____

DATES	SPEEDOMETER READING Out / In	LOCATION/POINTS VISITED	DETAILS OF SUBSISTENCE (Attach receipts of items $25 or more)				TOTAL	Do Not Use This Space FOR ACCT. DEPT.
			BREAKFAST	LUNCH	DINNER	LODGING		
6/1		Nashville/Chicago		18.00	56.80	240.93	315.73	
6/2		Chicago	12.00			240.93	252.93	
6/3		Chicago/Nashville	9.25	22.80	136.90		168.95	

NOTE: This statement must be submitted within 10 days of last date of travel for reimbursement.

DISTANCE TRAVELLED _____ KILOMETERS @ _____ CENTS A KILOMETER
(Must be supported by automobile travel record above.)

COMMON CARRIER: __X__ Taxi: _____ Limousine: _____ Airline: _____ Train: _____   42.00 / 328.00

MISCELLANEOUS EXPENSES: (telephone, postage, etc.):
Total here, itemize below   15.75

GRAND TOTAL OF TRAVEL EXPENSES   1123.36

List all miscellaneous expenses:

Explanation _____Telephone calls_____ Amount ____15.75____

Explanation _____ Amount _____

I certify that the above statements are true and I have incurred the described expenses in the discharge of my official duties for **NORTHSIDE MEDICAL CENTER, P.C.**

SIGNATURE _____ APPROVED _____ DATE _____

FIGURE 10–8 Travel expense form

```
                        Itinerary for Adam Anderson
                               Chicago, Illinois
                               April 1–3, 20–

Sunday, June 1   Nashville to Chicago

           8:40 AM        Leave Nashville on American Airlines flight #234. Snack on flight

           10:16 AM       Arrive at Chicago O'Hare Airport Room reservation at Marriott
                          Downtown (Confirmation attached)

           12:00 noon     Meet Dr. Allen Rorbach in Marriott dining room

           3:00 PM        Registration for AIDS CARE Conference, Grand Lobby

Monday, June 2  9 AM–5 PM       AIDS CARE Conference, Grand Ballroom

Tuesday, June 3  Chicago to Nashville

           9 AM–5 PM       AIDS CARE Conference continued

           5:00 PM        Dinner with Drs. Ceciol, Anthony, Matz. Reservations in Golden Inn
                          at airport

           7:50 PM        Leave Chicago O'Hare Airport United Airlines flight #692

           9:08 PM        Arrive Nashville, 9:30 PM. Taxi to your home
```

FIGURE 10–9   Airline itinerary

POSTAL AND DELIVERY SERVICES

Traditionally, the letters, x-rays, medical reports, and related materials going to and from a medical office were transmitted by first class or express mail via the U.S. Postal Service. However, private mailing and shipping services compete today with the postal service. Special attention must be paid to packaging x-rays and other laboratory materials to protect their contents. The categories of mail services are discussed below.

Private Mailing and Shipping Services

Several national and international delivery services such as Federal Express, UPS, and others compete with the U.S. Postal Service for delivery of mail and packages by picking up parcels to be shipped from the office. Speed is also an impor-tant factor, with private services often delivering faster than the post office. Taxicabs and bus service may also be used for delivery in small towns and cities. Big cities may offer door-to-door courier services via bicycle.

Domestic Mail Services

Domestic mail service can be categorized as follows:

- **Express Mail:** The fastest class of postal service. Items deposited at the post office by 5 PM are guaranteed for delivery by 10 AM the following day if the receiving post office has express service. In larger cities, special deposit boxes at some mail offices allow drop off until 7 PM. Letters, legal documents, or other items needing fast delivery may be sent through Express Mail. Express service is more expensive than other classes of mail service. Because postal fees change from time to time, check the post office or do an Internet search on the keywords "Postal Rates" for the current rate for Express Mail.

- **Priority Mail:** Second day delivery, not guaranteed for items weighing over 11 ounces. The maximum weight for priority mail is 70 pounds, and the maximum size is 100 inches combined length and girth. Charges are assessed according to zones, with the fee increasing as the distance increases. Priority mail is used for sending medical records when a former patient changes to a new physician in another city or when a package needs to be shipped by a fast method.

- **First Class:** Service includes items weighing up to 11 ounces, such as letters, laboratory reports, and medical reports. Items weighing over 11 ounces are considered priority mail. The charge for this service is by the ounce. First class is used for most of the printed communications leaving the office.

- **Second Class:** Printed newspaper and periodicals. Contact the local post office for second-class fees. Although medical offices receive a great deal of second-class mail, they rarely send items by this method.

- **Third Class:** Any material that does not fall in the categories of first-class or second-class mail and weighs less than 16 ounces, such as merchandise, printed matter, and keys. Bulk advertising material is third-class mail. Third-class mail is used for such mailings as a newsletter to patients.

- **Fourth Class:** The same as parcel post, including all mailable matter not in first, second, or third class that weighs 16 ounces or more. Rates are charged according to the weight of the parcel and the distance it will travel. Fourth-class mail is used for packages such as returned medical supplies or office supplies sent by the postal service.

Special Mail Services

Special mail services can be classified as follows:

- **Registered Mail:** First-class and priority mail of monetary value that must be guaranteed against loss or damage by the postal service. Fees are based on value of the contents.

- **Insured Mail:** Third- or fourth-class mail or priority mail with third- or fourth-class contents valued at $400 or less.

- **Return Receipt:** Evidence that mail was received by the Restricted Mail addressee. A return receipt should be requested and attached to the patient file any time a letter is mailed advising that the physician is withdrawing from a case. A return receipt is shown in Figure 10–10.

- **C.O.D.:** Merchandise for which the cost is collected at delivery. Merchandise ordered from a supplier with arrangements to pay the postal carrier when it is delivered is a C.O.D. item.

- **Certified Mail:** A record of delivery of a letter by the post office, attached to letters and other items that have no insured value but which need evidence that the item was actually delivered. Certified mail might be used on final collection notices before an account is turned over to a collection agency. A certified mail receipt is shown in Figure 10–11.

- **Special Delivery:** Immediate delivery by post office messenger to prescribed locations in a mailing area. X-rays might be sent by special delivery.

- **Special Handling:** Method of moving third- and fourth-class packages with first-class mail. Check the first-class rate for sending the package. It may be cheaper than special handling. Medical instruments are sometimes sent by special handling.

- **Metered Mail:** Postage that is affixed by a postage meter machine at the medical office, reducing handling time at the post office. Postage meters may be electronic, feeding, sealing, and stacking the stamped envelopes. The actual metering device maintains a record of postage expenditures and the number of pieces that have passed through the machine. Pitney Bowes is a major provider of postage meters (Figure 10–12).

Packaging and Sorting Mail

Some mail sent from medical offices requires special attention and packaging. For example, x-rays should be backed with cardboard and placed in a sufficiently large envelope so that

UNITED STATES POSTAL SERVICE

Official Business

PENALTY FOR PRIVATE
USE TO AVOID PAYMENT
OF POSTAGE, $300

U.S.MAIL

Print your name, address and ZIP Code here

Mr. B. J. Bunyon
618 Harris Drive
New Orleans, LA   70126-4178

SENDER:
- Complete items 1 and/or 2 for additional services.
- Complete items 3, and 4a & b.
- Print your name and address on the reverse of this form so that we can return this card to you.
- Attach this form to the front of the mailpiece, or on the back if space does not permit.
- Write "Return Receipt Requested" on the mailpiece below the article number.
- The Return Receipt will show to whom the article was delivered and the date delivered.

I also wish to receive the following services (for an extra fee):

1. ☐ Addressee's Address

2. ☒ Restricted Delivery

Consult postmaster for fee.

3. Article Addressed to:

Rene Hebert
7 Pease Hall
New Orleans, LA   70122-0161

4a. Article Number

4575231

4b. Service Type
☐ Registered   ☐ Insured
☒ Certified   ☐ COD
☐ Express Mail ☐ Return Receipt for Merchandise

7. Date of Delivery

3/11/20-

5. Signature (Addressee)

Rene Hebert

6. Signature (Agent)

8. Addressee's Address (Only if requested and fee is paid)

PS Form **3811,** December 1991   ☆U.S. GPO: 1993—352-714   **DOMESTIC RETURN RECEIPT**

Is your RETURN ADDRESS completed on the reverse side?

Thank you for using Return Receipt Service.

FIGURE 10–10   Return receipt

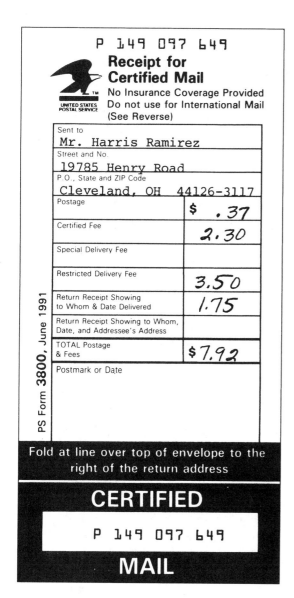

P 149 097 649

Receipt for Certified Mail

No Insurance Coverage Provided
Do not use for International Mail
(See Reverse)

Sent to Mr. Harris Ramirez	
Street and No. 19785 Henry Road	
P.O., State and ZIP Code Cleveland, OH 44126-3117	
Postage	$ .37
Certified Fee	2.30
Special Delivery Fee	
Restricted Delivery Fee	3.50
Return Receipt Showing to Whom & Date Delivered	1.75
Return Receipt Showing to Whom, Date, and Addressee's Address	
TOTAL Postage & Fees	$7.92
Postmark or Date	

PS Form 3800, June 1991

Fold at line over top of envelope to the right of the return address

CERTIFIED

P 149 097 649

MAIL

FIGURE 10–11   Certified mail receipt

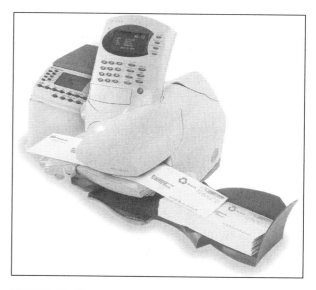

FIGURE 10–12   Postage scale and meter (Courtesy of Pitney Bowes)

Metered mail should be bundled and identified with the coding labels provided by the postal service. All mail for one state is identified by an orange label marked by an "S," and all mail from the same medical office is identified with a blue label marked "F," for "Firm." Delivery of an office's mail can further be expedited by separating the mail according to major zip code categories, such as local and out of town.

Recalling the Mail

Occasionally, a piece of mail may be sent in error. Mail that has been metered or stamped and mailed can be recalled if the sender acts quickly. First, an envelope identical to the one posted must be produced. The envelope must be taken to the local post office if the letter was mailed to the same zip code. The sender would have to call the local post office to determine where to take the envelope if the original was mailed out of town.

The sender would then complete a Sender's Application for Recall of Mail and give it and the duplicate envelope to a postal clerk. The original would be returned immediately if it were still at the local post office. If it had already been shipped to another zip code area, the postal clerk would contact the post office serving the area and attempt to have the letter returned. Letters that have already been delivered obviously cannot be recalled.

they will not be damaged, folded, or bent. An envelope containing x-rays should never be run through a postage meter. Instead, it can be hand stamped or postage meter tape can be attached to the envelope. When shipping medical records, the contents should be secured with rubber bands and cardboard backing and then placed in an envelope strong enough to contain the material.

Letters and packages should be clearly identified with the type of mail service desired. For example, "Registered" or "Special Handling" should be written with a felt tip pen in block letters under the stamp area on these items.

Processing Incoming Mail

The size of a medical practice determines the steps followed in processing incoming mail. Large physician groups usually have a mail room where one person receives and sorts all incoming mail and delivers it to the appropriate medical assistant. In smaller offices, the mail is typically delivered by a postal employee to the medical assistant who sorts it and delivers it to the appropriate people. The following section discusses how a medical assistant should process mail once it is delivered.

Follow five basic steps to process incoming mail — sorting, opening, reading and annotating, expediting, and distributing. Use these procedures for each step.

Procedures for Processing Incoming Mail

Sorting Mail

1. Separate the mail according to class. Place special delivery, express, registered, certified, and first-class mail in one stack. Place second- and third-class newspapers and magazines in another stack. Place fourth-class parcels and packages in still another stack.

2. Organize the special classes and first-class mail according to what appears to be most important. Place letters together in one group, medical reports in another, and items in their own groups according to their content. Sometimes several items for one patient will arrive from different laboratories. Organize all materials concerning one patient in a group and paper clip together.

Opening Mail

1. Leave any envelopes or packages marked "Personal" or "Confidential" to be opened by the persons to whom they are addressed. *Do not* open these letters or envelopes unless you have been specifically requested to do so by the addressee. If you open a personal letter by mistake, reinsert the letter in the envelope, tape the opened edges of the envelope, and write "Sorry, Opened by Mistake" on the front.

   Be alert for any letters that look personal or confidential even if they are not identified as such. In a medical office, this is a challenge, because patients often handwrite the envelopes in which they send payment for their accounts. Enclosing a pre-addressed envelope with the bills helps with this problem.

2. Collect these supplies for opening the mail: a letter opener, stapler, paper clips, tape, and a date and time stamp.

3. Open the most important-looking material first and scan the contents to see if you need to keep the mailing envelopes. If so, paper-clip the envelope to the contents. Repair any damaged items. Envelopes should be kept in the following situations:

   a. Look in the envelope for enclosures. If the letter refers to enclosures and none are found, underline the enclosure notation and write "No" beside the notation. Attach the envelope missing the enclosure to the letter.

   b. Paper-clip all checks to the envelopes in which they were received.

   c. Determine if the date on the letterhead matches the date on the envelope. If a major discrepancy exists, attach the envelope to the document and write a note about the date difference.

   d. Attach all envelopes that hold legal documents to the document. The envelope may be needed for evidence in the future.

4. Discard remaining envelopes unless office policy dictates otherwise.

5. Date and time stamp all mail, either with a commercial date/time stamp or by hand. This is very important in a medical office when a question arises regarding an insurance payment, a legal paper, the date a document was mailed, or any other controversial matter. Some offices maintain a log of all incoming mail as documentation in the event of legal problems.

6. Open packages after first-class mail has been processed.

Reading, Underlining, and Annotating Mail

1. Read all the first-class mail unless the employer requests otherwise. Most physicians expect medical assistants to read their mail.

It is not necessary to read the medical reports pertaining to individual patients.

2. Make calendar notations and notes based on the contents of the letters.
3. Highlight or underline words and phrases that will speed the physician's understanding of the message and add notes where helpful. Use a highlighter or pen in a color that contrasts with the paper and print of the letter. Check before marking up letters as some physicians prefer to read a "fresh" letter.
4. Make filing notations or follow-up comments if the letter may be returned for additional filing or processing.

Expediting Mail

1. Determine whether background information, previous correspondence, a medical record, or other information is needed for understanding a specific piece of mail. If so, attach the necessary information.

   For example, a consulting physician may ask the primary care physician to answer a question about the patient's previous history. In this case, retrieve the medical record and paper-clip the consulting physician's letter to the folder or file before giving the letter to the physician.
2. Prepare an action slip for materials that are routinely handled in a particular way. For example, laboratory reports often need to be filed in the medical record without further action from the physician. An action slip can be attached to the lab report before giving it to the physician; the physician can then simply pass the report back to the medical assistant when it is ready for filing. An action slip is shown in Figure 10–13.
3. Fill out a routing slip and attach it to materials that the physician may send to others. For example, magazines often are routed among the staff or used in the lobby after the physician has read them. Time can be saved by attaching a routing slip to the magazine before giving it to the physician. (Figure 10–14).

Distributing Mail

1. Distribute mail to the individual to whom it is addressed after sorting materials that need

Action Slip

_____ File in the medical record.

_____ Send to bookkeeping.

_____ Please make _____ copies.

_____ Please follow up.

_____ Please record in tickler.

FIGURE 10–13 Action slip

Please pass the attached periodical to the next name on the list after you finish reading it.

_____ Dr. Mallaney

_____ Dr. Ricardo

_____ Ellyn Kincaid

_____ Dr. Henry Plunkett

FIGURE 10–14 Routing slip

only to be filed, "junk" mail, and magazines to be placed in the waiting room. Stack all the mail for each individual into categories according to importance.
a. To be answered immediately
b. To be answered routinely
c. To be answered by someone else
d. To be read for information
e. To be filed
f. To be forwarded
g. To be discarded
2. Distribute mail addressed to the practice to its proper destination. For example, all checks should be sent to the bookkeeper even though they are addressed in care of the practice name.
3. Return all mail that was delivered incorrectly. Write an appropriate comment, "Not at this address," or "Delivered to the wrong address."

IN YOUR OPINION

1. Under what circumstances might a letter need to be recalled?
2. If you are in charge of sorting the mail, how can you save time for recipients of the mail?
3. In what ways might procedures for processing mail in a medical office be different from the procedures used in a business office?

INTERNET ACTIVITIES

Go to the *Orbitz* Web site at http://orbitz.com and search for the best schedule for a physician who will travel from New York City to Chicago on November 18 and return on November 20. Create an itinerary showing the times of each flight. What is the cost of the ticket?

STUDENT STUDY CHECKLIST

Workbook

1. Complete Chapter 10 exercises in the workbook.
2. Complete Chapter 10 simulations in the workbook that access the CD-ROM in the back of the book.

Administrative Skills CD-ROM

1. Go the Library on the CD-ROM and play the interactive games for Chapter 3.

REFERENCES

Lindh, Wilburta Q., Marilyn S. Pooler, and Carol D. Tamparo. *Administrative Medical Assisting*, 2nd ed. Clifton Park, NY: Delmar Learning, 2002.

Pusins, Dolores Wells and Ann-Peele Ambrose. *Computer Concepts*. Cambridge, MA: Thomson Learning/Course Technology, 2001.

CHAPTER ACTIVITIES

PERFORMANCE-BASED ACTIVITIES

1. What type of postal or communication service do you recommend in each of the following situations, and why?

   Situation   *Service Recommended*

   a. *Letter advising that the physician will no longer treat a patient*

   b. *Letter from you renewing a magazine subscription*

   c. *X-rays needed across the country tomorrow*

   d. *Final collection letter to a patient*

   e. *Letter to a consulting physician*

   f. *Letter announcing a new partner*

   g. *Newsletter to all patients*

2. Using the Internet, develop information for trips that include the following information. Do not actually SEND the reservations; you do not want to pay for it.

   a. A round-trip flight to New York City, Chicago, or Los Angeles from the closest airport to your home

   b. A stay for three nights at a Marriott, Hilton, or Sheraton in Milwaukee, WI

   c. Travel to Burlington, VT, for the weekend by plane or car from Boston

   Make an itinerary and list costs of air, hotels, and rental cars.

   AIR:

   Carrier: _____

   Flight Number: _____

   Originating Departure Time: _____

   Originating Arrival Time: _____

   Return Departure Time: _____

   Return Arrival Time: _____

   Cost: _____

   HOTEL:

   Name of hotel: _____

   Cost: _____

   Description of accommodations: _____

   TRAVEL TO BOSTON:

   Method: _____

   Cost: _____

3. Conduct a search over the Internet on one of these topics: teen pregnancy, breast cancer, AIDS prevention, or another topic approved by your instructor. Print copies of five articles. Find the names, addresses, and phone numbers of at least two organizations or associations that can provide information on the topic.

EXPANDING YOUR THINKING

1. Interview someone about giving instructions. Write a short paper describing how patients are instructed and informed concerning one of the following:
   a. A chronic illness such as asthma, kidney disease, diabetes, or arthritis
   b. An acute illness or injury such as a heart attack, stroke, amputation, or bone fracture
   c. A major life change such as pregnancy, adolescence, menopause, or aging
   d. A psychological condition such as depression or anxiety
   e. Addiction, alcoholism, or obesity

2. Choose one of the following situations and compile a list of questions you would ask if you were a patient in one of these circumstances:
   a. Your sister-in-law is pregnant and a cocaine addict
   b. Your father has bleeding ulcers
   c. Your mother is scheduled for heart bypass surgery
   d. You have just been diagnosed with breast cancer
   e. Your brother has been diagnosed with a genetic disorder and you are planning to have children.

3. Interview three people who travel frequently. Ask each to describe their worst travel experience. Make a list of the responses and note how many times each factor was mentioned by a different person. As a class, compile all of the lists and present the results in a chart or graph.

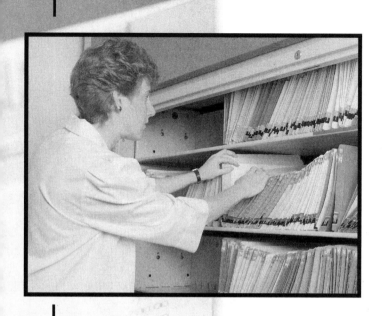

CHAPTER 11

Managing Medical Records

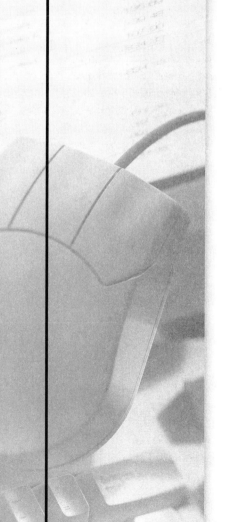

BOISE, IDAHO

Making certain that medical records are complete, up-to-date, and accurate is at the heart of any successful medical practice. Good records enable the doctors to perform better. This is because the quality of information in a patient's record can be critical in determining what an appropriate next step should be in the patient's treatment plan.

Without good records, the practice I work for would have difficulty in obtaining reimbursement from insurance companies, because they won't pay a claim if supporting medical data is missing. The work can be challenging because attention to detail makes the difference in whether a practice gets paid. If I don't place lab reports and summaries from consulting physicians in the correct patient folders, patients might receive improper treatment, and my job would be in jeopardy.

For instance, when I read over a doctor's notes before putting them in the patient's file and see that an important detail has been left out, I call it to the doctor's attention. As she tells me, that kind of critical eye helps both the patient and the practice. Each of the medical assistants rotates through the records responsibility. In our office, it's a sign of confidence when the medical staff allows a new medical assistant to take on the medical records task.

Nathan Randall
Medical Assistant

PERFORMANCE-BASED COMPETENCIES

After completing this chapter, you should be able to:
1. Explain the importance of maintaining accurate and up-to-date medical records.
2. Describe a method for maintaining progress notes.
3. Maintain medical records.
4. Determine needs for documentation and reporting.
5. Identify each type of document stored in a typical medical record.

VOCABULARY

Assignment of benefits   Signing over benefits from an insurance payment to a third party.

Blood tests   Analysis of blood to determine whether infection is present, excessive urea is evident, or glucose or other substances are present in too high or too low a concentration.

Capitation   Basing a physician's salary on the number of members enrolled in an insurance plan, no matter how many times each person is seen.

Case history   Analysis of the patient's complaint, examination results, lab results, diagnosis, prescribed treatment, and family and personal history.

Clearinghouse   Centralized location where claims are received, reviewed, and distributed electronically to insurance companies.

Closed files   Medical records of patients who are no longer under the physician's care because they have moved, changed doctors, or died.

Coordination of benefits   A clause in an insurance contract that limits the insurer's financial responsibility to 100% of cost.

Co-payment   The amount the policyholder must pay for each visit or medical service received.

Dependents   Individuals covered under a policyholder's insurance contract, including children and spouse.

Disability   An illness or injury that affects an individual's ability to continue in the job held previously.

Doctor's notes, or progress notes   Doctor's comments that are added to the medical record each time the patient is treated.

Electrocardiogram   Graphic illustration of the heart's activity.

Elimination period   Period of time after the onset of a disability for which no benefits are made.

Exclusions   Services that are not paid under the terms of an insurance contract.

Explanation of benefits (EOB)   A report from an insurance company that is sent with claim payments to provide details about the reimbursement.

Extended benefits   Supplemental coverage to a basic hospital plan, sometimes includes diagnostic x-rays and laboratory examinations.

Inactive files   Medical records of patients who have not visited the physician for an extended period.

Laboratory request   Test to be administered and the name of the attending physician.

Pathology and cytopathology   Field of laboratory testing that shows the results of studies of body tissue and body cells.

Patient health questionnaire   Questions about the patient's previous health and surgical history and family history.

Patient information form   Completed by a patient immediately on arriving at the medical office for the initial visit.

Problem-oriented medical record   Patient's complaints identified in list form.

Shingling   Method of filing small reports.

SOAP   Method of reporting patient's diagnosis and treatment plan: subjective examination (S), objective test results (O), doctor's assessment (A), and treatment plan (P).

Source-oriented medical record   Information grouped according to its source.

Urinalysis   Routine laboratory test of urine often requested by physicians.

X-rays, CAT scans, and ultrasound   Diagnostic tests to determine whether any unusual medical condition, such as a tissue mass, is present in the body.

A medical record is a permanent document giving a complete account of a person's illnesses or injuries and the services rendered by medical professionals. Usually, the medical record contains the patient's medical history, results of physical examinations, doctor's notes, laboratory reports, prescriptions, medical instructions, and other relevant medical information.

The level of detail required on medical records is substantial. If records are not clear and legible, or if they do not accurately reflect actual proceedings, the practice may not be fully reimbursed by insurance companies or other third-party providers. Complete accurate records also protect the practice against malpractice claims. Medical assistants who understand record-keeping requirements and actively seek missing information enhance the financial security of the practice.

Accurate medical records benefit the patient, the physician, and the public. They are used for research, insurance claims, and legal actions. The government and insurance companies use medical records to evaluate the quality and cost of medical and surgical procedures in different parts of the country.

For the patient, the medical record serves as a quick reference that aids the physician with diagnosis and treatment. An accurate, up-to-date records allows a physician to tell at a glance what previous conditions, illnesses, or allergies to medication may contribute to the patient's present problem and what future treatment is appropriate. For example, a medical record showing that a patient is allergic to penicillin alerts the physician to prescribe a sulfa drug or other antibiotic, instead of a penicillin-based drug, for a bacterial infection.

Complete medical records can protect the physician from liability during medical malpractice claims by outlining the course of treatment the physician prescribed for an illness or accident. A lawsuit can turn in a physician's favor if the medical record shows documentation of proper treatment or, in contrast, can turn against a physician when documentation is not present or incomplete. For example, if a physician is being sued for malpractice because a patient believes that her baby was harmed because he was delivered too early by cesarean section, the physician can show sonogram results proving that the actual delivery date was warranted by the sonogram.

Medical records serve the public because researchers can perform statistical analyses of data contained in them. Researchers may discover from a confidential analysis of many patients' medical records a common factor or factors present in many or all patients who suffer from the same medical problem. For example, information from medical records helped scientists conclude that Reye's syndrome, a rare childhood disease of the liver and central nervous system, develops while a child is recovering from a mild viral illness, such as chicken pox or influenza, or from taking aspirin after a viral illness. Several treatments for acquired immunodeficiency syndrome (AIDS) are based on analyses of the medical records of previous AIDS patients.

With the vast number of medical records that must be maintained in today's medical offices, accurate filing of patient charts is the only method by which a facility can efficiently track information vital to patient care. The soaring number of medical malpractice lawsuits requires every medical office to use great diligence and a well-trained staff to maintain medical records.

METHODS FOR KEEPING RECORDS

The physicians' preferences determine the methods that are used for keeping records. When several physicians practice in the same office, more than one method may be used.

1. **The physician enters the data**, either by hand or by a computer terminal placed in the examining room. Because handwriting will be read by others, it must be legible so it will be read correctly. This is especially important when others are dispensing or giving medications based on the handwritten record.
2. **The medical assistant enters the data** based on a checklist, form, or template developed for use with common health problems and procedures. The assistant completes the form in the examining room as the physician dictates. The physician reviews the forms before leaving the room or at a later time.
3. **The physician dictates** the notes while in the examining room or as soon after as possible. A transcriptionist enters the data in a computer terminal for later review by the physician.

TRENDS AND ISSUES IN MEDICAL RECORD KEEPING

Case histories and documentation of medical examinations are becoming more complex and detailed because of the requirements of insurance companies. The fees insurance companies pay are determined by the *Current Procedural Terminology* (CPT) code assigned to the treatment or procedure and the *International Classification of Diseases* (ICD) code assigned to the diagnosis. The medical record must precisely match the CPT and ICD codes submitted. Medical Office assistants are required to collect, sort, store, and retrieve records in an organized way. In Chapter 13 you will learn about CPT and ICD codes and the requirements for each.

Standardization of formats for medical records is one way to manage the cost and complexity of record keeping. Hospitals, physicians, insurance companies, and government agencies each have their own formats and data requirements for medical records. The medical assistant wastes a great deal of time when information has to be reformatted to match the requirements of each agency. The chance for error is also increased.

Standardization of Forms

Many barriers to standardization exist. The greatest barrier is the modification or replacement cost to almost every medical practice, hospital, insurance company, and health agency in the country. The problems of fully automating medical records nationwide, or even worldwide, are policy issues, not technological issues. For example, if all records are in a computer, how does the physician "sign" them? Most states presently prohibit "electronic signatures" and would have to change their laws to permit this practice. Technology is available for each physician to "sign" an electronic document with a voice-activated code or password when laws permit their use.

Legal Issues

One barrier to full automation is protection of records from undocumented changes. Anyone who has worked with word processing software knows how easy it is to change text. To change a medical record, however, one cannot simply open the file and change a patient's height from 6'1" to 5'10", or age from 22 to 42. Changes and corrections must be made by adding notes to the record, never by changing or deleting information already recorded. Therefore, to meet legal requirements, software for medical record keeping must include security measures that prevent the editing of previously entered materials. These and other issues have created a demand for consultants who specialize in medical record keeping.

Computers play an important role in the storing of medical records for statistical purposes and for retrieval and review, for example, when a physician wants to evaluate data on the effectiveness of a treatment plan or follow the course of several patients who have the same diagnosis. Confidentiality of the medical information must be safeguarded. Some states have laws that require human immunodeficiency virus (HIV) test results to be entered in the medical record, whereas other states do not.

CREATING A MEDICAL RECORD

A medical record is kept for each patient under a physician's care. The first time the patient visits the doctor, the medical assistant creates the record based on information the patient supplies. Each time the patient returns, the record is updated by adding medical reports, test results, and other data. Most medical offices continue to maintain traditional paper records in file folders, because this is convenient to the physician who can quickly review the entire record if desirable during a patient examination.

Color Coding the Folder

The first step in creating a paper medical record is to prepare a folder to hold the medical information. Commercial color-coded labels placed on the folder tab to form color patterns are widely used on medical record folders. When folders are filed alphabetically on a shelf, large patterns of color blocks are created (Figure 11–1). An out-of-place file breaks the color pattern, making incorrectly filed records easy to detect (Figure 11–2).

A partial color coding chart is shown in Figure 11–3. Notice that combination of letters form color patterns. In the name Caton, for example, the "C" is represented by orange and the "a" by brown. Folders for other patients whose names start with "Ca" also show orange and brown in positions three and four. If a folder showing orange and blue in the third and fourth positions (representing "Ce") is filed incorrectly with the "Ca" folders, it is easily visible because the color pattern is interrupted. A colored strip can be used in position two to separate folders according to primary physician when more than one physician shares an office. For example, a green strip may represent all the patients for Physician No. 1, and a red strip may represent all the patients for Physician No. 2.

In the same way that different colors can represent letters of the alphabet, different colors can

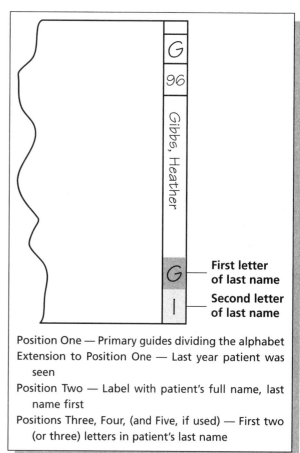

Position One — Primary guides dividing the alphabet

Extension to Position One — Last year patient was seen

Position Two — Label with patient's full name, last name first

Positions Three, Four, (and Five, if used) — First two (or three) letters in patient's last name

FIGURE 11–2   Color-coding systems

Letter Represented	Color
A	Brown
B	Yellow
C	Orange
D	Light Blue
E	Blue
F	Pink
G	Green
H	Purple
I	Grey
J	Red

FIGURE 11–3   Partial color-coding chart

also represent the numbers zero through nine in a numeric system. Patient numbers are color-coded in positions one through five, creating large blocks of color when folders are filed

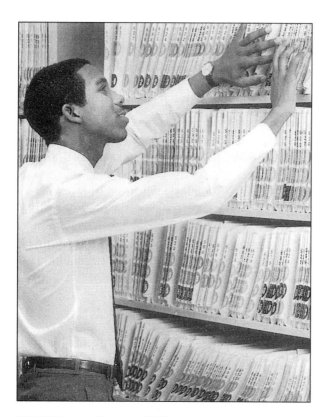

FIGURE 11–1   Open-shelf filing systems are commonly used to store color-coded medical records

correctly. Some medical offices use color codes to identify the year a patient last came to the office. For example, patients who were seen in 2003 might have red color codes on their records.

Contents of the Medical Record

The medical record contains various forms and reports, some completed by the patient and others completed by the physician. Initially, the medical record includes two questionnaires completed by the patient: the patient information form and the patient health questionnaire. It also includes a history and physical form that the physician completes during an interview with the patient. Laboratory reports, examination findings, consulting reports, and other medical documents are added during the course of treatment. Several typical forms are discussed and illustrated in the next section.

Patient-Completed Forms

Patient Information Form   Patients are asked to arrive early for the first visit to complete a patient information form (Figure 11–4). It includes the name, address, and telephone number of the patient; the name, address, and telephone number of the person responsible for payment (if different from the patient); all insurance company names and policy numbers; and other

---

Patient Information

Please Print Clearly   DATE ___SEPT. 9, 20–___

NAME ____NATHAN LEE____ AGE __45__ SEX __M__

__12/7/41__ ☐ SINGLE ☐ MARRIED ☐ WIDOWED ☒ DIVORCED
BIRTH DATE

ADDRESS ____1071 FULTON DR.____

CITY ___ATLANTA___ STATE ___GEORGIA___ ZIP __30312-1768__

PHONE __555-0542__ OCCUPATION ___SALES REPRESENTATIVE___

EMPLOYED BY ____FEZCO, INC.____

CITY ___ATLANTA___ STATE ___GEORGIA___ ZIP __30316-9502__

SPOUSE'S NAME __NA__

EMPLOYED BY __NA__

CITY __NA__ STATE __NA__ ZIP __NA__

PHONE __NA__ OCCUPATION __NA__

REFERRED BY ____DR. ABNER DOWARKSIK____

MEDICAL INSURANCE? ☒ YES ☐ NO SURGICAL? ☒ YES ☐ NO

MEDICAL INSURANCE GROUP NO. __GA66951__ CERTIFICATE NO. __475__

COMPANY ____STONE MOUNTAIN GENERAL____

SURGICAL INSURANCE GROUP NO. __1765__ CERTIFICATE NO. __818__

COMPANY ____UNITED SURGICAL PLAN____

NAME ____NATHAN LEE____
(PERSON RESPONSIBLE FOR PAYMENT)

ADDRESS ____1071 FULTON DR.____

CITY ___ATLANTA___ STATE ___GEORGIA___ ZIP __30312-1768__

FIGURE 11–4   Patient information form

information needed to set up an accounting record for the patient. The patient information form often is taped to the left side of the folder where it is visible each time insurance information is needed.

Patient Health Questionnaire   The patient health questionnaire, as shown in Figure 11–5, asks questions about the patient's previous health and surgical history and the patient's family history, both personal and medical. This information gives the physician an overview of factors that may influence or help determine current treatment.

Physician-Completed Forms

Case History   The physician may dictate the case history for the medical assistant to transcribe after the patient's initial visit (Figure 11–6).

	DATE		SUBSEQUENT VISITS AND FINDINGS
MO.	DAY	YR.	
12	20	--	*Laceration of third finger left-hand p.i.p. joint*
			Good movement, no tendon damage
			3, r-0 prolene sutures

CASE NO. _____

FIGURE 11–5   Patient health questionnaire

Patient Case History

Lance Glasser
930-03
August 14, 200x

CHIEF COMPLAINT
Mild chest discomfort

PRESENT ILLNESS
Patient, a 44-year-old white male, occasionally experiences mild chest pain. Two weeks ago he felt a tightness across his chest, equating it with a feeling of an air bubble. He has missed no work and enjoys an active life.

PAST HISTORY
The patient says his general health is good and that he exercises moderately on a home weight-training machine thirty minutes three times a week. He experiences periodic sinusitis and evidences mild osteoarthritis. He undergoes a complete physical each year with his company physician.

FAMILY HISTORY
Patient is married and has four children, ages 7–12. The youngest child, age 7, is mentally handicapped. Patient's mother died at 81 of Lou Gehrig's disease, and his father, in apparent good health, died in an automobile accident at 72. One sister, 35, and one brother, 47, both in good health.

PERSONAL HISTORY
Patient leads an active life. He is employed as a regional sales manager of a national corporation and considers himself to be a "workaholic." He suffered a mild myocardial infarction two years ago and asserts sensitivity to any potential health problems. He presents as emotionally stable and secure and has had no other major illnesses since childhood.

REVIEW OF SYSTEMS
GENERAL: BP normal, pulse normal, temperature normal
HEENT: Occasional headaches, primarily when glasses are dirty, no deafness or earaches
CR: No tachycardia, shortness of breath, or wheezing
GI: Appetite normal, frequent gas, no constipation
GU: No dysuria, hematuria, or pyuria
CNS: No dizziness, fainting, seizures, or loss of balance

PHYSICAL EXAMINATION
Routine examination reveals a well-developed, well-nourished male in apparent good health. The patient is overweight and is trying to lose the weight through an exercise program.

Height, 5'10". Weight, 180. Blood pressure, 130/85. Temperature, 98.2. Pulse, 80. Respirations, 20.

LABORATORY TESTS
Chest x-ray revealed evidence of inflammation of the pleura. An ECG revealed evidence of a prior myocardial infarction.

DIAGNOSIS
1. Unstable arteriosclerotic heart disease, prior myocardial infarction, and recent heart irregularity.
2. Essential hypertension.
3. Probable pluerisy

TREATMENT
Ampicillan, 500 mg q.i.d. by mouth
Recheck in two weeks

REMARKS
Patient may continue working but should take rest breaks twice a day.

Susan Reilly, M.D.

FIGURE 11–6 Patient case history

The case history describes (1) the patient's complaint or physical problem, (2) past history, (3) family history, (4) personal history, (5) review of systems, (6) physical examination, (7) laboratory tests, (8) diagnosis, (9) treatment, and (10) remarks.

Doctor's Notes Doctor's notes, or progress notes, are added to the medical record each time the patient is treated (Figure 11–7). Comments about the condition, diagnosis, and treatment are listed as well as prescription information, telephone consultations, and other related information. The person who writes the notes, usually the physician, initials them.

Laboratory Request

A laboratory request indicating the name of the test to be administered and the name of the attending physician is completed when a test is required. A copy is stored in the medical record (Figure 11–8).

Laboratory reports are often small and irregular in size; therefore, they can be easily lost if not permanently secured to the folder. Shingling is a method of affixing small reports in chronological order to a standard size sheet of paper. The earliest report is taped to the bottom of the sheet of paper, the second earliest report is taped on top of the first about one inch above the

---

Laboratory Request

John H. Sparks, M.D.   555-0078
8504 Capricorn Drive
Atlanta, GA 30033-7775

Date _____ 4/16/-- _____

To _____ Rachel Morgan _____

_____ Briarcliff Labs _____

Re _____ Susanne Snoffer _____

Please perform the following tests:
- ☐ Culture of _____
- ☐ C S F for _____
- ☐ Feces for _____
- ☐ E K G _____
- ☐ B M R _____
- ☐ Pregnancy _____
- ☑ Urinalysis _____
- ☐ H P N _____
- ☑ Blood Sugar _____
- ☐ R H Factor & Blood Type _____
- ☐ SED Rate _____
- ☑ W B C & Diff _____
- ☐ R B C & H G D _____
- ☐ Other _____

John H. Sparks, M. D.
Signature

FIGURE 11–8 Laboratory request

5	18	--	*URI — stuffy nose, sore throat, sleeplessness*	
			Ampicillin #20 t.i.d. till gone	
8	10	--	*Warts on hand — removed with liquid nitrogen. Return in*	
			2 week for reevaluation.	

NAME *Marvin Connelly*

FIGURE 11–7 Physician's progress notes

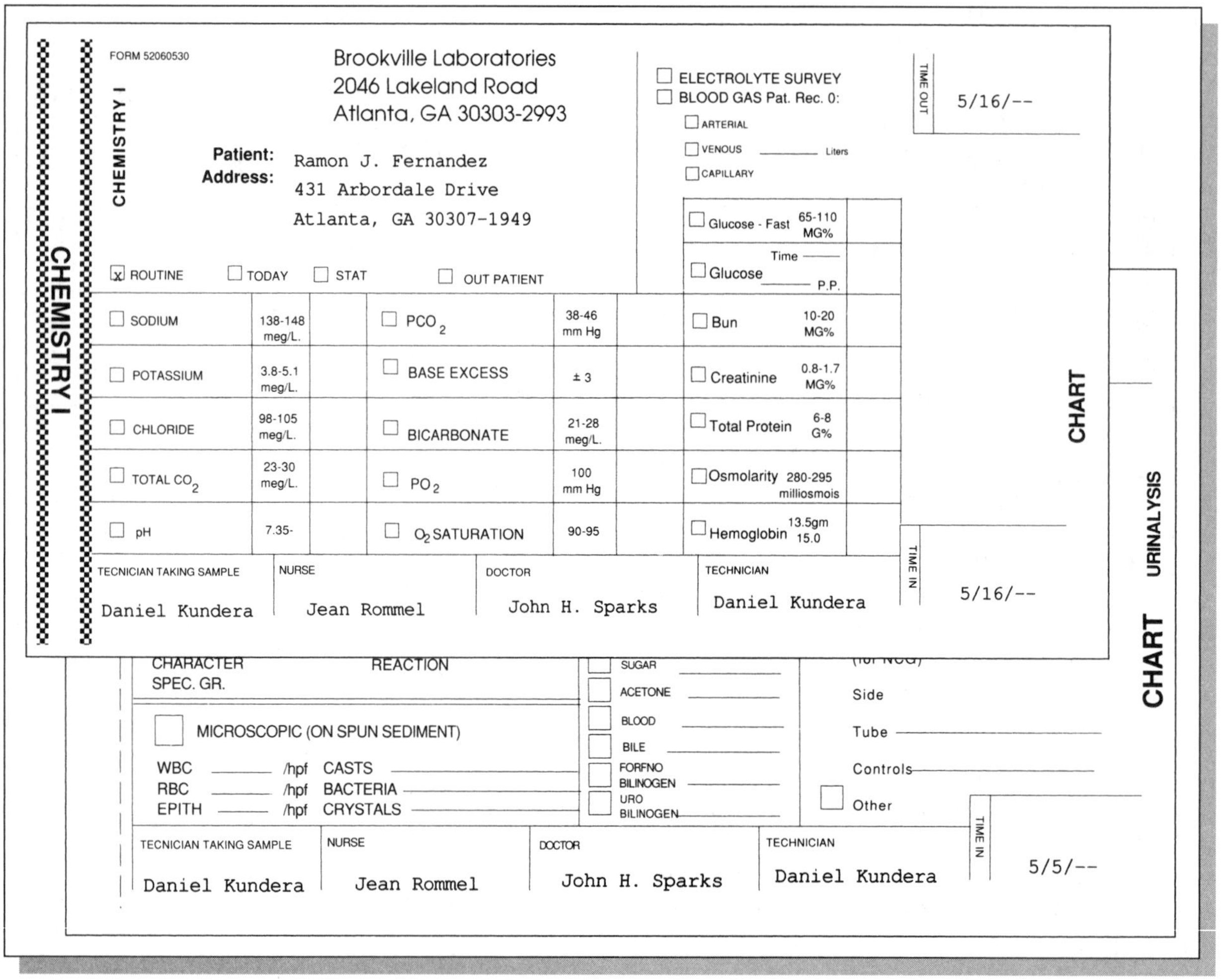
CHEMISTRY I

FORM 52060530

Brookville Laboratories
2046 Lakeland Road
Atlanta, GA 30303-2993

Patient: Ramon J. Fernandez
Address: 431 Arbordale Drive
Atlanta, GA 30307-1949

[x] ROUTINE ☐ TODAY ☐ STAT ☐ OUT PATIENT

☐ ELECTROLYTE SURVEY
☐ BLOOD GAS Pat. Rec. 0:
☐ ARTERIAL
☐ VENOUS ______ Liters
☐ CAPILLARY

TIME OUT 5/16/--

☐ SODIUM	138-148 meg/L.		☐ PCO_2	38-46 mm Hg		☐ Glucose - Fast	65-110 MG%	
						☐ Glucose	Time ___ ___ P.P.	
☐ POTASSIUM	3.8-5.1 meg/L.		☐ BASE EXCESS	± 3		☐ Bun	10-20 MG%	
☐ CHLORIDE	98-105 meg/L.		☐ BICARBONATE	21-28 meg/L.		☐ Creatinine	0.8-1.7 MG%	
☐ TOTAL CO_2	23-30 meg/L.		☐ PO_2	100 mm Hg		☐ Total Protein	6-8 G%	
☐ pH	7.35-		☐ O_2 SATURATION	90-95		☐ Osmolarity	280-295 milliosmois	
						☐ Hemoglobin	13.5gm 15.0	

TECNICIAN TAKING SAMPLE	NURSE	DOCTOR	TECHNICIAN
Daniel Kundera	Jean Rommel	John H. Sparks	Daniel Kundera

TIME IN 5/16/--

CHART

URINALYSIS

CHARACTER REACTION
SPEC. GR.
☐ MICROSCOPIC (ON SPUN SEDIMENT)
WBC ______ /hpf CASTS
RBC ______ /hpf BACTERIA
EPITH ______ /hpf CRYSTALS
☐ SUGAR
☐ ACETONE
☐ BLOOD
☐ BILE
☐ FORFNO BILINOGEN
☐ URO BILINOGEN
Side
Tube
Controls
☐ Other

TECNICIAN TAKING SAMPLE	NURSE	DOCTOR	TECHNICIAN
Daniel Kundera	Jean Rommel	John H. Sparks	Daniel Kundera

TIME IN 5/5/--

CHART

FIGURE 11–9 Shingled laboratory reports

bottom, and so on up the page. Shingled laboratory reports are shown in Figure 11–9.

Typical Laboratory Tests

Urinalysis A urinalysis is a routine laboratory test often requested by physicians. From urine tests, physicians can determine whether infection is present in the body, as well as a variety of other conditions. A urinalysis report is shown in Figure 11–10.

Electrocardiogram An electrocardiogram (ECG), a graphic illustration of the heart's activity, is used to test heart conditions (Figure 11–11). Taken at intervals such as every six months or every year, ECGs are compared to determine whether a change in heart activity has occurred since the last test.

Blood Test Blood tests reveal whether infection is present in the body, urea is elevated in the blood, or glucose or other substances are present in too high or too low a concentration in the blood (Figure 11–12).

Radiology Report X-rays, CT scans, and ultrasound examinations are diagnostic tests analyzed by radiologists to determine whether any unusual medical condition, such as a tissue mass, is present in the body. The radiologist prepares a report of the findings for the medical record (Figure 11–13); the actual x-rays are stored in another location because they are large and bulky.

Pathology and Cytopathology Report Pathology and cytopathology reports are prepared to show the results of studies of body tissue and body

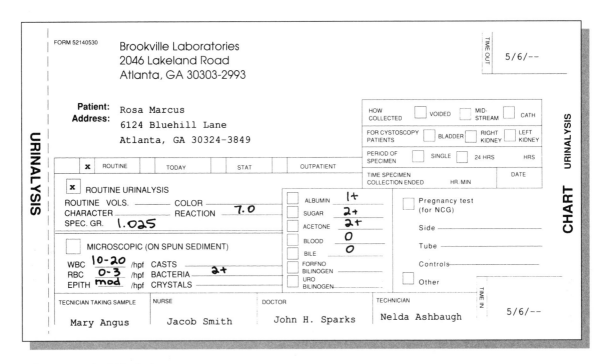

FORM 52140530

Brookville Laboratories
2046 Lakeland Road
Atlanta, GA 30303-2993

TIME OUT 5/6/--

Patient: Rosa Marcus
Address: 6124 Bluehill Lane
Atlanta, GA 30324-3849

HOW COLLECTED	☐ VOIDED	☐ MID-STREAM	☐ CATH
FOR CYSTOSCOPY PATIENTS	☐ BLADDER	☐ RIGHT KIDNEY	☐ LEFT KIDNEY
PERIOD OF SPECIMEN	☐ SINGLE	☐ 24 HRS	HRS
TIME SPECIMEN COLLECTION ENDED	HR./MIN		DATE

| ☒ | ROUTINE | TODAY | STAT | OUTPATIENT |

☒ ROUTINE URINALYSIS

ROUTINE VOLS. _____ COLOR _____
CHARACTER _____ REACTION __7.0__
SPEC. GR. __1.025__

☐ MICROSCOPIC (ON SPUN SEDIMENT)

WBC __10-20__ /hpf CASTS _____
RBC __0-3__ /hpf BACTERIA __2+__
EPITH __mod__ /hpf CRYSTALS _____

☐ ALBUMIN	1+
☐ SUGAR	2+
☐ ACETONE	2+
☐ BLOOD	0
☐ BILE	0
☐ FORFNO BILINOGEN	
☐ URO BILINOGEN	

☐ Pregnancy test (for NCG)

Side _____
Tube _____
Controls _____
☐ Other _____

| TECNICIAN TAKING SAMPLE | NURSE | DOCTOR | TECHNICIAN | TIME IN |
| Mary Angus | Jacob Smith | John H. Sparks | Nelda Ashbaugh | 5/6/-- |

URINALYSIS   CHART URINALYSIS

FIGURE 11–10 Urinalysis report

cells. A Pap smear is an example of a cytopathology report (Figure 11–14).

PROBLEM-ORIENTED AND SOURCE-ORIENTED MEDICAL RECORDS

Two different formats are used for recording information in the patient's medical record. The problem-oriented medical record, developed in the 1970s, identifies the patient's complaints in a problem list. The source-oriented medical record groups information according to its source; for example, from laboratories, examinations, nurse's or doctor's notes, consulting physicians, and other sources.

Problem-Oriented Medical Record

The problem-oriented medical record (POMR) came into use as a way to organize medical information in an orderly and easy-to-understand manner. In a POMR, the patient's complaints are seen as a series of problems, which are identified from the initial case history, the physical examination, and the results of diagnostic tests and procedures. Each problem is given a number, which is used when referring to the treatments and procedures the physician performs to correct the problem. Each time the patient returns for treatment of a recurring problem, the reference number for the problem is written before the doctor's notes about the visit. If more than one problem is identified, the number of each problem is listed, along with the treatment and procedures. If a patient describes a new complaint, it is added to the problem list and given its own number. The problem list is stored in a prominent location in the medical record so that anyone reviewing the record can locate it quickly.

The POMR is most useful in settings where several different people must refer to records. For example, in an ambulatory clinic staffed by several physicians on a rotating basis, a patient may see a different physician on each visit. With

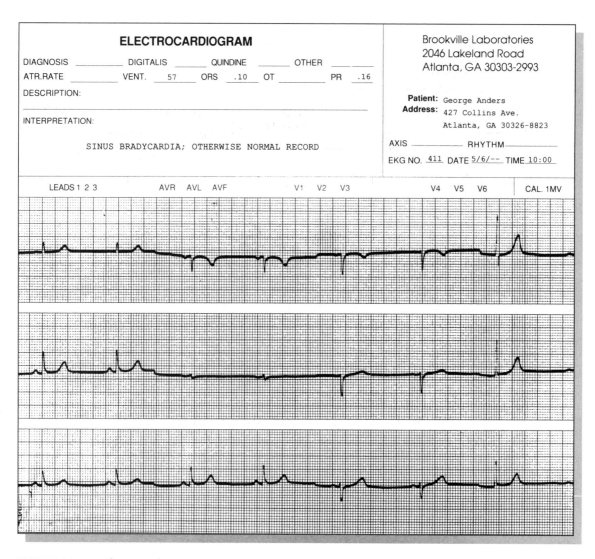

FIGURE 11–11 Electrocardiogram

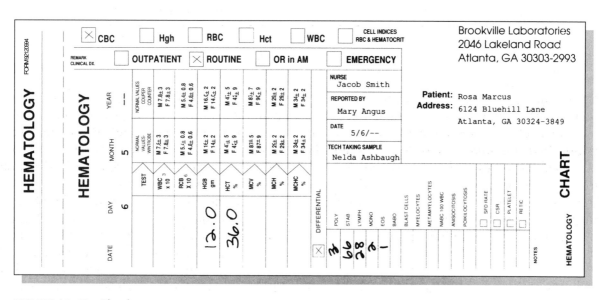

FIGURE 11–12 Blood test report

DEPARTMENT OF RADIOLOGY
NUCLEAR MEDICINE REPORT

Patient's Name   Jennifer Alexander
Hosp. No.
Room No.
Ref. Physician

Date 3/15/--	Nuclear Medicine No.: 005375	Pregnant:

Examination:	Isotropic Compound:	Dose:	Ancillary Studies:
Thyroid Scan I 131 Uptake	Sodium I 131		

The patient has had a thyroidectomy for hyperthyroidism. A 24-hour radioactive iodine uptake is .08% reflecting the surgical removal of the thyroid.
A small area of functioning thyroid tissue is seen to the right of the midline probably in the region of the upper pole of the thyroid. There is no evidence of activity in the lower left midline neck in the region of the palpable nodule.

Dr. Sabina Gwyn

NUCLEAR MEDICINE REPORT

FIGURE 11–13   Radiology report

the POMR method, the physician can quickly scan the charts to review the patient's progress.

The doctor's notes for a POMR follow an established formula called SOAP. After the physician identifies and numbers the problem, the doctor's notes are organized and dictated using the initials S-O-A-P, which stand for Subjective, Objective, Assessment, and Plan. Figure 11–15 explains the SOAP formula.

Source-Oriented Medical Record

The source-oriented medical record (SOMR) stores similar forms and reports together. For example, all laboratory reports are shingled and stored in one section; all consultation reports are stored in another; and all doctor's notes, nurse's notes, consulting reports, and other reports are grouped according to their source and stored in separate locations in the folder. When a specific report is needed, the physician must flip through the entire medical record to find it. As a result, the SOMR format means that the physician must look through the folder several times during a patient's visit to obtain all the necessary information from various sources.

FIGURE 11–14 Pathology and cystology report

The form contains:

Brookville Laboratories
2046 Lakeland Road
Atlanta, GA 30303-2993

METROPOLITAN HOSPITAL
ATLANTA, GA **CYTOLOGY**

☒ GENITAL   ☐ NON GENITAL

☒ CERVICAL

☐ VAGINAL

☐ MATURITY INDEX

☐ LAB USE ONLY

Patient: Rosa Marcus   Age 45
Address: 6124 Bluehill Lane
         Atlanta, GA 30324-3849

☐ SPUTUM   ☐ GASTRIC
☐ URINE   ☐ SMALL INT.
☐ BREAST   ☐ LARGE INT.
☐ PLEURAL   ☐ OTHER
☐ PERITONEAL
☐ BRON. WASH
☐ BRON. BRUSH
☐ C S F
☐ ESOPH

CLINICAL INFORMATION:
LAST MENSTRUAL PERIOD:
         6/31/--

PREVIOUS SMEARS _____ 19 ____
DIAGNOSIS *NEGATIVE*
PREGNANT ☐ YES ☒ NO
YEARS POSTMENOPAUSAL

Date: 6/24/--

CHART COPY

CONSULTATION REPORT: REMARKS:
☐ UNSATISFACTORY   ☐ POSITIVE
☒ NEGATIVE   ☐ IN SITU
☐ NO ENDOCERVICALS ☐ INVASIVE
☐ ATYPICAL BENIGN   ☐ OTHER
☐ DYSPLASIA

CYTOTECHNOLOGIST   PATHOLOGIST

S	Subjective	Information based on the patient's feelings and symptoms (feels bad, no energy, headaches). The examiner writes the subjective analysis in the patient's own words and includes the chief complaint or reason for the visit.
O	Objective	Information based on the results of diagnostic tests and procedures. These are symptoms that can be seen or proved (bruises, high blood pressure, fever).
A	Assessment	Diagnosis of the problem based on subjective and objective data.
P	Plan	Manner in which the problem will be managed. The plan usually consists of three parts: (1) medical management, including medication, diet, and therapy; (2) diagnostic follow-up, including x-rays and additional lab tests; and (3) patient education, including reinforcement of the physician's instructions by the medical assistant.

FIGURE 11–15 SOAP formula

Progress Notes

Each time the patient returns to visit the doctor, progress notes or chart notes are made in the medical record. If possible, the note should be computer printed and not handwritten. Progress notes are shown in Figure 11–7. The medical assistant should check with the physician to see which patients have been seen outside the office, at the hospital, or at a nursing home, so those records can be pulled and brought up to date with progress notes.

Progress notes contain information about every encounter, other than personal, between the patient and physician, whether in the office or another setting. If the patient is referred for consultation, the consulting physician's name and the reason for the consultation are recorded. Appointment cancellations or no-shows and refusal of patients to cooperate with the treatment plan are also shown.

For legal protection, the notes must be accurate, legible, and up to date. They should have no omissions and should be signed or initialed by the physician. Abbreviations used in recording patient care are shown in Table 11–1.

TABLE 11–1
Patient Care Abbreviations

A	allergy; abortion	CBC	complete blood count	DPT	diphtheria, pertussis, tetanus (vaccine)
AB	antibiotic	cc	cubic centimeter	Dr.	Doctor
abdom	abdomen	CC	chief complaint	drsg	dressing
abt	about	CDC	calculated date of confinement	Dx, Dg, dx	diagnosis
Acc, acc	accommodation	CHF	congestive heart failure	E	emergency
AD, a.d.	right ear	chr	chronic	ECG	electrocardiogram; electrocardiograph
adm	admit; admission; admitted	CI	color index	ED	emergency department
adv	advice	cm	centimeter	EDC	estimated date of confinement; due date for baby
aet.	at the age of	CNS	central nervous system		
AgNO₃	silver nitrate	CO, C/O	complains of	EEG	electroencephalogram; electroencephalograph
AIDS	acquired immuno-deficiency syndrome	CO₂, CO2	carbon dioxide		
		comp	comprehensive	EENT	eye, ear, nose, and throat
alb	albumin	compl	complete	EKG	electrocardiogram; electrocardiograph
ALL	allergy	Con, CON, Cons	consultation	epith.	epithelial
a.m., AM	before noon	Cont.	continue	ER	emergency room
AMA	American Medical Association	COPD	chronic obstructive pulmonary disease	ESR	erythrocyte sedimentation rate
ant	anterior	CPX, CPE	complete physical examination		
ante	before	C section	cesarean section	est.	established; estimated
AP	anterior posterior; anteroposterior	CT	computed tomography	etiol.	etiology
AP & L	anteroposterior and lateral	CV	cardiovascular	EU	etiology unknown
		CVA	costovertebral angle; cardiovascular accident; cerebro-vascular accident	Ex, exam.	examination
approx	approximate			exc.	excision
apt	apartment			ext	external
ASA	acetylsalicylic acid	CXR	chest x-ray	F	Fahrenheit; French (catheter)
asap, ASAP	as soon as possible	Cysto	cystoscopy		
ASCVD	arteriosclerotic cardio-vascular disease	D & C	dilatation and curettage	FACP	Fellow, American College of Physicians
ASHD	arteriosclerotic heart disease	dc	discontinue		
		DC	discharge	FACS	Fellow, American College of Surgeons
asst	assistant	del	delivery		
auto	automobile	Dg, Dx, dx	diagnosis		
Ba	barium	diag.	diagnosis, diagnostic	FH	family history
Bl	biopsy	diam.	diameter	FHS	fetal heart sounds
BM	bowel movement	diff.	differential	fluor	fluoroscopy
BMR	basal metabolic rate	dilat	dilate	ft	foot; feet
BP, B/P	blood pressure	disch.	discharged	FU	follow-up
Brev	Brevital	DNA	does not apply	Fx	fracture
BUN	blood urea nitrogen	DNS	did not show		
Bx, BX	biopsy	DOB	date of birth	G	gravida (number of pregnancies)
C	cervical; centigrade, celsius	DPM	Doctor of Podiatric Medicine		
C & S	culture and sensitivity				
Ca, CA	cancer, carcinoma				
Cauc	caucasian				

continues

TABLE 11–1 *(continued)*

g, gm	gram	int, INT	internal	O₂, O2	oxygen
GA	gastric analysis	intermed	intermediate	OB	obstetrical, obstetrics
GB	gallbladder	interpret	interpretation	OC	office call
GC	gonorrhea	IPPB	intermittent positive pressure breathing	occ	occasional
GGE	generalized glandular enlargement			O.D., o.d.	right eye
		IQ	intelligence quotient	ofc	office
GI	gastrointestinal	IV, I.V.	intravenous	OH	occupational history
GU	genitourinary	IVP	intravenous pyelogram	O.L.	left eye
Gyn, GYN	gynecology			OP, op.	operation, operative, outpatient
H	hospital call	JVD	jugulovenous distention	OPD	outpatient department
HA	headache			OR	operating room
HBP	high blood pressure	K35	Kollmann (dilator)	orig.	original
HC	hospital call; hospital consultation	KUB	kidneys, ureters, bladder	O.S., o.s.	office surgery; left eye
HCD	house call, day			OT	occupational therapy
HCl	hydrochloric acid	L	left; laboratory; living children; liter	OTC	over the counter
HCN	house call, night			OV	office visit
hct	hematocrit	lab., LAB	laboratory		
HCVD	hypertensive cardio-vascular disease	L&A, l/a	light and accommodation	P	pulse; preterm parity or deliveries before term
HEENT	head, eyes, ears, nose, and throat	L&W	living and well		
		lat, LAT	lateral	PA	posterior anterior, posteroanterior
Hgb, Hb	hemoglobin	lbs	pounds		
hist	history	LLL	left lower lobe	P&A	percussion and auscultation
H₂O, H2O	water	LLQ	left lower quadrant		
hosp	hospital	LMP	last menstrual period	PAP, Pap	Papanicolaou (test)
H & P	history and physical	lt., LT	left	Para I	woman having borne one child
HPI	history of present illness	ltd.	limited		
		LUQ	left upper quadrant	PBI	protein-bound iodine
hr, hrs	hour, hours			PC	present complaint
HS	hospital surgery	M	medication; married	PD	permanent disability
Ht, ht	height	MA	mental age	PE	physician examination
HV	hospital visit	med., MED	medicine	perf.	performed
HX	history	mg	milligram(s)	PERRLA, PERLA	pupils equal, round, react to light and to accommodation
HX PX	history and physical examination	MH	marital history		
		ml	milliter(s)		
I	injection	mm	millimeter(s)	pH	Hydrogen ion concentration
I&D	incision and drainage	MM	mucous membrane		
IC	initial consultation	mo	month(s)	PH	past history
i.e.	that is			Ph ex	physical examination
IM	intramuscular	N	negative	phys.	physical
imp., IMP	impression	NA, N/A	not applicable	PI	present illness
inc	include	NaCl	sodium chloride	PID	pelvic inflammatory disease
inf, INF	infected	NAD	no appreciable disease		
inflam., INFL	inflammation	neg.	negative	p.m., PM	after noon
		NPN	nonprotein nitrogen	PMH	past medical history
init	initial	N&V	nausea and vomiting	PND	postnasal drip
inj., INJ	injection	NYD	not yet diagnosed		

continues

TABLE 11–1 *(continued)*

PO, P Op	postoperative; phone order	SH	social history	URI	uppery respiratory infection
pos.	positive	SLR	straight leg raising	UTI	urinary tract infection
post.	posterior	slt	slight	VD	veneral disease
postop.	postoperative	Smr, sm.	smear	VDRL	Veneral Disease Research Laboratory (test for syphilis)
preop.	preoperative	SMWD	single, married, widowed, divorced		
prep	prepare, prepared	SOB	shortness of breath		
PRN, p.r.n.	as necessary	sp gr	specific gravity	W	work; white
prog	prognosis	SQ	subcutaneous	WBC, wbc	white blood cell or count; well baby care
P&S	permanent and stationary	SR	sedimentation rate		
PSP	phenolsufonphthalein	STAT, stat.	immediately	WF	white female
Pt, pt	patient	STD	sexually transmitted disease	wk.	week; work
PT	physical therapy	strab	strabismus	wks	weeks
PTR	patient to return	surg.	surgery	WM, W/M	white male
PX	physical examination	Sx.	symptoms	WNL	within normal limits
				WR	Wassermann reaction
R	right; residence call; report	T	temperature; term parity or deliveries at term	wt	weight
RBC, rbc	red blood cell			X	x-ray(s); multiplied by
rec	recommend	T&A	tonsillectomy and adenoidectomy	XR	x-ray(s)
re ch	recheck	Tb, tbc, TB	tuberculosis		
re-exam, reex	reexamination	TD	temporary disability	yr	year
reg.	regular	temp.	temperature		
ret, retn	return	TIA	transient ischemic attack	**Symbols**	
rev	review	TMs	tympanic membranes	*	birth
Rh–	Rhesus negative (blood)	TPR	temperature, pulse, respiration	c̄, /c, w/	with
RHD	rheumatic heart disease	Tr.	treatment	P̄	after
RLQ	right lower quadrant	TTD	total temporary disability	s̄, /s, w/o	without
RO, R/O	rule out	TURB	transurethral resection of bladder	c̄c, c̄/c	with correction (eyeglasses)
ROS	review of systems	TURP	transurethral resection of prostate	s̄c, s̄/c	without correction (eyeglasses)
rt.	right	TX, Tx	treatment	+	positive
RT	respiratory therapy			–	negative
RTC	return to clinic	U	unit	ō	negative
RTO	return to office	UA, U/A	urinalysis	Ⓛ	left
RUQ	right upper quadrant	UCHD	usual childhood diseases	ⓜ	murmur
Rx, RX, ℞	prescription; any medication or treatment ordered	UCR	usual, customary, and reasonable	Ⓡ	right
		UGI	upper gastrointestinal	♂	male
S	surgery	UPJ	ureteropelvic junction or joint	♀	female
SD	state disability	UR, ur	urine	μ	micron
SE	special examination			±	negative or positive; indefinite
sed rate	sedimentation rate				
Sep.	separated				

FILE MANAGEMENT

Databases of paper medical records are standard in most medical practices today. Offices that do use medical record software tend to store only a capsule portion of each record on disk and continue to maintain paper files as well.

Paper Files

Most offices that use traditional paper medical records store them on open shelves and in file cabinets. As a medical assistant, you will use either an alphabetic or a numeric filing method for filing records.

Active Files

Open-shelf filing cabinets with stationary or pull-out open shelves are commonly used for storing active files. The folder tabs, which extend beyond the side of the folders, show the caption or name of the folder (Figure 11–16). Three-, four-, and five-position folders with color coding make retrieval of records easy and fast.

Inactive and Closed Files

When a patient has not visited the physician for an extended period, the medical record is moved to the inactive files. Most physicians consider a patient to be inactive after two to three years. Inactive files are usually stored in an out-of-the-way location to conserve space for active files.

Closed files contain the medical records of patients who are no longer under the physician's care because they have moved, changed doctors, or died. Because malpractice suits may be filed several years after the disputed treatment, inactive files and closed files are kept indefinitely. The laws of each state specify how long after a disputed action a claim can be made. The statute of limitations in a state determines how long medical records must be kept and the number of years that may pass before a claimant may no longer file a suit.

Microfiche or microfilm is often used to store inactive and closed records. Because a sheet of microfiche is about the size of a 3" × 5" card and holds 96 pages of information, records for several patients can be filmed on one microfiche sheet and stored in less space than would be necessary for conventional records.

Miscellaneous Correspondence

Letters, memos, reports, and other documents not directly related to patients are filed alphabetically in individual folders according to subject in a separate file labeled "Miscellaneous Correspondence." Follow these procedures for filing material in the Miscellaneous Correspondence file.

1. Clip together all correspondence by subject and arrange it in chronological order with the most recent in front.
2. Prepare an individual folder for a single subject when more than five items are clipped together.
3. Transfer these materials to a folder.
4. File the new folder alphabetically with the other individual folders in the Miscellaneous Correspondence file.
5. File the remaining materials alphabetically by subject in a folder. Store the folder at the back of the individual folders.

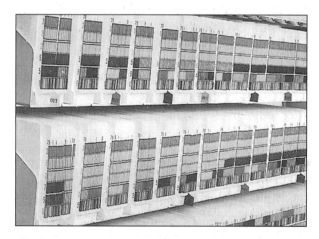

FIGURE 11–16 Color-coded labels of folder tabs are widely used to make incorrectly filed records easier to detect.

IN YOUR OPINION

1. Does a POMR or SOMR make more sense to you? Why?
2. Can security be more easily maintained for paper records or computerized records?
3. What things should a medical assistant check when receiving a file back from a physician after a patient's visit?

RULES FOR FILING

Medical records, ledger cards, general correspondence, research reports, tax records, and magazine articles related to the physician's specialty are typical documents that you will file in a medical office. The alphabetic and numeric filing methods are commonly used for filing patient records; the alphabetic, numeric, geographic, and subject methods are used for other materials.

Alphabetic Indexing

The alphabet is basic to all four methods of filing: alphabetic, numeric, subject, and geographic. Several standard rules apply for filing by the alphabetic method.

Standards for Alphabetic Filing

Rule 1: Order of Indexing Units For filing purposes, the parts of an individual's name are called **indexing units**. The surname, or last name, is identified as the first indexing unit; the first name or initial is identified as the second unit; and the middle name or initial is identified as the third unit. For example, you would index the name *Samuel Arthur Clark* like this: *Clark* (first unit); *Samuel* (second unit); and *Arthur* (third unit).

Rule 2: Names of Businesses Names of businesses, institutions, and organizations are indexed in the order in which the name is written. Abbreviations such as *Co.*, *Inc.*, and *Ltd.* are also indexed as written. Therefore, the business name *Clinical Supply Company* would be alphabetized exactly as it is written, using *Clinical* as the first indexing unit.

Rule 3: Symbols and Coordinating Words Symbols and coordinating words like *a, an, and, the, in, of, #*, and *&*, that are part of a name are also considered as indexing units. For example, you would index the business name *Palmer & Palmer Labs* like this: *Palmer* (first unit); *and* (second unit); *Palmer* (third unit); and *Labs* (fourth unit). Notice that *&* is written out as *and*.

In addition, if a business name begins with *The*, that word becomes the last indexing unit. For example, the name *The Sands Ambulance Service* would follow this system. *Sands* (first unit); *Ambulance* (second unit); *Service* (third unit); and *The* (last unit).

Rule 4: Initials and Abbreviations Initials and abbreviations of business and personal names are indexed as written. Hyphens, periods, or parentheses are ignored in the indexing order. For example, in the name *A B C Radiology Co.*, *ABC* is treated as one indexing unit, and in the name *C & D Drug Co.*, *C* and *D* are treated as three separate indexing units.

Rule 5: Possessives The apostrophe is not considered when indexing possessives. Therefore, *Harper's* is indexed as *Harpers* and *Manns'* is indexed as *Manns*.

Rule 6: Titles A person's title is considered as the last indexing unit. For example, you would consider the title *Dr.* in the name *Dr. Ester Diaz* as the last indexing unit. However, if a title appears with the last name only, you index the name and title as written. To illustrate, with the name *Professor Mendel*, *Professor* would be the first indexing unit, and *Mendel* would be the second unit.

Rule 7: Married Women A married woman's name is indexed as used, whether she continues to be known by her maiden name or by her husband's name. Some married women use their husbands' last names and their own first names, and middle names or initials. Others use their husbands' last names, first names, and middle names or initials. In either case, the last name is the first indexing unit; the first name is the second unit; the middle name or initial is the third unit; and the title *Mrs.* or *Ms.* is the last unit. Therefore, the name *Mrs. Alice Marie Lunkin* is indexed like this: *Lunkin* (first indexing unit); *Alice* (second part); *Marie* (third unit); and *Mrs.* (last unit).

If a married woman uses a combination of her own last name and her husband's last name, you should consider the compound name as one indexing unit. For example, in the name *Ms. Althea Sanders-Smith*, the first indexing unit is *Sanders Smith*. Notice that the hyphen is omitted. When a married woman is known by more than one name, all forms of the name are cross-referenced.

Rule 8: Foreign Language Prefixes A foreign language prefix is considered to be a part of the business name or personal name that follows it. Capitalization or spacing between the prefix and the root word does not influence the indexing order. Examples of foreign language prefixes include *De*, *Di*, *Du*, *L'*, *Las*, *O'*, *Van*, and *Van Der*. Therefore, you would consider the surname *Di George* as one indexing unit, *DiGeorge*. Similarly, you would index the business name *William Van Hook Optical Co.* like this: *William* (first unit); *VanHook* (second unit); *Optical* (third unit); and *Co.* (last unit).

Rule 9: Identical Names When several names of individuals or businesses are the same, you must use the address for filing. Addresses are indexed alphabetically first by city, then by state (if the city name is duplicated), then by street name and address or building number. Addresses and building numbers are indexed in ascending order, meaning that the numbers go from smaller to larger.

In the same way, the seniority designations *Junior* (Jr.) and *Senior* (Sr.) are considered in alphabetic order. The seniority designations II, III, and IV are put into numeric order. Therefore, *Francisco Toros II*'s name would be listed before *Francisco Toros III*.

Rule 10: Numerals in Business Names A numeral that is part of a business name is written as a single word and indexed as a single unit. For example, *9th Avenue Garage* is filed as *9* (first unit); *Avenue* (second unit); and *Garage* (third unit). In addition, all Arabic numerals and Roman numerals are filed sequentially before alphabetic characters.

Rule 11: Organizations and Institutions Names of organizations and institutions are indexed exactly as they are written. For example, *National Association of Radiologists* is filed like this: *National* (first unit); *Association* (second unit); *of* (third unit); and *Radiologists* (last unit).

Rule 12: Separated Single Words Separate parts of words that the dictionary treats as a single word are indexed as written in the business name. Therefore, if the word is separated in the business name, it should be indexed as separate units. For example, even though the word *interstate* is normally considered one word, for the name *Inter State Listing Service*, *Inter* and *State* would be treated as separate words.

Rule 13: Compound Names Parts of compound business names separated by a space are indexed as individual units. Hyphens are disregarded and the parts are considered as a single unit. Forms of the word *Saint*, such as *San* and *Sainte*, are considered prefixes and are indexed as part of the names that follow. (See Rule 8.)

Rule 14: Coined Words, Unusual Words Coined or unusual words are indexed as written and hyphens are disregarded. For example, the first word of *Shur-Fit Optical* is indexed as *ShurFit*.

Rule 15: Government Names All government agencies, both domestic (in the United States) and foreign, are indexed according to political divisions. Sometimes the words *United States Government* are understood to be part of a name but are not written in the name. They should always be considered as units 1, 2, and 3 for filing purposes. The name of the government body is indexed first (country, state, city) and is followed by the other units in descending order of importance (department, bureau, division, agency). The words *Bureau of*, *Department of*, *County of*, etc., are eliminated unless they are needed for clarity.

For example, the name *State of Georgia Department of Human Resources* would be indexed exactly as it is written. But the name *U.S. Department of Health and Human Services* would be indexed like this: *United States Government* (first, second, and third units), followed by *Health and Human Services, Department of*.

Cross-Referencing

A cross-reference card is used when a name might be indexed in more than one way. Foreign names, names of married women, unusual business names, hyphenated names, multiple business names, abbreviated or single letter names, and names that may be spelled several ways are examples of situations in which a cross-reference card should be made. The original card lists the name that is the most likely means of identification. A second, and perhaps a third card, is used to show other names by which the individual, firm, or agency might be identified.

Alphabetic Filing Guides and Tabs

Primary file guides made of heavy cardboard or plastic are used to identify the broad categories of a file. In an alphabetic file, primary guides usually divide the alphabet into twenty-six sections, one for each letter of the alphabet. The primary guides are placed in the first position of the file shelf (at the top) or file drawer (at the far left). Secondary guides subdivide the alphabet into smaller parts; for example, the primary guide *A* may be subdivided into *Aa–Al* and *Am–Az*. These are placed in second position of the file shelf or drawer. File folders with their individual captions often are placed in third position. For the medical office that wishes to further subdivide folders, guides are available for fourth and fifth positions. File dividers can also be color-coded, thus reducing the need for some of the secondary guides used in the past.

Procedures for Alphabetic Filing

Follow these procedures to ensure easy retrieval of materials filed by alphabetic method.

1. Code the document by underlining the indexing units or by writing the code name in the upper right corner.
2. Cross-reference the document as needed.
3. Locate the correct alphabetic guides in the filing system.
4. File the document and any cross-references.
5. Retrieve the file folder as needed.

Numeric Filing

Numeric filing is a method of filing by number instead of by letter. The numeric method is used in many medical offices to maintain the confidentiality of patient records. A number on a folder tab does not reveal a patient's identity as easily or as directly as the person's name does. In large medical centers and hospitals with many folders, the numeric method is used to make files easier to retrieve.

The Accession Book or Patient Identification Ledger

The **accession book** or **patient identification ledger** provides a conservative record of the numbers and names of all patients. When a new patient visits the medical office, the next available number in the accession book is assigned to that patient, and the person's name is written beside the number. This number identifies the patient and is written on each paper associated with the patient before the paper is filed. For example, lab reports, case histories, letters, or other documents that refer to the patient are coded with the patient's number.

Numeric procedures can also be used in subject and geographic filing systems. Subjects or geographic names are assigned a number; then a list is maintained for each folder name and its identifying number.

Alphabetic Card File

An alphabetic card file containing a card for each patient is an essential part of numeric and alphabetic filing system. Each card lists the patient's full name, address, telephone number, and patient number. Alphabetic cards are stored in a rotary card holder, a card tray, or a card box in alphabetic order according to the patient's last name. When a patient's folder must be retrieved, the patient's card can be located, the patient number identified from the card, and the folder matching the number in the patient files can be located.

In addition, most medical offices maintain a separate file for miscellaneous alphabetic cards. These cards list the names, addresses, and telephone numbers of hospitals, ambulance services, police, research organizations, professional organizations, suppliers, and other physicians.

Numeric File Guides and Tabs

Numeric file guides break numeric files into manageable sections. Folders may be divided into number groups of 1–99, 100–199, 200–299, and so on. Secondary guides placed in second position may be used to subdivide the numbers further. The tabs of individual folders are usually shown in third position. Fourth- and fifth-position folders are available for medical offices requiring them. To maintain confidentiality, the folder tab usually lists only the patient's number, although in some offices the patient's name is also listed. Folders are stored in ascending order with the smaller number in the front.

Miscellaneous Correspondence File

When a numeric system is used for filing medical records, an alphabetic correspondence file is usually maintained for materials not related to patients. These materials contain general information pertaining to the practice, professional organizations, or research. The alphabetic caption on each folder identifies the contents. A separate folder labeled *Miscellaneous* or *Miscellaneous Correspondence* is stored at the back of the file or shelf to hold miscellaneous materials or correspondence involving fewer than five items about a single subject. When five related items accumulate, the medical assistant should prepare a new folder with an appropriate tab caption and then merge it in alphabetic order with the other folders. This is different than with a patient file, which must be made up immediately.

Procedures for Numeric Filing

Follow these procedures when a new patient visits a medical office that uses numeric filing:

1. Assign the next unused number in the accession book to the patient.
2. Complete an alphabetic card for the patient.
3. Prepare a file folder listing the patient number on the tab.
4. Store the folders in ascending order with the other patient folders.

Follow these procedures to retrieve a file:

1. Locate the patient's name in the alphabetic card file and identify the patient's number.
2. Look for the patient's number on the folder tabs of the medical records. Remove the appropriate medical record from the files.
3. Return the folder to the files when there is no further need for it.

Subject Filing

Subject filing is a method of filing by subject titles instead of by individuals' names. Subject titles are used in medical offices to identify diseases, research, treatments, drugs, and other areas of interest to the physician. For example, a physician researching children's diseases may use the titles *Diabetes*, *Muscular Dystrophy*, *Heart Disease*, or others. Letters, memos, research reports, and other items from many different sources are stored in the folders.

The business-related activities of a medical office also lend themselves to subject filing. For example, a medical office may have folder tabs labeled *Medicare*, *Medicaid*, *Workers' Compensation*, *Blue Cross/Blue Shield*, or others. Usually subject files are stored alphabetically; however, a number may be assigned to each subject so the folders can be filed by the numeric method.

Materials filed by subject often need to be cross-referenced because all individuals do not think in the same terms. For example, a letter about research on skin disease might be filed by the subject title. *Skin Disease* and cross-referenced under the letter writer's name.

Geographic Filing

Geographic filing is a method of filing by geographic area instead of by a person's name or by a subject. Often geographic and subject methods are used together. Although most medical offices do not use geographic files, they are useful in medical research centers to identify regions of the country in which research is being conducted. For example, the geographic method might be used to identify states or regions in which research into allergies is being conducted. Geographic materials may be stored by the alphabetic or numeric methods.

Cross-referencing is also important to the geographic system. This is because all individuals who use the materials may not think in terms of the same geographic areas.

Research Files

Medical research is filed according to either the subject or geographic methods. Research about allergies, for example, might be filed according to the name of the allergy, such as *hay fever* or *poison ivy*, or according to the geographic areas of the country where the allergy is found. Sometimes both the subject and geographic methods are used in a research file. Whichever method is used, the categories are arranged in alphabetic order.

THE MEDICAL ASSISTANT'S ROLE IN RECORD KEEPING

Managing a system of medical records that meets medical, administrative, ethical, and legal requirements is a very important task. If you are the medical assistant entrusted with this responsibility, you must conscientiously maintain complete, accurate, and up-to-date records. Follow these procedures for managing patients' records:

1. Chart or file all information about patients every day.
2. Show all new information to the physician for reading and initialing.
3. Shingle records less than 8.5" × 11".
4. File all materials in the correct file.
5. Place correspondence about patients in their medical records and unrelated correspondence in the *Miscellaneous Correspondence* file.

IN YOUR OPINION

1. How is a paper file system similar to a computer database?
2. Why is cross-referencing essential?
3. How would the filing needs of a general practice and a research institution differ?

INTERNET ACTIVITY

Log on to the Internet and locate a supplier of alphabetic and numeric filing systems. Summarize the system's attributes. If special supplies or cabinets are required, list the requirements.

STUDENT STUDY CHECKLIST

Workbook

1. Complete Chapter 11 exercises in the workbook.
2. Complete Chapter 11 simulations in the workbook that access the CD-ROM in the back of the book.

Administrative Skills CD-ROM

1. Go to the Library on the CD-ROM and play the interactive games for Chapter 11.
2. Go to the Medical Records area of the office and click on the medical records folder on the desk. Perform the exercises.
3. Explain how the four elements of the SOAP progress record work together to give physicians a quick overview of a patient's status.

REFERENCES

Fordney, Marilyn T. and Joan J. Follis. *Administrative Medical Assisting*, 4th ed. Clifton Park, NY: Delmar Learning, 1998.

Lindh, Wilburta Q., Marilyn S. Pooler, and Carol D. Tamparo. *Administrative Medical Assisting*, 2nd ed. Clifton Park, NY: Delmar Learning, 2002.

Rowell, JoAnn C. and Michelle A. Green. *Understanding Health Insurance*, 6th ed. Clifton Park, NY: Delmar Learning, 2002.

CHAPTER ACTIVITIES

PERFORMANCE-BASED ACTIVITIES

1. Refer to the sample color coding system in Figure 11–3. On 3" × 5" cards, color code the names of the following patients. Use colored markers to produce the colors needed. Then file the cards in correct alphabetic order.

   a. Jeff Ramsey Hight

   b. Cynthia Givens

   c. Mrs. William (Marian) Highers

   d. Gregory Eaton, Jr.

   e. Samuel Higgens

   f. Tara Handley

   g. Melinda Headley

   h. Saratina Handley

   i. Tina Hardley

   j. Gregory Eaton, Sr.

2. Log on to the Internet and find an article about numeric filing in a medical office. Write a summary of why you think numeric filing is popular.

3. Summarize an article from the Internet about trends in medical record keeping.

EXPANDING YOUR THINKING

1. Keeping in mind the type of information maintained today in paper medical records and the type of information stored in computerized medical records, indicate with a "P" or "C" the following items most likely to be found in a paper record or computerized record where stored.

   Information

   a. The names of all children given a particular drug.

   b. The insurance policy numbers of several patients.

   c. A patient's blood pressure reading from the previous visit.

   d. The results of a urine test.

   e. The zip codes of all patients.

   f. A letter to a consulting physician about a specific patient.

2. What three groups of people are served by well-maintained medical records? How is each served?

3. What is the significance of alphabetic filing in a numeric filing system?

4. Determine the correct filing order for the following names.

Susan Van der Croft

V. Crandell

Victoria Crandell

Darlene Vanderbilt

Darlene Vandercroft

V. Anderson

Van Andrews

PART IV

Automating Medical Office Financial Management

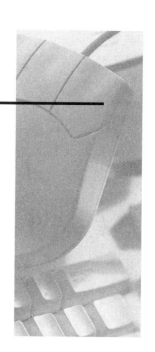

inancial management is a challenge for many physicians. They generally go into the practice of medicine to provide healing services and treatments, yet they operate their practices in a competitive, fee-driven business climate where large insurance companies frequently control what they can charge.

This difficult financial climate combined with the rapidly accelerating cost of medical malpractice insurance puts physicians in the uncomfortable position of trying to serve two masters: the patient and the financial system.

CHAPTER 12

Pegboard Accounting and Computerized Account Management

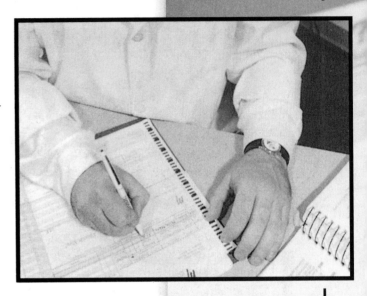

ANNAPOLIS, MARYLAND

Whenever my friends ask why I enjoy my bookkeeping responsibilities as a medical assistant, I tell them my work is absolutely vital to the success of the practice. If we don't know how much money we have to spend or if we don't keep proper payroll records to pass along to the Internal Revenue Service, we will be in trouble.

Another reason that I find working with the books so satisfying is that the work is organized, neat, and comprehensible. Reconciling the books every month can range from being a five-minute exercise of filling in the blanks and adding and subtracting until my figure and the bank's figure agree; or it can be twenty minutes of playing detective to see why there's a difference. Figuring out the mystery is a reward itself — like a crossword puzzle with numbers.

At the same time, I enjoy the precision of keeping our payroll system up to date and working with our accountant. In a way, I think I've got the best of both worlds. I'm definitely working in a field I love — medicine — but I'm also learning basic accounting principles that already have helped me in my personal life. Don't turn your head on numbers. They're important, and being able to handle them helps a medical assistant make an important contribution to the practice.

Jack O'Hara
Medical Assistant

PERFORMANCE-BASED COMPETENCIES

After completing this chapter, you should be able to:
 1. Describe pegboard bookkeeping system.

2. Describe the process of financial management in a medical office.
3. Apply bookkeeping principles.
4. Document and maintain accounting and banking records.
5. Process payroll.
6. Follow federal, state, and local legal guidelines.

VOCABULARY

Balance   The amount of money in a checking account at any given moment.

Charge slip   Receipt listing the typical examinations, procedures, treatments, and services a patient might have during one visit.

Check register   The record book in which all information about checks is recorded.

Current Procedural Terminology (CPT)   Industry coding standard recognized by most insurance companies and widely used in medical offices to identify procedures and services performed.

Daily log   The day's summary of patient transactions.

Electronic fund transfer   Using computer networks to move money from one bank account to another.

FICA   Federal Insurance Contribution Act; set up by the social security retirement system. Social Security deductions are called FICA deductions.

Form W-2   The form sent by every employer to every employee, with copies to the IRS and state government, summarizing the year's gross income, tax deductions, and net income.

Form W-4   The employee's withholding allowance certificate, filled out at the beginning of employment and whenever exemptions change, listing the exemptions from taxation that the employee is claiming.

ICD codes   Diagnosis codes from the *International Classification of Diseases*, Tenth Edition, used to identify the patient's medical problem.

Ledger card   Chronological listing of one family's financial activity with the practice.

Overdraft   A check written for an amount that exceeds the balance of the account the check is drawn on. When such a check is not honored — paid — by a bank, it is said to have bounced. A bounced check is an overdraft that comes back to the person who drafted it.

Pegboard accounting   Traditional method of maintaining accounts, named for the flat writing board on which accounting papers are prepared.

Practice analysis   Overview of procedures and treatments provided and income derived during a specified period.

Proof of posting   Verification of the calculation of columns in the daily log.

Reconciliation   The monthly task of ascertaining that the practice's determination of the amount of its account balance agrees with the balance arrived at by the bank.

PEGBOARD ACCOUNTING

The financial success of any practice depends on accurate and timely financial record keeping. If you are asked to handle patient accounts, you must have a good understanding of bookkeeping, a mind for details, and the ability to complete tasks on time.

The paper method of maintaining accounts is called pegboard accounting, named for the flat writing board with attached pegs on which accounting papers are prepared.

Pegboard accounting refers to a simple "write-it-once" method of record keeping. Carbonized or no-carbon-required accounting papers are placed on top of one another, so that any charge or payment posted one time with a hard-tipped ball point pen will imprint on all sheets beneath the original. Posting to several records in one writing reduces the probability of error and saves valuable employee time.

Pegboard Accounting Components

Pegboard accounting systems are available from most medical office supply companies. Although these systems vary slightly according to the manufacturer, all of them consist of the actual writing board and three basic components: (1) the patient charge slip, (2) the ledger card, and (3) the daily log. In addition, a check register accompanies most systems. A typical pegboard is a hard writing board with pegs along the side or top as shown in Figure 12–1. At the beginning of each day, a daily log is placed over the pegs to prepare for the first patient.

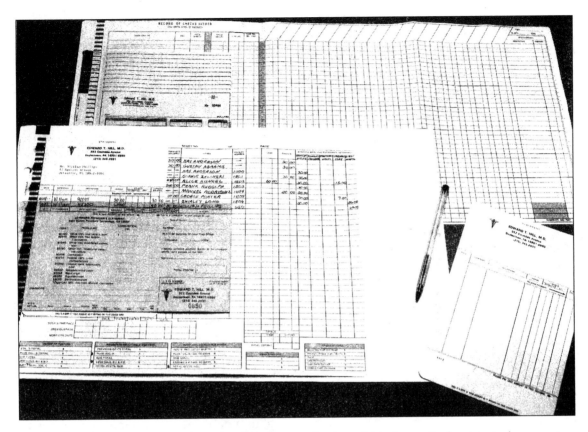

FIGURE 12–1 A good understanding of pegboard accounting is useful to the medical assistant who uses a computerized accounting system.

When a patient checks in, the medical assistant retrieves the person's ledger card from a file and places it on top of the daily log, then places a pad of sequentially numbered patient charge slips on the pegs. With three items in place on the pegs, the medical assistant writes the date, the patient's name, the previous balance, and the account number, if used, on the charge slip. All this information is automatically posted through the carbon to the ledger card and daily log beneath. This process is repeated each time a different patient registers for an appointment.

At the end of the day, the daily log lists transactions for all patients seen during the day. The ledger cards are up to date and a patient charge slip, which serves as a bill — or a receipt if the patient pays — has been given to each patient. The bank deposits and day totals can also be developed from the entries.

Charge Slip or Receipt

The charge slip or receipt lists the typical examinations, procedures, treatments, and services that match each *Current Procedural Terminology* code printed on the charge slip. Charge slips are individualized by specialty. The services and procedures codes shown for a family physician are different from the listings for a urologist, cardiologist, or other specialist. ICD *(International Classification of Diseases)* diagnosis codes are also printed on charge slips in some offices, because Medicare and most insurance providers require these codes to document claims. A patient charge slip is shown in Figure 12–2.

A comprehensive charge slip can be used to document an insurance claim. When accompanied by a partially completed claim form, it will be accepted in place of the fully completed form, saving time for both the patient and the medical assistant.

After a patient's name and other information are written on a charge slip, the slip is clipped to the medical record and follows the patient from the time of registration until after the examination is completed. During the examination, the physician marks (/) or circles the appropriate code on

				(f)		(g)		(h)		(a)		
2/11/--	Heather	NP, TT, VT, HT	128	00				128	00	0	00	Gibbs
DATE	PATIENT	PROFESSIONAL SERVICES	TODAY'S CHARGE		PAYMENT		CURRENT BALANCE		PREVIOUS BALANCE			NAME

PATIENT CHARGE SLIP

OFFICE CARE	CPT-4*	HYPO-THETICAL FEE
1. Brief Service	90040	
2. Limited Service	90050	
3. Intermediate Service	90060	
4. Extended Service	90070	
5. Comprehensive Service— Established Patient, Complete Examination	90080	
⑥ New Patient—Initial Care, Complete Examination	90020 (b)	75.00
7. Emergency—Acute Illness	99058	
8. Emergency—After Hours	99050	
9. Telephone Consultation	99013	
10. Prenatal Conference	99078	
11.		
12.		

HOSPITAL CARE		
thru		
15. Newborn—Initial Service	90285	
16. Limited Service	90250	
17. Extended Service	90270	
18. Comprehensive Service	90280	
19. Emergency Room	99062	
20.		
21.		

OFFICE PROCEDURES	CPT-4*	HYPO-THETICAL FEE
24. Diphtheria, Pertussis, Tetanus	90701	
25. Diphtheria, Tetanus	90702	
26. Trivalent Oral Polio	90712	
27. Measles, Mumps, Rubella	90707	
㉘ Tuberculin Tine	86585 (c)	8.00
29. Developmental Testing	90774	
30. Epinephrine Injection	90782	
31. Allergy Injection	95120	
32. Allergy Testing	95000	
㉝ Vision Testing	92002 (d)	20.00
㉞ Hearing Testing	92552 (e)	25.00
35. Tympanometry	92567	
36. Sutures		
37. Injection		
38.		
39.		

HOSPITAL CARE		
45. Urinalysis	81000	
46. Infant PKU—Thyroid	84030	
47. Hematocrit	85014	
48. Complete Blood Count	85022	
49. Throat Culture	87060	
50. Urine Culture	87086	
51.		

SYMPTOMS: _Red, watery eyes; nasal congestion_

DIAGNOSIS: _Allergic diathesis_

INSTRUCTIONS: _____

RETURN: _____ Days _____ Weeks _____ Months

PEDIATRIC ASSOCIATES, P.C.
8412 Northlake Professional Center
Atlanta, GA 30345-2691
(404) 823-2403

ELAINE H. LYNN, M.D.
Tax ID No. 21-0850852
SS No. 416-84-8948

8101

*Copyright 1985. Americal Medical Association

FIGURE 12–2 Patient charge slip

the charge slip to indicate the procedure or treatment performed and designates when the patient should return for a follow-up appointment. When the examination is complete, the physician gives the charge slip to the patient, nurse, or medical assistant. The medical assistant calculates the charges.

The charge slip is replaced in its original position on top of the daily log, then the ledger card is inserted between the charge slip and daily log. As the charges, payments, adjustments, and the current balance are recorded in the proper columns of the charge slip, the information is posted simultaneously to the ledger card and the daily log beneath.

Ledger Card

The ledger card is a summary of one family's account with the practice and lists chronologically all financial activity for the account over a period of time. Each time a family member visits the physician, the medical assistant retrieves the ledger card, inserts it between the charge slip and daily log on the pegboard, and records information about the visit on a new line of the card. When all the lines of a ledger card are filled, a new ledger card is stapled to the first so there is no break in the chronological listings.

The following information is automatically recorded on a ledger card when a charge slip is completed: (1) the date of service, (2) the patient's name, (3) the professional service rendered, (4) the charge, (5) any payment or adjustment credits, and (6) the new balance.

The medical assistant also records payments made by mail and charges for hospital visits on the ledger card.

In some small offices, the ledger card is also used as a billing statement, and the word "Statement" appears at the top of the card instead of the word Ledger Card. At the end of the billing period, a photocopy of the card is made and mailed to the responsible person. More often, however, payment is required at the time of the visit, or a computerized statement is developed and mailed by the physician's billing service. A partial ledger card is shown in Figure 12–3.

Daily Log

The daily log is a summary of the medical office's daily financial activity. A separate log is started every morning. During the day, as each charge

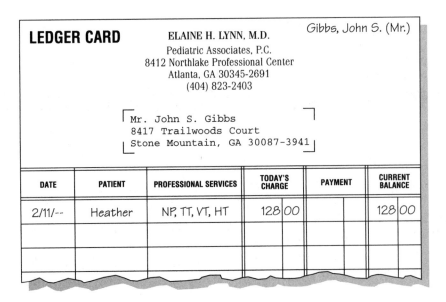

FIGURE 12–3 Partial ledger card

slip is aligned over the daily log and completed, information is transferred automatically to the daily log. In addition, mail payments and hospital charges are transferred to the daily log when they are recorded on the ledger card. At the end of each day, the daily log shows a complete picture of all charges, payments and adjustments, and outstanding balances for each patient. After each column is totaled, a summary of the day's

financial activity is provided. A partial daily log is shown in Figure 12–4.

Accounts Receivable Control

Accounts receivable provide a good measure of a practice's financial health because they show the amount of money its patients owe. When accounts receivable are too large, cash flow is

DAILY LOG

ELAINE H. LYNN, M.D.

DATE	PATIENT	PROFESSIONAL SERVICES	TODAY'S CHARGE		PAYMENT		CURRENT BALANCE		PREVIOUS BALANCE		NAME
2/11/--	Pat	OV, TOPV	34	00			34	00	0	00	O'Meara
2/11/--	Lucinda	OV	35	00			35	00	0	00	Jensen
2/11/--	Heather	NP, TT, VT, HT	128	00			128	00	0	00	Gibbs
2/5-2/11--	Matthew	HV	245	00			325	00	80	00	Wiley
TOTALS											

FIGURE 12–4 Partial daily log

low and the practice may have difficulty paying its bills. In this event, the practice must make a greater effort to collect a portion of the outstanding balances. Collection procedures are discussed in Chapter 13.

Daily Cash Paid-Outs

From time to time, the office will need cash for minor office expenses. A petty cash fund of $50 to $75 is usually set aside for this purpose. When money from petty cash is spent, a note should be made on the daily log indicating the amount and the purpose of the payment. Always keep receipts from purchases for tax purposes.

Cash Control

Maintaining a daily summary of cash collected and paid out is important, because cash that is unaccounted for can disrupt the office's financial records. All cash over the amount kept in the petty cash fund should be deposited in the bank each day. Individuals handling cash should be bonded. Ask your insurance carrier how you can become bonded; this is usually a matter of paying an additional insurance premium.

Business Analysis Summaries

Some daily logs provide space for business analysis summaries, allowing for a breakdown of fees according to service or procedure performed or according to the service's provider. For example, the information that was transferred from the patient's charge slips and the columns where the transactions are broken down according to the provider of the service could be reviewed. (Each transaction is probably listed under one of the physician's names.) In a group practice, this information provides a quick means of analyzing each physician's contribution to the practice in terms of daily fees. The breakdown can also show other summaries, for example, a summary of the services provided each day, including office visits, periodic examinations, laboratory, allergy injections, x-rays, surgery, and diagnostic services.

BANKING

Among the many vital tasks of medical office management are banking and payroll. A medical assistant needs to be able to manage a bookkeeping system that allows practice members to tell at a glance which services, treatments, and procedures are the most profitable and which are the least profitable. Monitoring cash flow is vital to the success of the practice. It lets the practice know how much money is available at any time to meet expenses.

The system will be successful if it is built with attention to detail. This means accounting for all checks written against the practice account as well as all deposits made into it. At years' end these records will provide a vital database for filing tax returns.

ACCEPTING CHECKS

Several guidelines should be followed when receiving checks. A list is provided for your information:

- Inspect the check for correct date, amount, and signature.
- Do not accept a third-party check from anyone other than an insurance company (a check made out to the patient from someone else).
- Call the bank that returns a check marked "Insufficient Funds." If funds are available, redeposit the check. If the check is returned a second time, alert the patient.

Daily Deposits

All checks and all cash in excess of the petty cash fund should be deposited in the bank each day. They should be endorsed "For Deposit Only" as soon as they are received. A deposit slip is shown in Figure 12–5.

Procedures for Preparing Deposit Slips

1. Count the currency and coins and compare the tally with the total from the Cash column of the daily log. Record the total amount of cash to be deposited in the Cash column of the bank deposit slip (for example, $85).

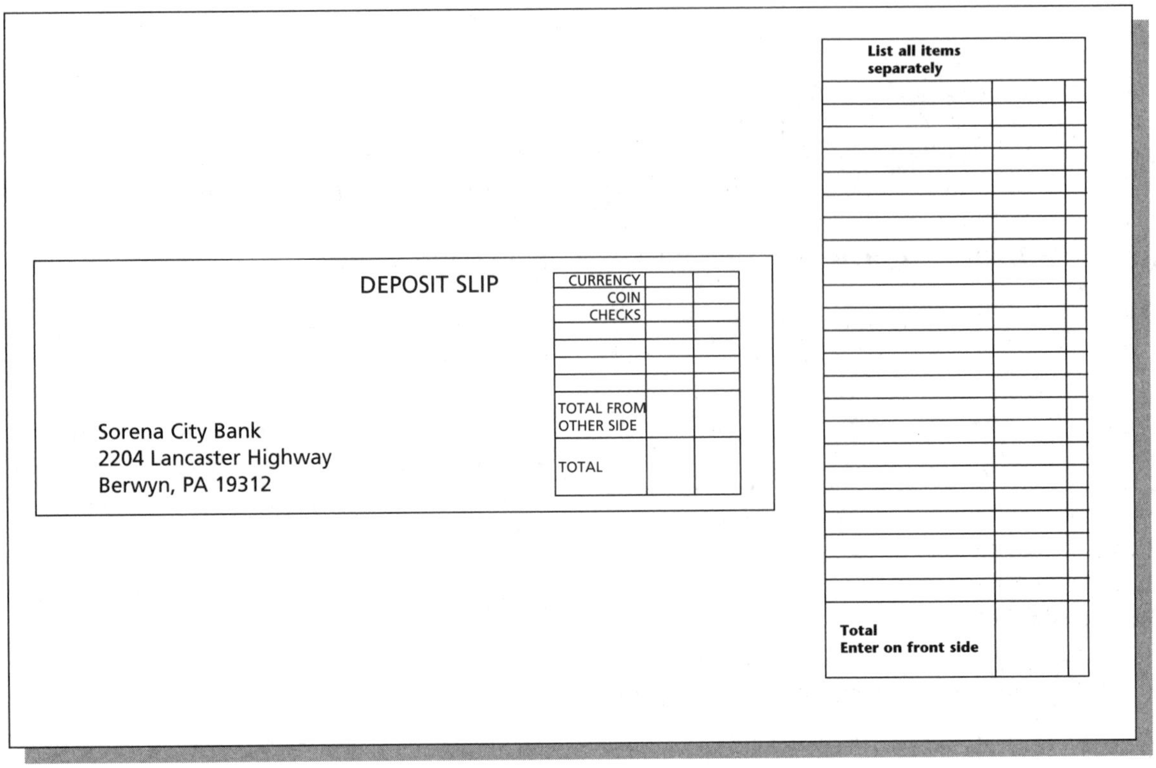
List all items separately

Total
Enter on front side

DEPOSIT SLIP

CURRENCY		
COIN		
CHECKS		
TOTAL FROM OTHER SIDE		
TOTAL		

Sorena City Bank
2204 Lancaster Highway
Berwyn, PA 19312

FIGURE 12–5 Deposit slip

2. Write the receipt number from the patient's charge slip for the first check to be listed. When there is no charge slip, write the name of the company or individual on whose account the check is drawn. Some physicians prefer to identify checks by the name of the person on whose accounts the check was drawn.
3. Write the American Banking Association (ABA) number that identifies the bank on which each check is drawn in the next column of the form. This number is usually printed in the upper right corner of checks and is the top number of a two-part number divided by a horizontal line.
4. Write the amount of each check.
5. Total the Cash and Checks column of the deposit slip. Compare this total with the Credits section from the daily log. If adjustments are shown for any patients, subtract them from the Credit section before the comparison is made, because adjustments are credits that do not involve an exchange of money. For example, an adjustment for an overcharge would not be included on the deposit slip.

Checks and Check Register Management

As a medical assistant you will be called on to prepare checks for the practitioner's signature and enter information about the check on the stub in the **check register**, as well as keeping a running tabulation of the balance of money remaining in the checking account. This is not a complicated procedure, but attention must be paid to details.

Get in the habit of always filling out the check stub first — before writing the check itself. That will make it impossible for you to make an error of omission — writing a check and forgetting to record it. Interruptions happen that can make you forget an important task like this; posting the check to the register as a first step protects against this.

With the exception of computing the new balance to be brought forward after the amount of the check has been subtracted, the information you will record in the register is the same as that which you place on the check. This allows you to look at the register and know everything about the check: its number, date, amount, who it is made out to, and what it is for. Most check registers are nothing but forms in which you fill in the blanks. Suppose that you are about to write a check to pay a bill of $822.24 from the Main Line Diagnostic Clinic. Suppose also that the balance of the checking account (the balance brought forward) is $5,280.88. To post the check in the ledger and to write the check, follow these steps, shown as completed in Figure 12–6.

Ledger Entries

- Enter the check number.
- Enter the date.
- From the previous transaction in the ledger, enter the Balance Carried Forward amount ($5,280.88) in the Balance Brought Forward line.
- On the Pay To line enter the name of the firm or person (the Payee) that the check is being written to (Main Line Diagnostic Clinic).
- Enter the purpose of the check on the For line (clinical testing services, month of July).
- Enter the amount of this payment.
- Subtract the amount of the check from the Total ($5,280.88 minus $822.24).
- Enter the new balance ($4,458.64) in the Balance Carried Forward line.

Check Entries

- Enter the check number, if it is not already printed on the check.
- Fill in the date line with the current date.
- On the "Pay to the Order of" line, put the name of the payee (Main Line Diagnostic Clinic).
- To guard against mistakes, the amount of the check is written twice, once as a number and once in words. So, next to the dollar sign, enter the amount of the check ($822.24), and then on the line ending in the word "Dollars," write out the amount of the check, expressing any change as a fraction of a dollar: "eight hundred twenty-two and 24/100." Draw a line to the word "Dollar" for security to prevent others from changing the amount.
- On the line beginning with For, write the purpose of the check (clinical testing services, July).

Many practices still rely on a hand-entered ledger system to maintain a record of income and expenses. But a growing majority rely on computer-driven systems that write checks, automatically debit appropriate bank accounts, post the debit to the ledger and, if it is a business expense, also post the debit to the tax preparation program for use when tax returns are prepared. Still other practices contract out all of their financial systems to expert consultants who handle everything from accounting for expenses and managing payroll.

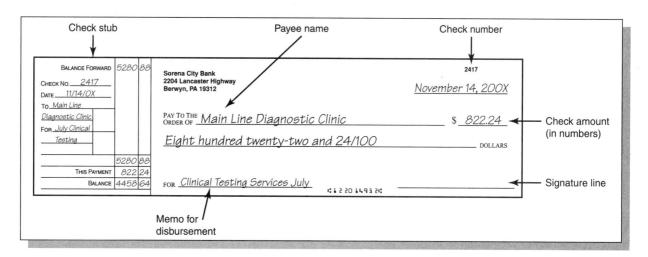

FIGURE 12–6 Check and check stub from check register

Whatever systems you encounter in your career, you will need basic grounding in the fundamentals that underlie financial management systems. These fundamentals include paying bills for rent, telephone, electricity, supplies, the Internet, lab tests, consults with other physicians, and equipment. All of these expenses need to be recorded and classified. And patients have to be billed. Maintaining patient's accounts on a current basis will likely occupy a majority of your time in the financial area; still, you may be called on to manage the practice's checkbook, including making deposits and reconciling office records of expenses and deposits with the bank's monthly statement.

Reconciling a Bank Statement

Reconciliation allows you to be confident, before you write a check (or draft, as it is sometimes called), of how much money is in the practice's account. The last thing you want to do is write an **overdraft**, where there are insufficient funds in the account to cover the amount of the check. Whatever money is in the account is called the **balance**.

The object of reconciliation is to ensure that the practice's assessment of the balance, and the bank's assessment, agree. Reconciling is done to eliminate differences — to determine the reasons for the differences. The statement received from the bank reflects the bank's assessment of the account balance as of a certain date. Money you have deposited after that date, and checks that have been written after it, are not included in the reconciliation of that month's statement; they will be part of the following month's reconciliation.

You will find that in the vast majority of cases where there is a discrepancy between the balance shown by the bank and the balance shown in the office check ledger, it is the bank that is correct. So, by and large, reconciliation is an opportunity for you (the practice) to learn where you have made an error — by not recording a check or a deposit, or by having recorded an amount incorrectly, or adding or subtracting incorrectly.

The practice you join, or the bank it deals with, will have a form designed to make reconciliation a matter-of-fact and simple process.

Basically, the process begins with your entering the current checkbook balance, which your records show. Then, any fees charged by the bank (shown on the bank's statement) are deducted from the checkbook balance. The new balance is called the Adjusted Checkbook Balance. Your job is to make the Adjusted Checkbook Balance and the Bank Statement Balance match. A reconciliation form is shown in Figure 12–7.

1. Start by writing the bank's Ending Balance from the front of the bank statement.
2. Add to it any deposits that have been made but which are not shown on the bank's statement.
3. Add these two amounts to obtain a Subtotal.
4. List all outstanding checks that have been written. Outstanding checks are those you have recorded in the ledger and have subtracted from the account balance but that had not been processed by the bank at the time the statement was issued.
5. Write the total of all outstanding checks. Subtract this total from the Subtotal in Item 3.
6. This new total is the Adjusted Bank Balance. If everything is well, the Adjusted Bank Statement Balance and the Adjusted Checkbook Balance will be the same amount and reconciliation has been successful.

Electronic Banking

Because the largest part of electronic banking is completed by computer programs, as a medical assistant you will not have to "operate" electronic banking procedures. You will have to understand the money transfer concepts underlying them, and be able use them. If you have a bank debit card that you can use at an automated teller machine (ATM), every time you use that card you are interfacing with a part of the electronic banking system.

As computer technology became increasingly sophisticated and efficient, it became apparent to people in the banking industry that it would be less costly to them to "move" money — transfer funds — from one account to another if it could be done electronically instead of using checks and other paper instruments. **Electronic fund transfers** (EFT) are at the heart of electronic

Front

Summary of Account Balance			Closing Date 1/15/0X		

Account # 1257-164013 — Ending Balance $8,347.62

Beginning Balance		$7,152.18
Total Deposits and Additions		$8,643.86
Total Withdrawals		$7,433.21
Service Charge		$ 15.24

Number	Date	Amount	Number	Date	Amount
201	12/18/0X	173.82	234	1/4/0X	96.31
223*	12/18/0X	44.12	235	1/4/0X	73.48
224	12/20/0X	586.00	236	1/6/0X	325.40
225	12/21/0X	24.15	237	1/7/0X	40.00
236	12/22/0X	33.90	238	1/8/0X	66.77
228*	12/23/0X	1250.00	241*	1/9/0X	15.55
229	12/24/0X	11.75	242	1/10/0X	12.45
230	12/24/0X	19.02	243	1/10/0X	4441.25
231	1/2/0X	43.80	244	1/10/0X	64.55
232	1/3/0X	39.00			
233	1/4/0X	71.50			

*Denotes gap in check sequence

Date	Deposit Amount	Date	Deposit Amount
18-Dec	361.75	4-Jan	825.00
19-Dec	586.00	5-Jan	1286.71
20-Dec	918.21	7-Jan	608.00
21-Dec	201.00	8-Jan	811.15
2-Jan	475.00	9-Jan	1092.68
3-Jan	1478.36.		

Reconciliation form

1. Enter Ending Balance from the front of this statement
$____8,347.62____

2. Enter deposit not shown on this statement
$____3,162.50____

3. Subtotal (add 1 & 2)
$____11,510.12____

4. List outstanding checks or other withdrawals here

Check #	Amount
222	37.89
227	161.15
229	11.50
240	92.12
245	835.17
246	21.75
247	586.00

5. Total outstanding checks
$____1,745.58____

6. Balance (subtract #5 from #3)
$____9,764.54____
This should equal your checkbook balance

FIGURE 12–7 Bank statement and reconciliation form

banking. EFT allows funds to be moved from one account to another (from your bank account, for instance, to the electric company).

Here is a thumbnail overview of four electronic banking systems that you may encounter in your work as a medical assistant.

1. *Automated teller machines.* ATMs are everywhere. By inserting or swiping a plastic card containing an electronically readable stripe and entering the personal identification number (PIN) associated with that card, the user can access her account to make a cash withdrawal, obtain the account balance as of that day, make a deposit, and make payments to companies that are part of the electronic banking system.

2. *Electronic deposits and payments.* More and more businesses, including medical practices, are using the electronic banking system for a variety of fund transfer tasks. If your bank and your practice's bank are linked on the system, it is possible for the practice to arrange to have your paycheck automatically transferred from the practice's account to yours at the end of every pay period. This automatic transfer eliminates checkwriting at the office, depositing the check by you, and handling it by the bank (most banks charge extra for person-to-person transactions). You will get a paper record of your pay and year-to-date history. Similarly, the practice may choose to pay monthly bills, such as for utilities and insurance, automatically. All of these transactions are recorded by the bank and appear in the monthly statement.

3. *Sale transfers.* If the practice needs supplies faster than an order can be placed and the delivery made, a medical assistant may be asked to go out, and using the practice's bank card and knowing the PIN, get the needed goods. Using the card in the store is a lot like using it at an ATM. Funds are automatically and instantly transferred from the practice's account to that of the vendor.

4. *Telephone payments.* Once in place, this system allows the user to telephone the bank and tell it to transfer funds from one account to another or to pay prearranged bills.

PAYROLL ACCOUNTING PROCEDURES

Whether the practice you join has computerized its payroll accounting process or still relies on a manual system, the principles involved remain the same. As a medical assistant, the odds are you will have some payroll responsibilities during your career. Under federal, state, and local tax laws employers are required to keep ongoing records of all of their own transactions, including the payroll records of each of its employees. These records provide the basis for income and Social Security tax assessments. Additionally, businesses are required to pay payroll taxes and withhold and manage the federal, state, and local withholding taxes of its employees.

Federal and State Withholding Taxes

Among the first things a new employee is asked to do on joining an organization is to fill out a **Form W-4** (Employee's Withholding Allowance Certificate Figure 12–8). The form allows the employee to claim exemptions from the withholding tax. The withholding mechanism is the government's way of making sure that the taxes that will be due at the end of the year are automatically set aside on a paycheck-by-paycheck basis. The amount of money withheld from anyone's salary is determined by a formula that is designed to take more taxes from high income earners and less taxes from low income earners. Each exemption claimed on Form W-4 allows the earner to exempt from income a sum of money for each dependent claimed. The wage earner can claim an exemption for herself, for a spouse (if the spouse is not employed), and for children.

It is the responsibility of the medical practice to handle the withholding. So, whenever the number of exemptions changes for an employee, the employer needs to obtain a revised Form W-4. The practice then files that form with the Internal Revenue Service. The practice also keeps a copy to be used when computing and recording payroll and taxes each pay period. Actually, the computing of taxes is more a matter of reading an Internal Revenue Service chart, "Circular E, Employer's Tax Guide." The guide is a series of tables that allow employers to identify an employee's tax liability based on earnings for the pay period and the number of deductions claimed. As the guide changes from year to year, request a current copy from the practice's accountant.

Social Security Taxes

Employers are also required to withhold Social Security payments from employees' paychecks. Social Security provides a base financial cushion for people who retire. It is contributed to equally by employees and employers, and once again the employer acts as the on-site tax collector. Social Security was established by the Federal Insurance Contributions Act, and so Social Security deductions from pay are often called **FICA** deductions. Employers report their FICA contributions on Form 941. Obtain a copy of the current FICA guide from the practice's accountant.

Miscellaneous Deductions

Other deductions may also be made to an employee's paycheck, if the employee has authorized it. Deductions can include health insurance, disability insurance, and retirement or pension contributions to a 401K or other plan. Here again, the practice manages the deducting and allocating of the money. Statements issued with paychecks itemize and explain the deductions.

The Payroll Register

Increasingly being handled by computer — in which case the medical assistant enters appropriate data — the payroll register is at the heart of payroll record keeping for any practice. The register lists each employee along with the person's pay, hours worked, and taxes and other deductions withheld. In this way, gross earnings, net earnings, and all taxes and deductions are accounted for the pay period (Figure 12–9). Typically, payroll registers are forwarded to the

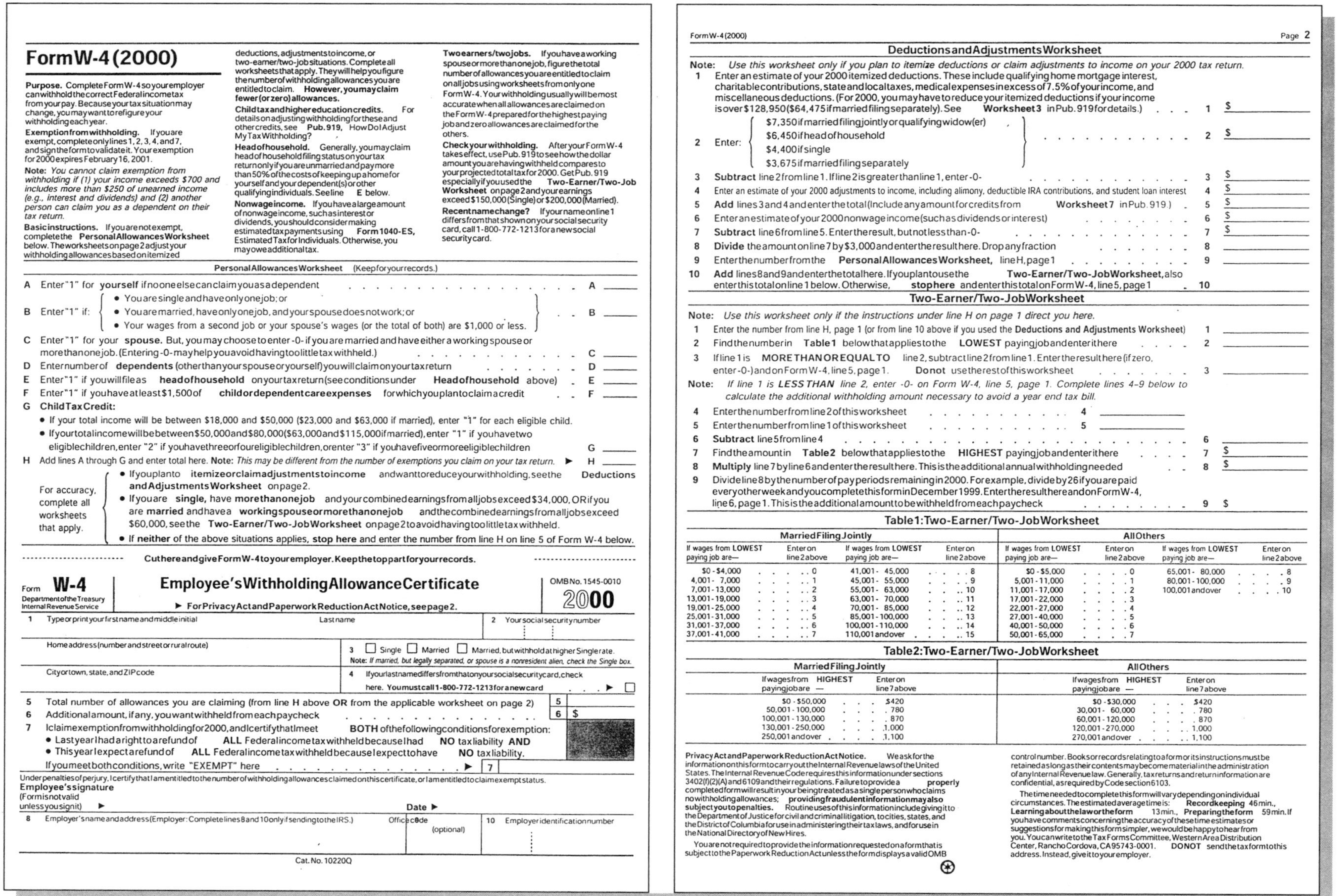

Form W-4 (2000)

Purpose. Complete Form W-4 so your employer can withhold the correct Federal income tax from your pay. Because your tax situation may change, you may want to refigure your withholding each year.

Exemption from withholding. If you are exempt, complete only lines 1, 2, 3, 4, and 7, and sign the form to validate it. Your exemption for 2000 expires February 16, 2001.

Note: *You cannot claim exemption from withholding if (1) your income exceeds $700 and includes more than $250 of unearned income (e.g., interest and dividends) and (2) another person can claim you as a dependent on their tax return.*

Basic instructions. If you are not exempt, complete the **Personal Allowances Worksheet** below. The worksheets on page 2 adjust your withholding allowances based on itemized deductions, adjustments to income, or two-earner/two-job situations. Complete all worksheets that apply. They will help you figure the number of withholding allowances you are entitled to claim. **However, you may claim fewer (or zero) allowances.**

Child tax and higher education credits. For details on adjusting withholding for these and other credits, see **Pub. 919,** How Do I Adjust My Tax Withholding?

Head of household. Generally, you may claim head of household filing status on your tax return only if you are unmarried and pay more than 50% of the costs of keeping up a home for yourself and your dependent(s) or other qualifying individuals. See line **E** below.

Nonwage income. If you have a large amount of nonwage income, such as interest or dividends, you should consider making estimated tax payments using **Form 1040-ES,** Estimated Tax for Individuals. Otherwise, you may owe additional tax.

Two earners/two jobs. If you have a working spouse or more than one job, figure the total number of allowances you are entitled to claim on all jobs using worksheets from only one Form W-4. Your withholding usually will be most accurate when all allowances are claimed on the Form W-4 prepared for the highest paying job and zero allowances are claimed for the others.

Check your withholding. After your Form W-4 takes effect, use Pub. 919 to see how the dollar amount you are having withheld compares to your projected total tax for 2000. Get Pub. 919 especially if you used the **Two-Earner/Two-Job Worksheet** on page 2 and your earnings exceed $150,000 (Single) or $200,000 (Married).

Recent name change? If your name on line 1 differs from that shown on your social security card, call 1-800-772-1213 for a new social security card.

Personal Allowances Worksheet (Keep for your records.)

A Enter "1" for **yourself** if no one else can claim you as a dependent . . . . . A ____

B Enter "1" if: { • You are single and have only one job; or • You are married, have only one job, and your spouse does not work; or • Your wages from a second job or your spouse's wages (or the total of both) are $1,000 or less. } . . B ____

C Enter "1" for your **spouse.** But, you may choose to enter -0- if you are married and have either a working spouse or more than one job. (Entering -0- may help you avoid having too little tax withheld.) . . . C ____

D Enter number of **dependents** (other than your spouse or yourself) you will claim on your tax return . . . D ____

E Enter "1" if you will file as **head of household** on your tax return (see conditions under **Head of household** above) . E ____

F Enter "1" if you have at least $1,500 of **child or dependent care expenses** for which you plan to claim a credit . . F ____

G **Child Tax Credit:**
- If your total income will be between $18,000 and $50,000 ($23,000 and $63,000 if married), enter "1" for each eligible child.
- If your total income will be between $50,000 and $80,000 ($63,000 and $115,000 if married), enter "1" if you have two eligible children, enter "2" if you have three or four eligible children, or enter "3" if you have five or more eligible children . G ____

H Add lines A through G and enter total here. **Note:** *This may be different from the number of exemptions you claim on your tax return.* ▶ H ____

For accuracy, complete all worksheets that apply.
- If you plan to **itemize or claim adjustments to income** and want to reduce your withholding, see the **Deductions and Adjustments Worksheet** on page 2.
- If you are **single,** have **more than one job** and your combined earnings from all jobs exceed $34,000, OR if you are **married** and have a **working spouse or more than one job** and the combined earnings from all jobs exceed $60,000, see the **Two-Earner/Two-Job Worksheet** on page 2 to avoid having too little tax withheld.
- If **neither** of the above situations applies, **stop here** and enter the number from line H on line 5 of Form W-4 below.

Cut here and give Form W-4 to your employer. Keep the top part for your records.

Form **W-4** — Department of the Treasury, Internal Revenue Service

Employee's Withholding Allowance Certificate

▶ For Privacy Act and Paperwork Reduction Act Notice, see page 2.

OMB No. 1545-0010 **2000**

1 Type or print your first name and middle initial — Last name — 2 Your social security number

Home address (number and street or rural route) — 3 ☐ Single ☐ Married ☐ Married, but withhold at higher Single rate.
Note: *If married, but legally separated, or spouse is a nonresident alien, check the Single box.*

City or town, state, and ZIP code — 4 If your last name differs from that on your social security card, check here. **You must call 1-800-772-1213 for a new card** . . . ▶ ☐

5 Total number of allowances you are claiming (from line H above **OR** from the applicable worksheet on page 2) 5

6 Additional amount, if any, you want withheld from each paycheck . . . 6 $

7 I claim exemption from withholding for 2000, and I certify that I meet **BOTH** of the following conditions for exemption:
- Last year I had a right to a refund of **ALL** Federal income tax withheld because I had **NO** tax liability **AND**
- This year I expect a refund of **ALL** Federal income tax withheld because I expect to have **NO** tax liability.

If you meet both conditions, write "EXEMPT" here . . . ▶ 7

Under penalties of perjury, I certify that I am entitled to the number of withholding allowances claimed on this certificate, or I am entitled to claim exempt status.
Employee's signature
(Form is not valid unless you sign it) ▶ **Date** ▶

8 Employer's name and address (Employer: Complete lines 8 and 10 only if sending to the IRS.) — 9 Office code (optional) — 10 Employer identification number

Cat. No. 10220Q

Form W-4 (2000) Page **2**

Deductions and Adjustments Worksheet

Note: *Use this worksheet only if you plan to itemize deductions or claim adjustments to income on your 2000 tax return.*

1 Enter an estimate of your 2000 itemized deductions. These include qualifying home mortgage interest, charitable contributions, state and local taxes, medical expenses in excess of 7.5% of your income, and miscellaneous deductions. (For 2000, you may have to reduce your itemized deductions if your income is over $128,950 ($64,475 if married filing separately). See **Worksheet 3** in Pub. 919 for details.) . . . 1 $ ____

2 Enter: { $7,350 if married filing jointly or qualifying widow(er) / $6,450 if head of household / $4,400 if single / $3,675 if married filing separately } . . . 2 $ ____

3 **Subtract** line 2 from line 1. If line 2 is greater than line 1, enter -0- . . . 3 $ ____

4 Enter an estimate of your 2000 adjustments to income, including alimony, deductible IRA contributions, and student loan interest 4 $ ____

5 **Add** lines 3 and 4 and enter the total (Include any amount for credits from **Worksheet 7** in Pub. 919.) . 5 $ ____

6 Enter an estimate of your 2000 nonwage income (such as dividends or interest) . . . 6 $ ____

7 **Subtract** line 6 from line 5. Enter the result, but not less than -0- . . . 7 $ ____

8 **Divide** the amount on line 7 by $3,000 and enter the result here. Drop any fraction . . . 8 ____

9 Enter the number from the **Personal Allowances Worksheet,** line H, page 1 . . . 9 ____

10 **Add** lines 8 and 9 and enter the total here. If you plan to use the **Two-Earner/Two-Job Worksheet,** also enter this total on line 1 below. Otherwise, **stop here** and enter this total on Form W-4, line 5, page 1 . 10 ____

Two-Earner/Two-Job Worksheet

Note: *Use this worksheet only if the instructions under line H on page 1 direct you here.*

1 Enter the number from line H, page 1 (or from line 10 above if you used the **Deductions and Adjustments Worksheet**) 1 ____

2 Find the number in **Table 1** below that applies to the **LOWEST** paying job and enter it here . . . 2 ____

3 If line 1 is **MORE THAN OR EQUAL TO** line 2, subtract line 2 from line 1. Enter the result here (if zero, enter -0-) and on Form W-4, line 5, page 1. **Do not** use the rest of this worksheet . . . 3 ____

Note: *If line 1 is **LESS THAN** line 2, enter -0- on Form W-4, line 5, page 1. Complete lines 4–9 below to calculate the additional withholding amount necessary to avoid a year end tax bill.*

4 Enter the number from line 2 of this worksheet . . . 4 ____

5 Enter the number from line 1 of this worksheet . . . 5 ____

6 **Subtract** line 5 from line 4 . . . 6 ____

7 Find the amount in **Table 2** below that applies to the **HIGHEST** paying job and enter it here . . . 7 $ ____

8 **Multiply** line 7 by line 6 and enter the result here. This is the additional annual withholding needed . . 8 $ ____

9 Divide line 8 by the number of pay periods remaining in 2000. For example, divide by 26 if you are paid every other week and you complete this form in December 1999. Enter the result here and on Form W-4, line 6, page 1. This is the additional amount to be withheld from each paycheck . . . 9 $ ____

Table 1: Two-Earner/Two-Job Worksheet

Married Filing Jointly				All Others			
If wages from LOWEST paying job are—	Enter on line 2 above	If wages from LOWEST paying job are—	Enter on line 2 above	If wages from LOWEST paying job are—	Enter on line 2 above	If wages from LOWEST paying job are—	Enter on line 2 above
$0 - $4,000	0	41,001 - 45,000	8	$0 - $5,000	0	65,001 - 80,000	8
4,001 - 7,000	1	45,001 - 55,000	9	5,001 - 11,000	1	80,001 - 100,000	9
7,001 - 13,000	2	55,001 - 63,000	10	11,001 - 17,000	2	100,001 and over	10
13,001 - 19,000	3	63,001 - 70,000	11	17,001 - 22,000	3		
19,001 - 25,000	4	70,001 - 85,000	12	22,001 - 27,000	4		
25,001 - 31,000	5	85,001 - 100,000	13	27,001 - 40,000	5		
31,001 - 37,000	6	100,001 - 110,000	14	40,001 - 50,000	6		
37,001 - 41,000	7	110,001 and over	15	50,001 - 65,000	7		

Table 2: Two-Earner/Two-Job Worksheet

Married Filing Jointly		All Others	
If wages from HIGHEST paying job are —	Enter on line 7 above	If wages from HIGHEST paying job are —	Enter on line 7 above
$0 - $50,000	$420	$0 - $30,000	$420
50,001 - 100,000	780	30,001 - 60,000	780
100,001 - 130,000	870	60,001 - 120,000	870
130,001 - 250,000	1,000	120,001 - 270,000	1,000
250,001 and over	1,100	270,001 and over	1,100

Privacy Act and Paperwork Reduction Act Notice. We ask for the information on this form to carry out the Internal Revenue laws of the United States. The Internal Revenue Code requires this information under sections 3402(f)(2)(A) and 6109 and their regulations. Failure to provide a **properly** completed form will result in your being treated as a single person who claims no withholding allowances; **providing fraudulent information may also subject you to penalties.** Routine uses of this information include giving it to the Department of Justice for civil and criminal litigation, to cities, states, and the District of Columbia for use in administering their tax laws, and for use in the National Directory of New Hires.

You are not required to provide the information requested on a form that is subject to the Paperwork Reduction Act unless the form displays a valid OMB control number. Books or records relating to a form or its instructions must be retained as long as their contents may become material in the administration of any Internal Revenue law. Generally, tax returns and return information are confidential, as required by Code section 6103.

The time needed to complete this form will vary depending on individual circumstances. The estimated average time is: **Recordkeeping** 46 min., **Learning about the law or the form** 13 min., **Preparing the form** 59 min. If you have comments concerning the accuracy of these time estimates or suggestions for making this form simpler, we would be happy to hear from you. You can write to the Tax Forms Committee, Western Area Distribution Center, Rancho Cordova, CA 95743-0001. **DO NOT** send the tax form to this address. Instead, give it to your employer.

FIGURE 12–8 Form W-4

PAYROLL REGISTER FOR PERIOD ENDING: August 31, 20--

EMPLOYEE NAME				EARNINGS			DEDUCTIONS							
	No. of Exempts	Hours Worked	Hourly Rate	Reg. Pay	Over-time	Gross Pay	FICA	Fed Inc. Tax	State Inc. Tax	SDI	Medicare	TOTAL DEDUC.	Check No.	NET PAY
Mary Jo Davis	1-S	90	13.	1144	39.	1183.	73.35	145.	36.51	—	17.15	259.97	554	910.99
Beverly Woo	0-S		Salary	1200		1200.	75.64	145.	39.30	—	17.40	277.34	555	922.66
Harold Bohrn	2-M	88	12.	1056		1056.	65.47	84.	23.46	—	15.31	188.24	556	867.76
Joan Gonzalez	1-M		Salary	1000		1000.	62.00	92.	23.85	—	14.50	192.35	557	807.65

FIGURE 12–9 Payroll register sheet

practice's accounting firm for use in maintaining the practice's books.

Employee Earnings Records

The employee earnings record is a pay period-by pay period, as well as a cumulative record, of each employee's pay history. It is required and is used to provide information for tax returns and Social Security payment contributions. It needs to be updated at the close of every pay period. By January 31 each employer is required to mail out federal Form W-2 to employees and federal and state tax authorities. This form displays an employee's gross and net pay and federal and state tax and Social Security contributions. The employee earnings record is the basis for computing this information. Employees use it as the basis for computing their final federal taxes when they submit their tax returns in April. A W-2 form is shown in Figure 12–10.

IN YOUR OPINION

1. What do you think are the advantages of a computer-based banking/accounting system compared to one that is manually based? Would errors be easier to detect in one compared to the other?
2. What effect do you think an overdraft might have on reconciliation?
3. Do you think electronic banking is desirable or undesirable for a medical practice? Explain your answer.

COMPUTERIZED ACCOUNT MANAGEMENT

Account management is the most widely used computer application in medical offices. Software is used to prepare the patient charge slip, develop medical reports, complete billing statements, and prepare insurance claim forms.

Computerized management of patient accounts can save a medical practice thousands of dollars a year by eliminating costly human errors, accelerating the collection process, and handling routine clerical and accounting activities. Medical assistants are relieved of routine, time-consuming activities such as posting, billing, and collecting.

Patient Accounts

Account management programs automatically create a patient charge slip at the time of each patient's visit and calculate the charges after the physician's examination. The programs also create and update the ledger card, add new names to the list of patients and to the daily log, and transfer data to produce insurance forms, statements, a list of checks received each day, and deposit slips. In addition, the programs age accounts at each billing cycle and create billing statements; usually when patient accounts are computerized, practice collections increase.

On a patient's first visit to the medical office, the individual is asked to complete a personal

a Control number	TAXABLE YEAR		**Copy B To Be Filed With Employee's FEDERAL Tax Return**	
			This information is being furnished to the Internal Revenue Service.	
b Employer's identification number			1 Wages, tips, other compensation	2 Federal income tax withheld
c Employer's name, address, and ZIP code			3 Social security wages	4 Social security tax withheld
			5 Medicare wages and tips	6 Medicare tax withheld
			7 Social security tips	8 Allocated tips
d Employee's social security number			9 Advance EIC payment	10 Dependent care benefits
e Employee's name, address, and ZIP code			11 Nonqualified plans	12 Benefits included in Box 1
			13 See Instrs. for Box 13	14 Other
			15 Statutory employee Deceased Pension plan Legal rep. Deferred compensation	

16 State Employer's state I.D. No.	17 State wages, tips, etc.	18 State income tax	19 Locality name	20 Local wages, tips, etc.	21 Local income tax

Form **W-2** Wage and Tax Statement

Department of the Treasury—Internal Revenue Service
OMB No. 1545-0008

FIGURE 12–10 Form W-2

---

information form (Figure 12–11). This includes the name and address of the person responsible for payment of the account, the name and address of the responsible person's insurance company, and the policy number. Other information, such as whether the account should receive credit messages and finance charges is also entered into the computer. All of this information can be entered quite quickly. After this initial information, charges, payments, and adjustments will be entered as they occur during the course of the patient's care.

Daily Activities

The computer is also useful for managing an office's daily activities. Each day several activities must be completed to ensure that the practice operates efficiently. These activities include:

(1) preparing a daily list of appointments; (2) completing a charge slip, a ledger card, and a portion of the daily log for each patient; and (3) preparing a daily cash and check register.

The Daily List of Appointments

Medical offices that are computerized use software for appointment scheduling. Software can generate a daily list of appointments automatically. If scheduling software is not available, the medical assistant will prepare a daily list of appointments at the end of each day by entering the names and the reason for the appointment from the appointment book in the computer. When the medical assistant enters the first patient's name, the computer supplies the account number, the name or identification number of the physician, and the balance due on the account. A list of the appointments for each physician or

Patient Registration Form

Neil Bliven and Associates • 28 Carpenter Street • Wellings, CO 28495   TODAY'S DATE 2/20/0X

Walson	Randy	R	215-555-0199	215-555-0126
RESPONSIBLE PARTY LAST NAME	FIRST NAME	MI	(AREA CODE) HOME PHONE	(AREA CODE) WORK PHONE

2206 Swede Road	415-00-6214	M	8/04/1951
MAILING ADDRESS	SOCIAL SECURITY NUMBER	SEX	DATE OF BIRTH

Patchwork Iron
EMPLOYER NAME

STREET ADDRESS (IF DIFFERENT)

Radnor	PA	19087	103-B Wayne Lane
CITY	STATE	ZIP CODE	EMPLOYER ADDRESS

Sue Lorelai, MD	Radnor, PA 19087	610-555-0144
REFERRED BY:	EMPLOYER (CITY, STATE, & ZIP)	PHONE

IF YOU HAVE DEPENDENTS WHO ARE ALSO BEING SEEN AS PATIENTS, PLEASE FILL IN:

Bernice Walson	Luanne Walson
FIRST DEPENDENT'S NAME	SECOND DEPENDENT'S NAME

4/2/??	F	Wife	813-00-7182	9/10/1990	F	Daughter	813-00-9062
DATE OF BIRTH	SEX	RELATIONSHIP	SOC. SECURITY #	DATE OF BIRTH	SEX	RELATIONSHIP	SOC. SECURITY #

Worthline Foods	215-555-0199	Wenn School	610-555-0190
EMPLOYER OR SCHOOL	PHONE	EMPLOYER OR SCHOOL	PHONE

Frazer, PA 19301	212 Lincoln Lane, Radnor, PA 19087
ADDRESS OF EMPLOYER OR SCHOOL	ADDRESS OF EMPLOYER OR SCHOOL

INSURANCE INFORMATION: (YOU DO NOT NEED TO FILL IN ADDRESS IF YOUR INSURANCE IS MEDICARE, MEDICAID, CHAMPUS, OR BC/BS)

Metropolitan Ins.	MI-246-9012	62401
NAME OF PRIMARY INSURANCE COMPANY	IDENTIFICATION #	GROUP NAME AND/OR #

1043 West End Ave.	NY	NY	10023	212-555-0147
ADDRESS	CITY	STATE	ZIP CODE	PHONE

Rainey Walson				
INSURED PERSON'S NAME (IF DIFFERENT FROM THE RESPONSIBLE PARTY)	ADDRESS (IF DIFFERENT)	CITY	STATE	ZIP

415-00-6214	215-555-0199	Self
SOCIAL SECURITY #	PHONE	WHAT IS THE RESPONSIBLE PARTY'S RELATIONSHIP TO THE INSURED?

SECONDARY INSURANCE

NAME OF SECONDARY INSURANCE COMPANY	IDENTIFICATION #	GROUP NAME AND/OR #

ADDRESS	CITY	STATE	ZIP CODE	PHONE

INSURED PERSON'S NAME (IF DIFFERENT FROM THE RESPONSIBLE PARTY)	ADDRESS (IF DIFFERENT)	CITY	STATE	ZIP

SOCIAL SECURITY #	PHONE	WHAT IS THE RESPONSIBLE PARTY'S RELATIONSHIP TO THE INSURED?

FIGURE 12–11 Patient registration form

a master list showing appointments for several physicians in a practice can be printed. If appointment scheduling is completely computerized, the computer will generate a daily list of appointments automatically, which eliminates the need for the above procedure.

Computerized Patient Charge Slip

When a patient arrives for treatment, the medical assistant enters the name in the computer and a patient charge slip prints automatically. This slip is attached to the medical record and taken to the examination room. As in a pegboard system, the physician or nurse circles the treatment or treatment code and enters only the services not listed by CPT code. Next, the charge slip is returned to the medical assistant, who enters the diagnosis codes and procedure codes in the computer. The program calculates the day's charges and an ending balance. Finally, a copy of the completed patient charge slip is presented to the patient as a receipt. This slip gives information about the patient's account and serves as a reminder of any overdue balance. It can be used for insurance documentation. A computerized patient charge slip is shown in Figure 12–12.

Computerized Patient Ledger

As information is entered from the patient charge slip, the computer automatically updates the ledger by adding a description of each procedure and procedure code and each diagnosis and diagnosis code. It automatically posts the charges and calculates the balance after credits and adjustments are entered.

The ledger may be viewed on the computer screen or printed at any time. If a patient calls with a question regarding an account, the medical assistant can view the ledger on the screen by entering the patient's name. When a correction is needed, it can be made on the screen and stored. Figure 12–13 shows a posted ledger account produced by computer.

Computerized Daily Log

The daily log is generated from information posted to accounts each day. The computer produces a daily log that reports payments, charges, and adjustments by patient name and account number. These reports usually show the total number of patients seen each day and the day's total billings, collections, and adjustments. You can also post broken appointments and "no-shows." Including these appointments explains the broken sequential numbering on the patient charge slips. The daily log can be customized according to the financial reporting needs of a practice, whether it is run by a single physician or by a large group.

VICTORIA McHUGH, M.D.	STATEMENT DATE	08/29/--	
102 FREDERICKS RD.	PATIENT NUMBER	113	
NEW YORK, NY 10012-0000	PREVIOUS BALANCE	$0.00	OFFICE PHONE: (404) 555-0078

DATE	CODE	DESCRIPTION	AMOUNT	STATEMENT DATE 08/29/--	
02/12/--	00000	BALANCE FORWARD	23.00	CURRENT	0.00
02/16/--	71020	CHEST X RAY, 2 VIEWS	40.00	OVER 30-DAYS:	52.00
03/14/--	81000	URINALYSIS	20.00	OVER 60-DAYS:	75.00
04/22/--	85022	CBC	12.50	OVER 90-DAYS:	1.85
06/13/--	99221	INIT. HOSP. EXAM, EXTENSIVE	75.00	BALANCE DUE	$128.85
07/05/--	93040	RHYTHM STRIP	17.00		
07/26/--	93000	ELECTROCARDIOGRAM	35.00		
08/29/--	PMT	PERSONAL CHECK	-93.65 CR		
				THANK YOU FOR YOUR PAYMENT.	
		BALANCE DUE	$128.85		
				113	

OFFICE CLOSED SEPTEMBER 5TH. NEW CHARGES HAVE BEEN SENT TO YOUR INSURANCE CARRIER(S).	VICTORIA McHUGH, M.D. 102 FREDERICKS RD. NEW YORK, NY 10012-0000	LINDA B. HAYLEY 532 5TH STREET ATLANTA, GA 30033-2385

FIGURE 12–12 Computerized patient charge slip

```
                          PATIENT LEDGER
                          ================


   Patient #218           WALRATH, MARY              Date: 06/24/-
                          206 COL. DE WEES DRIVE
                          WAYNE, PA 19087            PHONE: (610) 555-6123


            Insured #1                    Insured #2

            SAME                          WALRATH, FRANCIS
                                          206 COL. DE WEES DRIVE
                                          WAYNE, PA 19087


   Insurance #1:  PRUDENTIAL    Policy #:  987654321    Group #:  987700
   Insurance #2:  BLUE CROSS     Policy #:  321654907    Group #:  123456987


   ======================================================================

   01/26/-     59400     TOTAL OBSTETRICAL CARE                    1200.00
   01/26/-     99202     INTERMEDIATE EXAM, NEW PT.                  30.00
   01/26/-     88150     PAPANICOLAOU SMEAR                          18.50
   01/26/-     PMT        DEPOSIT OB CARE                          -250.00
   02/18/-     PMT        Insur. Pmt.   01/26/-    90015            -20.00
   02/18/-     ADJ        Adj. Cat. #1  01/26/-    90015            -10.00
   02/25/-     85022     CBC                                         12.50
   02/25/-     99212     LIMITED EXAM, ESTAB. PT.                    15.00
   02/25/-     PMT        Cash Pmt.     01/26/-    94000            -75.00
   04/26/-     85022     CBC                                         12.50
   04/26/-     99212     LIMITED EXAM, ESTAB. PT.                    15.00
   04/26/-     76805     DIAGNOSTIC ULTRASOUND                       55.00
   04/26/-     88150     PAPANICOLAOU SMEAR                          18.50
                                                                   _____

                         Balance for MARY WALRATH               $1,022.00
```

FIGURE 12–13 Computerized patient ledger card

Cash and Check Register

In addition to the capabilities already discussed, the computer can also be used to make a daily listing of all cash and checks received. The program searches through all the transactions completed for each patient during the day and calculates the amount of cash received and the amount paid by check. Then a check register showing each check number, the American Banking Association number, the amount of the check, and the patient's name and account number can be printed. A check register can be printed for one physician or for several physicians in a practice. The check register can be attached to a bank deposit slip, thereby requiring no further manual work.

Practice Management

Computer systems allow the medical office to develop a wide variety of reports in a minimum amount of time. These reports can show how physician and staff time is spent, what procedures are used most often, and how income is generated from the practice. Each computer system can generate different types of reports.

Practice Analysis

A practice analysis provides a quick overview of the procedures and treatments provided daily, weekly, monthly, or yearly, and the amount of income they produce. The analysis shows how income is derived; whether from cash, personal checks, insurance payments, or government-related programs. It also shows adjustments and payments.

Cross-Posting Report

A computer system can track the application of fees for group practices when the physicians provide service for one another's patients. Fees can be reported on a daily, weekly, or monthly basis by means of a cross-posting report.

IN YOUR OPINION

1. How can a background in pegboard accounting help with computerized accounting?
2. Will the introduction of computerized accounting in medical offices result in the addition or loss of jobs for medical assistants who are no longer needed for pegboard accounting? Explain your answer.
3. What steps can be taken to make the transition from a pegboard system to a computerized system easier for staff members?

INTERNET ACTIVITY

Search on the keywords "medical practice banking, daily banking, banking procedures or other similar words to locate an article about banking procedures preferred by medical offices. Write a brief summary of what you learned.

STUDENT STUDY CHECKLIST

Workbook

1. Complete Chapter 12 exercises in the workbook.
2. Complete Chapter 12 simulations in the workbook that access the CD-ROM in the back of the book.
3. Assume you are the manager of a medical office who has to explain to a new employee how the various payroll forms are used. Prepare a paragraph of explanation.

Administrative Skills CD-ROM

1. Go the Library on the CD-ROM and play the interactive games for Chapter 12.
2. Go to the Finance area of the office and click on the Payroll Forms folder. Work through the exercises.

REFERENCES

Fordney, Marilyn T. and Joan J. Follis. *Administrative Medical Assisting,* 4th ed. Clifton Park, NY: Delmar Learning, 1998.

Humphrey, Doris D. *Pediatric Associates, P.C.* Cincinnati, OH: South-Western, 1998.

Lindh, Wilburta Q., Marilyn S. Pooler, and Carol D. Tamparo. *Administrative Medical Assisting,* 2nd ed. Clifton Park, NY: Delmar Learning, 2002.

CHAPTER ACTIVITIES

PERFORMANCE-BASED ACTIVITIES

1. Set up a summary for a daily log. In the columns "Office Visit," "Laboratory," "Injections," and "Emergencies," list the medical fees given here. Then analyze the summary to determine the types of service performed most often. Based on the summary, which staff members do you think are busiest?

Brook Raines	Level IV Office Visit, New Patient, $125; Urinalysis, $16; Complete Blood Check, $15
Martin Omar	Level III Office Visit, Established Patient, $58; Allergy Injection, $35
Majik Bonak	Level IV Office Visit, Established Patient, $87; DPT shot, $35
Michelle Chung	Emergency Visit, $150
Charles Victor	Level III Office Visit, Established Patient, $58; Throat Culture, $26
Susan Ankar	Emergency Hospital Visit, $60
Barbara Ross	Allergy Injection, $30
Ashley Wilson	Level III Office Visit, New Patient, $83
Lawrence Rawley	Emergency Visit, $120
Santigo Mendez	Level III Office Visit, Established Patient, $58

Patient Identification	Office Visit	Laboratory	Injections	Emergencies
1. _____	_____	_____	_____	_____
2. _____	_____	_____	_____	_____
3. _____	_____	_____	_____	_____
4. _____	_____	_____	_____	_____
5. _____	_____	_____	_____	_____
6. _____	_____	_____	_____	_____
7. _____	_____	_____	_____	_____
8. _____	_____	_____	_____	_____
9. _____	_____	_____	_____	_____
10. _____	_____	_____	_____	_____

2. Following the procedures outlined in this chapter, determine the current balance for each of these patients (use the form on the following page):

	Old Balance	Today's Charges	Today's Payment
David Sebert	0	$60, 22, 16	$85
Rawley Ashburn-Myers	$16	$48, 38, 16	$75
Nancy O'Grady	$323	$46, 75, 18	$125
Tishee Bryant	$86	$46, 34, 22	$135
Carmen Sanchez	0	$70, 36, 20, 18	$120
Roulff Berquest	$122	$85, 25, 18	$175

Old Balance + Today's Charges – Today's Payment = New Balance

Patient	Old Balance	Today's Charges	Today's Payment	New Balance
1. _____	_____	_____	_____	_____
2. _____	_____	_____	_____	_____
3. _____	_____	_____	_____	_____
4. _____	_____	_____	_____	_____
5. _____	_____	_____	_____	_____
6. _____	_____	_____	_____	_____

3. Complete the following chart by filling in the correct responses.

Situation	Action/Answer
An established patient has arrived at the medical office. Trace the path of his computerized charge slip from creation to end of visit.	
On days the computerized monthly billing is prepared, the computer is tied up so frequently that patients must wait for their charge slip. Develop a correction for this problem.	
Your employer, who was out of town for several days, asked another physician to treat her patients. Now your employer wants to know the dollar amount of fees that were applied to other physicians. Explain how you will develop this information.	

EXPANDING YOUR THINKING

1. Reviewing Form W-4, determine how many dependents you would claim if you took a medical assisting position at this time.

2. What recommendations would you make to a new medical assistant who says that a background in financial operations is unimportant because the practice's accountant is responsible for financial matters?

CHAPTER 13

Billing and Collection

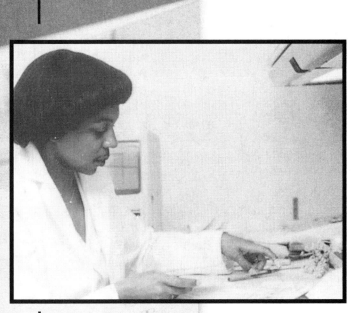

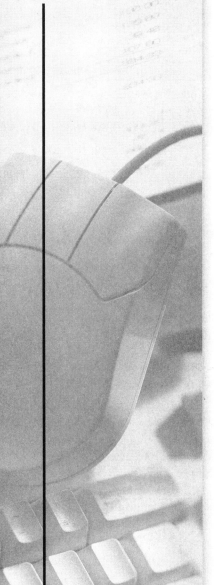

SOMERSET, NEW JERSEY

This is a fairly affluent town, twenty miles from Princeton and in easy commuting distance of the big money jobs in New York. Still, even though most of our patients are in financially comfortable situations — or so it would seem — we have our share of slow-pays and no-pays. That struck me as odd when I first joined this practice, after moving here from Philadelphia. My practice there was not as upscale as this, so, understandably, people who had trouble paying could point to pressing problems, such as heat or electricity due to be shut off.

I think what I've learned is that people at all income levels have problems with finances. Sometimes the problems are not really financial. We have half a dozen patients who I know have the ability to pay but who always procrastinate — postpone their payments until the last possible minute, usually when they're three months past due. I guess I'm suggesting that there's a rhythm and a flow to collections and after a while you get a feel for it. That doesn't remove the need to have a system in place that automatically ages accounts, alerting you to send out an appropriate reminder or request for payment. Often, a telephone call to the person, just after the first reminder has been sent and received, inquiring if everything is all right, will get things moving. Of course, I don't always have time for that. Time is always the MA's enemy. There's always so much to do.

Most people are well-intentioned when it comes to debt, I've found. It's just a matter of getting them to make the connection between their intentions and their checkbooks or credit cards. Collection procedures is an entire field of study and far more sophisticated than our needs, although when our patients bills become "hopeless," we turn them over to a collection agency. They sometimes have success.

Perhaps the most difficult thing, for me at least, is like what happened last week. Mrs. Walters, who is in her seventies and comfortably well-off, came in for a minor complaint. She also was three months past due on a bill of several hundred dollars. My job was to welcome her, go over her complaint, and decide how to bring up the matter of the missing money. What I did, worked. Just before I got up, after I had told her the doctor would see her shortly, I leaned forward and asked, quietly, "Is everything all right? We've been worried about your account and wondered if something was wrong or in dispute; you know it's so long past due. Is there any chance you could take care of it now?" Well, she could and did. It doesn't always work that well, but being courteous always helps.

Barbara Schults
Medical Assistant

PERFORMANCE-BASED COMPETENCIES

After completing this chapter, you should be able to:
1. Compare the advantages of internal billing and external billing.
2. Evaluate different methods of internal billing.
3. Manage the collection process.

VOCABULARY

Account aging   Method for reporting how long an account has been due.

Balance   Amount remaining owed.

Billing   Reminding patients that money is owed to the practice.

Collection   Process for expediting overdue accounts.

Cycle billing   Process for spreading billing over the whole month instead of sending all bills at the same time.

Invoice   Statement of services.

Payables   Amount of money owed by a practice to those from whom it purchases goods and services.

Receivables   Amount of money owed to a practice by those who purchase its services.

Third-party payers   Insurance companies or others who will pay the patient's bill.

Patient billing may take many forms, from the simplest to the complex. Whatever method is used, it must be managed efficiently and expeditiously if a medical practice is to succeed. If patients do not pay *their* bills, the practice will not be able to pay *its* bills, including the salaries of the physicians and the staff. An organized, standard billing system combined with accurate, complete records makes billing a relatively simple task.

If patients do not pay at the time of service, a routine statement of services mailed during the regular billing cycle usually suffices to collect patient accounts. When patients fail to pay their bills, the practice must attempt to collect. Collection can take many forms, from a series of letters, to personal telephone calls, to the services of a collection agency. If all of these efforts fail, the medical office can take a patient to court for nonpayment. Collection by means of a lawsuit is a costly procedure, however, and should be avoided when possible. Often this expensive process can be forestalled by simply calling the person responsible for the bill and asking if he understood it, if the bill is accurate, and if a payment plan needs to be established.

When a pegboard accounting system is used to maintain financial records, billing and collection activities are completed by hand. If the office uses a computer system, the computer produces billing statements, aging reports, and collection notices.

BILLING PATIENTS

Billing may be handled internally by a medical assistant who devotes some portion of the day or perhaps even the entire day to accounts control, or it may be contracted through an external service that manages billing for several different clients for a monthly or annual fee. In either case, the medical assistant must be knowledgeable about the process needed to manage the office's billing and collection. If you as a medical assistant are asked to handle the billing for the practice, you will be required to concentrate, to work for large blocks of uninterrupted time, and to have a clear understanding of the account aging process. Because you will usually work alone without much supervision, organizational skills and maturity are important.

Internal Billing

Billing can be as simple as requiring payment at the time of service or as complex as cycle billing that spans several days each month. The best billing system is the simplest one that meets the needs of the individual practice — the simpler the system, the better. Although some practices require complex billing systems, complexity itself does not always guarantee better payment results. Several methods of billings from simple to complex are discussed in the next section. Each practice must determine which method is best suited for its size, financial objectives, and patient load.

Charge Slip as Statement at Time of Service

The best opportunity for collection of an account is at the time of service, and it is becoming increasingly common for practices to require payment at the end of each visit. The charge slip, which is given to each patient at that time, serves as the first statement and eliminates the expense of preparing and mailing a statement of immediate payment. Another advantage is that the prac-

tice earns interest if the money is deposited in an interest-bearing account. To encourage payment, some medical offices accept major credit cards, as well as cash and checks, making it possible for almost everyone to pay immediately. Old balances can often be collected at the same time with a bit of subtlety and tact. While handing the charge slip to a patient, a medical assistant might make one of the following comments:

- "Here is your charge clip, Mrs. Mara. The charge is $88. Do you want to write a check or pay cash for today's visit?"
- "If it's helpful, Ms. Riegert, we take VISA and MasterCard as well as cash or a check."
- "Mr. Itani, today's charge is $54, and you have a balance of $28 from the last visit. Would you like to pay the entire account today?"

One way to prompt people to pay is by placing a small plaque or sign at the check-out window. A sample is shown in Figure 13–1.

Billing Statement

The practice that mails a billing statement has two options: (1) mailing a copy of the manually prepared or computerized ledger card as a statement, which is faster, or (2) sending a special statement form, which is time-consuming but looks more professional (Figure 13–2). In either

We would appreciate your payment at the end of your appointment today.

FIGURE 13–1   Small sign to prompt payment

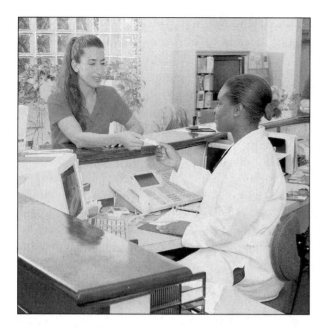

FIGURE 13–2 Some medical offices require payment at the time of service.

case, a self-addressed return envelope should be enclosed to make payment simple.

Ledger Card as Statement

If a practice uses the ledger card as a statement, the medical assistant should copy all the ledger cards with outstanding balances once during each billing cycle, enclose each in a window envelope, and mail the statement to the person responsible for the account. Because the ledger card shows the history of all the account's charges, credits, and adjustments, in addition to the patient's name and address, minimal time will be spent on billing. To eliminate the need to check each card individually, all ledger cards showing outstanding balances can be coded with colored strips doubled over the top of the cards so the color is visible as shown in Figure 13–3. When an account is paid in full, the colored strip is removed.

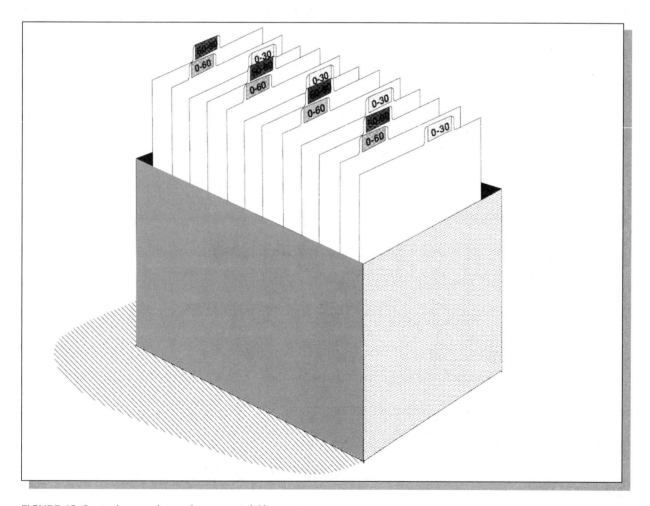

FIGURE 13–3 Ledger card stored in a special filing section

Another method to identify accounts with outstanding balances is to store the past due ledger cards in a special "Unpaid" or "Balance Due" section of the file as shown in Figures 13–3 and 13–4. There is, however, one disadvantage to using ledger cards as statements. Because the information on the ledger card is handwritten and transfers through carbon when the charge slip is completed, the copied ledger card is not an attractive method of billing.

Special Statement Form

A special printed statement form mailed in a window envelope looks more professional and attractive than a ledger card. The statement lists most of the same information shown on a ledger card; however, only the services performed since the last statement, along with any previous balance, are shown. This method is less efficient, but it makes a better impression for the practice. A special statement form is shown in Figure 13–5.

Computerized Statement

Using computer software, during each billing cycle the medical assistant will direct the program to search the patient database and print statements for patients with outstanding balances (Figure 13–6). The program automatically ages accounts at the same time. For overdue accounts, the computer can also print a series of prewritten collection letters to remind patients of their balances.

The medical assistant can process the billings while attending to other duties by entering the beginning and ending account numbers and instructing the computer to print. Look at the computerized sample monthly statement in Figure 13–6. The top of the form is perforated, so the patient can tear it off and return it to the medical office. Because the top shows the account name and number, the amount currently due, and the statement date, all the necessary posting information will be received when the patient returns the top with the payment.

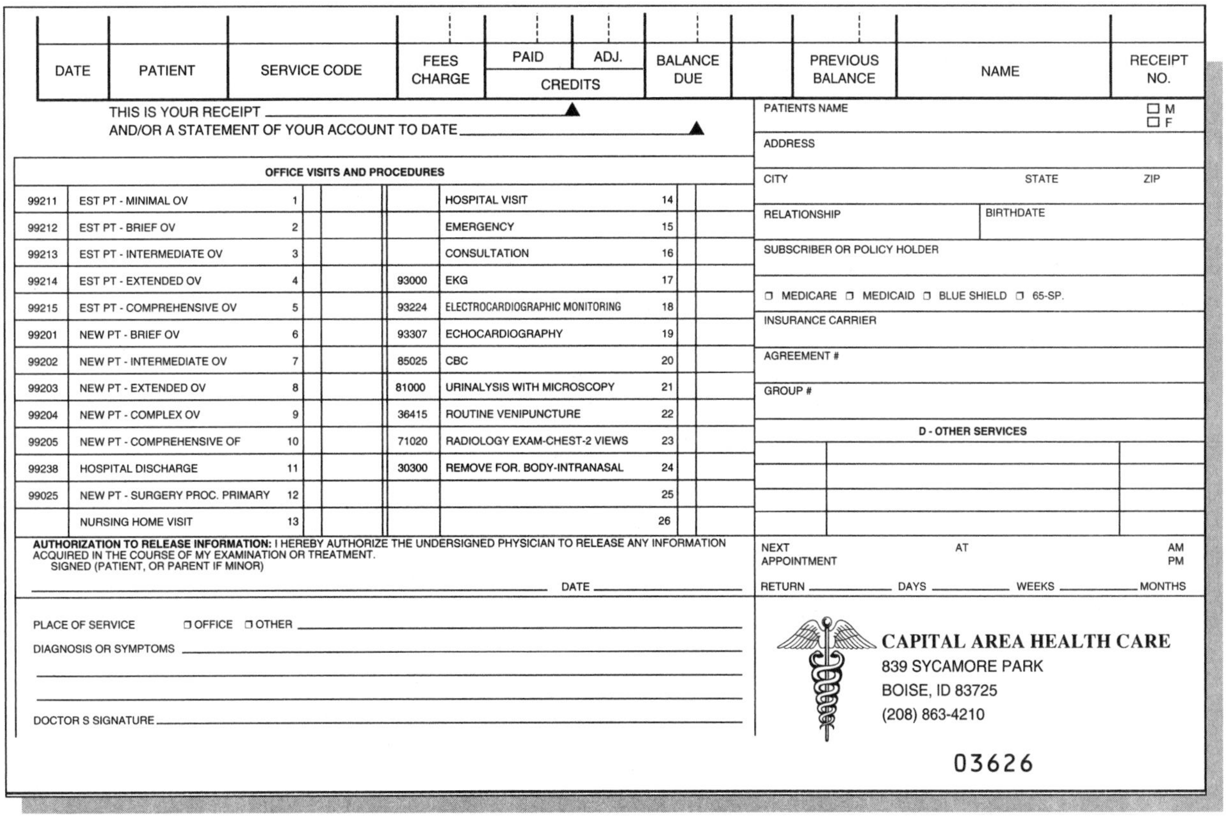

DATE	PATIENT	SERVICE CODE	FEES CHARGE	PAID (CREDITS)	ADJ. (CREDITS)	BALANCE DUE	PREVIOUS BALANCE	NAME	RECEIPT NO.

THIS IS YOUR RECEIPT
AND/OR A STATEMENT OF YOUR ACCOUNT TO DATE

PATIENTS NAME ☐ M ☐ F
ADDRESS
CITY STATE ZIP
RELATIONSHIP BIRTHDATE
SUBSCRIBER OR POLICY HOLDER
☐ MEDICARE ☐ MEDICAID ☐ BLUE SHIELD ☐ 65-SP.
INSURANCE CARRIER
AGREEMENT #
GROUP #

OFFICE VISITS AND PROCEDURES

99211	EST PT - MINIMAL OV	1		HOSPITAL VISIT	14
99212	EST PT - BRIEF OV	2		EMERGENCY	15
99213	EST PT - INTERMEDIATE OV	3		CONSULTATION	16
99214	EST PT - EXTENDED OV	4	93000	EKG	17
99215	EST PT - COMPREHENSIVE OV	5	93224	ELECTROCARDIOGRAPHIC MONITORING	18
99201	NEW PT - BRIEF OV	6	93307	ECHOCARDIOGRAPHY	19
99202	NEW PT - INTERMEDIATE OV	7	85025	CBC	20
99203	NEW PT - EXTENDED OV	8	81000	URINALYSIS WITH MICROSCOPY	21
99204	NEW PT - COMPLEX OV	9	36415	ROUTINE VENIPUNCTURE	22
99205	NEW PT - COMPREHENSIVE OF	10	71020	RADIOLOGY EXAM-CHEST-2 VIEWS	23
99238	HOSPITAL DISCHARGE	11	30300	REMOVE FOR. BODY-INTRANASAL	24
99025	NEW PT - SURGERY PROC. PRIMARY	12			25
	NURSING HOME VISIT	13			26

D - OTHER SERVICES

AUTHORIZATION TO RELEASE INFORMATION: I HEREBY AUTHORIZE THE UNDERSIGNED PHYSICIAN TO RELEASE ANY INFORMATION ACQUIRED IN THE COURSE OF MY EXAMINATION OR TREATMENT.
SIGNED (PATIENT, OR PARENT IF MINOR)
DATE

NEXT APPOINTMENT AT AM PM
RETURN DAYS WEEKS MONTHS

PLACE OF SERVICE ☐ OFFICE ☐ OTHER
DIAGNOSIS OR SYMPTOMS
DOCTOR S SIGNATURE

CAPITAL AREA HEALTH CARE
839 SYCAMORE PARK
BOISE, ID 83725
(208) 863-4210

03626

FIGURE 13–4 Sample charge slip used to document health insurance claims

STATEMENT

Telephone
615-555-8726

Alyson Malik, M.D.
423 West Main Street
Lebanon, TN 37087-0000

Mr. Amrit Singh
2203 Van Loan Drive
Lebanon, TN 37087-0000

| DATE | FAMILY MEMBER | PROFESSIONAL SERVICE | CHARGE | CREDITS | | BALANCE |
				PAYMTS	ADJ.	
			BALANCE FORWARD			
3/27	Michael	EV, S, HV				192 —
		We have received payment from your insurance company. Please pay the remaining amount.				
		WE NOW ACCEPT VISA/MASTERCARD FOR YOUR CONVENIENCE.				
		LAST BILL BEFORE COLLECTIONS				

PAY LAST AMOUNT IN THIS COLUMN

FIGURE 13–5 Special statement form

The bottom portion of the statement, which the patient keeps, shows the old balance, the date of service, the family member treated, each procedure and charge, any payments, and the current amount due.

After all statements are printed, they can be inserted in window envelopes and mailed to the responsible parties.

Monthly Billing and Cycle Billing

The size of a practice usually determines the billing schedule. In a single-physician or small group practice, monthly billing may be the most efficient method. However, in a large practice, the flexibility of cycle billing offers certain advantages.

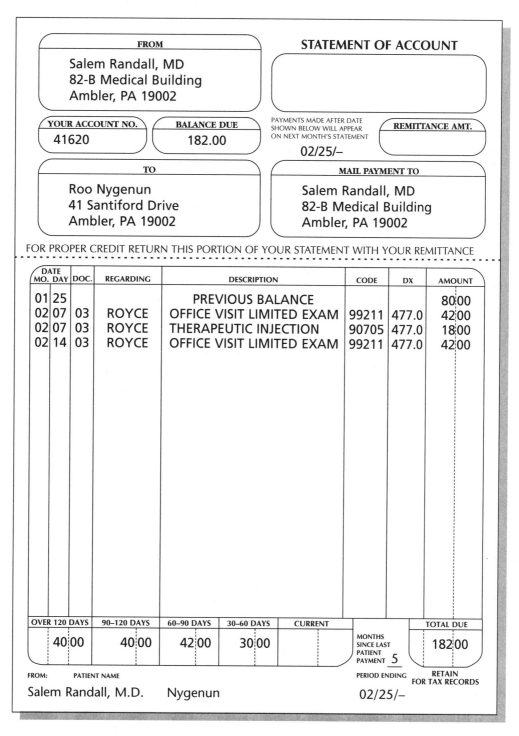

FROM

Salem Randall, MD
82-B Medical Building
Ambler, PA 19002

STATEMENT OF ACCOUNT

YOUR ACCOUNT NO.	BALANCE DUE
41620	182.00

PAYMENTS MADE AFTER DATE
SHOWN BELOW WILL APPEAR
ON NEXT MONTH'S STATEMENT

02/25/–

REMITTANCE AMT.

TO

Roo Nygenun
41 Santiford Drive
Ambler, PA 19002

MAIL PAYMENT TO

Salem Randall, MD
82-B Medical Building
Ambler, PA 19002

FOR PROPER CREDIT RETURN THIS PORTION OF YOUR STATEMENT WITH YOUR REMITTANCE

DATE MO. DAY	DOC.	REGARDING	DESCRIPTION	CODE	DX	AMOUNT
01 25			PREVIOUS BALANCE			80:00
02 07	03	ROYCE	OFFICE VISIT LIMITED EXAM	99211	477.0	42:00
02 07	03	ROYCE	THERAPEUTIC INJECTION	90705	477.0	18:00
02 14	03	ROYCE	OFFICE VISIT LIMITED EXAM	99211	477.0	42:00

OVER 120 DAYS	90–120 DAYS	60–90 DAYS	30–60 DAYS	CURRENT		TOTAL DUE
40:00	40:00	42:00	30:00		MONTHS SINCE LAST PATIENT PAYMENT 5	182:00

FROM: PATIENT NAME		PERIOD ENDING	RETAIN FOR TAX RECORDS
Salem Randall, M.D. Nygenun		02/25/–	

FIGURE 13–6 Computerized statement

Monthly Billing

In a monthly billing system, all accounts are billed at the same time, usually near the end of the month. This means that the medical assistant will devote one or two days to the billing task and mail all statements at the same time. Monthly billing offers the advantage of flexibility, allowing the assistant to plan other responsibilities around the billing schedule.

The disadvantage of monthly billing is that a medical assistant may neglect other activities during this billing time, or become overworked and harassed. To avoid these problems, billing statements can be prepared intermittently over a one- or two-week period and stored until the mailing date. However, if several days pass between the time statements are prepared and mailed, a message to "Disregard if payment has already been made" should be printed on the form. Patients become annoyed if a statement arrives several days after payment has been made.

Cycle Billing

Cycle billing offers a feasible alternative for practices that cannot devote the full services of a medical assistant to billing for one or more days each month. With this system, the alphabet is divided into sections and patients are billed according to where the first letter of their last name falls in the alphabet. Each month statements are prepared on the same schedule. Then they are mailed as they are completed, or held and mailed at one time. A typical cycle billing schedule is shown below. The system can be varied as needed by the individual practice:

1. Divide the alphabet into four sections: A–F, G–L, M–R, S–Z.
2. Prepare statements for patients whose last names begin with A through F on Monday and mail them on Tuesday of Week 1.
3. Prepare statements for patients whose last names begin with G through L on Monday and mail them on Tuesday of Week 2.
4. Prepare statements for patients whose last names begin with M through R on Monday and mail them on Tuesday of Week 3.
5. Prepare statements for patients whose last names begin with S through Z on Monday and mail them on Tuesday of Week 4.

External Billing Service

An outside billing service can be hired to manage patient accounts. The service maintains all ledger cards, posting debits and credits from copies of charge slips provided by the medical office. It prepares monthly statements, usually by computer, and mails them with a request for payment to be returned to the billing service. In addition, the billing service makes deposits directly to the practice's bank account and pre-pares a report outlining all transactions. External billing services are for small practices with limited staff and practices with a large number of patients. When a medical office uses a billing service, the medical assistant is responsible for coordinating activities between the two groups.

IN YOUR OPINION

1. In your opinion, is monthly billing or cycle billing preferable?
2. Why is it important to age accounts on a regular basis?
3. In addition to time savings, what advantages does computer billing offer over manual billing?

THE COLLECTION PROCESS

According to one study by the American Medical Association, 90–95% of patients pay their medical bills on time; 5–10% are slow to pay; and about 2% have no intention of paying. The collection process is geared to the patients who are slow to pay. Other measures, such as taking the patient to court, are used for the patients who do not intend to pay. Once a collection agency becomes involved with a patient's account, the medical assistant refers all calls regarding the account to the agency.

The purposes of the collection process are: (1) to determine if there are errors on the bills, (2) the remind patients of their overdue balances, (3) to encourage patients to pay their bills, and (4) to help patients find a way to pay their bills if they have financial difficulties. As a medical assistant, you may manage collections. The practice also can contract to have collections made by a private service. Collection agencies are expensive, only large, long-overdue accounts should be given over. Usually, accounts of more than $100 that are six months or more overdue are turned over to an agency, while the medical assistant manages routine collections.

Filing a lawsuit for nonpayment is the ultimate collection procedure. Typically, however, collection is attempted first by letter or telephone or by a combination of the two methods. The initial contact comes through letters, and telephone collections are instituted only after an account ages and the patient has made no response to letters.

Aging Accounts

A process called account aging identifies how long an account is overdue. In an aging system, past due accounts are coded according to the length of time they have been unpaid. In a pegboard accounting system, color-coded strips are attached to the ledger cards to show the age of an account, or the cards can be stored behind a color-coded divider in an "Unpaid" file. For example, a red code might be used for accounts one month overdue, a blue code for accounts two months overdue, and other colors for additional months overdue. A written code such as "OD2/6/18/–" should be written on the ledger card to indicate when the overdue notice was mailed, meaning "Overdue notice No. 2 mailed on June 18."

Computer account aging is simple. By giving the appropriate commands, the medical assistant can instruct the computer system to automatically age the accounts at the end of each month before printing billing statements. Most programs can age accounts according to several criteria, for example, by past due balance, zero balance, or credit balance. Accounts can also be aged by government agency category or by insurance carrier. Therefore, all Medicare or Medicaid accounts could be aged separately from other accounts.

The practice may also wish to have an accounts receivable report showing each overdue account, the balance overdue, and a breakdown of the length of time the account is overdue. This breakdown is usually divided into:

- 0–30 days overdue
- 31–60 days overdue
- 61–90 days overdue
- 90 days or more overdue

The computer also generates other reports from the accounts receivable report, for example, a report showing accounts that are delinquent for more than 90 days or accounts that are delinquent by more than a certain dollar amount.

Review the accounts receivable report shown in Figure 13–7. Notice the following items:

1. Seven accounts are past due by 31–60 days
2. Four accounts are past due by 61–90 days
3. Four accounts are past due by more than 90 days
4. One Medicaid account is past due by 61–90 days
5. In the delinquent accounts portion of the report, four patients are shown as delinquent in payment. According to the report, these regular accounts are overdue by $100 since May 30, 20–

The addresses and telephone numbers of the responsible parties are listed, so you may contact the person to begin the collection process.

Aging systems differ according to the type of patient served. For example, a private patient's account is aged differently from a Medicare patient's account. This occurs because federal reimbursement takes time, and the patient may be unprepared to pay without the reimbursement. In a computerized billing system, the accounts are automatically aged, and the aging code is shown on the computerized ledger card. A typical aging code for a private patient follows:

- **C:** Charge slip given to patient at time of visit.
- **1:** Itemized statement mailed when account is past due one month.
- **2:** Itemized statement with overdue notice mailed when account is past due two months.
- **3:** Letter stating, "We have not received payment for your account," when account is past due three months.
- **4:** Letter stating, "Your account is overdue" when account is past due four months; or
- **4T:** Telephone call reminding patient of overdue account and offering to help arrange a payment schedule.
- **5** or **5T:** Letter or telephone call stating, "Your account will be turned over to a collector," when account is past due five months.
- **6:** Certified letter stating, "Your account was turned over to a collection agency," when account is past due six months. No further telephone calls are necessary, because they might antagonize the patient and leave the medical assistant open to verbal abuse.
- **7:** Collection agency attempts to collect.
- **8:** Lawsuit filed.

ACCOUNTS RECEIVABLE REPORT   07/06/-

NAME	BALANCE	CURRENT	0–30	31–60	61–90	OVER 90
Mason	325.00	50.00	118.00	70.00	12.00	75.00
Tiebot	68.00	0.00	0.00	44.00	24.00	0.00
Rohn	483.00	0.00	0.00	435.00	0.00	48.00
Rosa	53.00	0.00	0.00	53.00	0.00	0.00
Bradshaw	358.00	40.00	0.00	34.00	24.00	260.00
South	273.00	0.00	200.00	73.00	0.00	0.00
Capowitz	350.00	138.00	0.00	212.00	0.00	0.00
Adam	282.00	0.00	35.00	0.00	227.00	20.00
	2,192.00	228.00	353.00	921.00	287.00	403.00

Medicaid   Accounts Receivable Report   07/06/-

NAME	BALANCE	CURRENT	0–30	31–60	61–90	OVER 90
Myers-Brooke	12.00	0.00	0.00	0.00	12.00	0.00
	12.00	0.00	0.00	0.00	12.00	0.00
	2,204.00	228.00	353.00	921.00	299.00	403.00

REGULAR   DELINQUENT ACCOUNTS MORE THAN $200.00   NO PAYMENT SINCE 05/30/-

ACCOUNT NAME AND ADDRESS	DATE	AMOUNT	BALANCE	31–60	61–90	OVER 90
Ms. Suzanne Rohn P.O. Box 360 Cincinnati, OH 45249	00/00/- none	0.00	483.00	435.00	0.00	48.00
Mr. Matthew Bradshaw 1914 Galen Drive Blue Ash, OH 45236	04/14/- Cash 555-3083	40.00	358.00	34.00	24.00	260.00
Ms. Patricia Capowitz 890 Tower Place Cincinnati, OH 45242	04/14/- Personal Check 555-4581	60.00	350.00	212.00	0.00	0.00
Mr. Arthur Adam 601 Springfield Terr. Montgomery, OH 45249	02/21/- Insurance Payment 555-8412	65.00	282.00	0.00	227.00	20.00
Totals			1,473.00	681.00	251.00	318.00

FIGURE 13–7   Computerized accounts receivable report

Collection Letters Series

Medical offices send collection letters to encourage patients and third-party carriers to pay overdue balances. The series of letters to the patient begins after two statements are mailed with no response and to third-party carriers after sixty days have passed.

Collection Letters to Patients

Lack of payment is not considered serious until after sixty days. When the patient has not responded to the charge slip, to the statement, or to the statement with an "Overdue" remark at the end of sixty days, a series of collection letters begins. A typical collection letter is shown in Figures 13–8 through 13–11.

Collection Letters to Third-Party Carriers

Patients are not the only source of late payment. Often private and government insurance groups also need to be reminded of overdue balances. Because the claims units of insurance companies and government agencies are large, with many employees of varying levels of experience, the delay can be caused by an overburdened claims department, by a form that has been lost in transit, by a misfiled form, by an inexperienced employee, or several other reasons. The claims units are concerned with hundreds or thousands of claims, and one misfiled form from a private practice is of little consequence. As a medical assistant, if you maintain a current claims register or tickler and take firm control of the practice's collection procedures, you can get receipt of payment sooner.

Many patients have private medical plans or qualify for government insurance; therefore, the medical assistant may need to write these carriers. In offices where the medical assistant files claims for patients, a follow-up collection policy is important to maintain strong cash flow. When agencies do not pay in full or question or deny a claim, the assistant will have to determine the nature of the problem and notify the patients. Figures 13–12 through 13–17 illustrate several kinds of correspondence relating to insurance claims.

Salem Randall, M.D.
82-B Medical Building
Ambler, PA 19002

June 14, 20–

Mr. Roo Nygenun
41 Santiford Drive
Ambler, PA 19002

Dear Mr. Nygenun:

Your account with our office is three months past due, and you have not responded to our previous requests for payment. Please pay your balance of $152 at this time, or contact us with an explanation of why you cannot pay.

Please call me at 555-7823 if you have a question about your account. Otherwise, we expect your payment immediately.

Sincerely,

Casey Husted
Accounts Manager

FIGURE 13–8 First collection letter to a patient

Salem Randall, M.D.
82-B Medical Building
Ambler, PA 19002

July 15, 20–

Mr. Roo Nygenun
41 Santiford Drive
Ambler, PA 19002

Dear Mr. Nygenun:

Your son, Royce, was seriously ill in March when he came to Dr. Randall for treatment. Dr. Randall was pleased to use her experience and education to treat Royce, and it was in this same spirit of cooperation that we expected you to pay your account within a reasonable amount of time.

Four months have passed and you have still not remitted the $152 outstanding balance on your account. We cannot continue to keep your unpaid account on our books. If you are experiencing financial difficulties, please call the office so we can arrange a payment schedule that is agreeable to both of us.

Sincerely,

Casey Husted
Accounts Manager

FIGURE 13–9 Second collection letter to a patient

Salem Randall, M.D.
82-B Medical Building
Ambler, PA 19002

August 14, 20–

Mr. Roo Nygenun
41 Santiford Drive
Ambler, PA 19002

Dear Mr. Nygenun:

You have not replied to our previous notices regarding your unpaid balance of $152. Unless we hear from you personally within 14 days, your account will be given to the Ambler Medical Collection Service.

Do not wait any longer to contact me at 555-7823 if you wish to maintain your previous good credit record with Dr. Randall. As previously suggested, we will cooperate in arranging a suitable payment schedule if needed.

Sincerely,

Casey Husted
Accounts Manager

FIGURE 13–10 Third collection letter to a patient

Salem Randall, M.D.
82-B Medical Building
Ambler, PA 19002

September 17, 20–

CERTIFIED MAIL

Mr. Roo Nygenun
41 Santiford Drive
Ambler, PA 19002

Dear Mr. Nygenun:

This is our final attempt to collect your account of $152, which is six months past due. You have ignored all our previous letters [or letters and phone calls], so we have no alternative but to turn over your account to a collection company.

Your account is being assigned to Ambler Medical Collection Service, which will pursue whatever legal means is necessary to collect this debt. If you contact me at 555-7823 within seven days, we will retrieve your account from the collection service to protect your credit rating.

Sincerely,

Casey Husted
Accounts Manager

FIGURE 13–11   Fourth collection letter to a patient

Salem Randall, M.D.
82-B Medical Building
Ambler, PA 19002

June 15, 20–

Mrs. Sarika Javis
7823 Midland Circle
Paoli, PA 19301

Dear Mrs. Javis:

Medicaid has notified us that no payment will be made on your account with Dr. Randall because you no longer qualify for the program. When a government agency does not pay, the patient is responsible for the account.

Please pay your outstanding balance of $286 within the next thirty days or, if you prefer, call me at 555-7823, so we can arrange a payment plan that will be satisfactory for both you and Dr. Randall.

Sincerely,

Casey Husted
Accounts Manager

FIGURE 13–12   Letter to patient regarding Medicare's refusal to pay

Salem Randall, M.D.
82-B Medical Building
Ambler, PA 19002

June 15, 20–

Miss Lisa Izzo
982-B Chesterbrook Boulevard
Wayne, PA 19087

Dear Miss Izzo:

Your personal record in our office is incomplete and does not provide the information necessary for us to file a claim with your insurance company. If you will answer the questions below that apply to you and return the letter to this office within ten days, we will be happy to submit the necessary paperwork to collect payment.

1. Medicare number
2. Medicaid number
3. Blue Cross/Blue Shield Group Number
4. Blue Cross/Blue Shield Contract Number
5. Name of Blue Cross/Blue Shield Subscriber
6. Other Insurance, HMO, or PPO Name and Address
7. Other Insurance, HMO, or PPO policy or identification number

Thank you for your cooperation. We will contact you as soon as we hear from your carrier.

Sincerely,

Casey Husted
Accounts Manager

FIGURE 13–13 Letter to patient asking for insurance information

---

Salem Randall, M.D.
82-B Medical Building
Ambler, PA 19002

June 17, 20–

Mr. Todd Ingram
78 Lenape Drive
Berwyn, PA 19312

Dear Mr. Ingram:

Metropolitan Insurance has informed us that the annual deductible on your health insurance policy has not been met, and they will not pay for Dr. Randall's services on May 2. Because payment of an account is the patient's responsibility, we would appreciate your sending us a check for the outstanding balance of $98.

Please contact your insurance carrier directly if you have a question about their denial of payment. If I can be of further help, please call me at 555-7823.

Sincerely,

Casey Husted
Accounts Manager

FIGURE 13–14 Letter informing patient of carrier's refusal to pay

Salem Randall, M.D.
82-B Medical Building
Ambler, PA 19002

June 17, 20–

The Travelers
90 Merrick Avenue
East Meadow, NY 11554

Ladies and Gentlemen:

Patient Name: Holly Sparkman
Insured Name: John Sparkman
Contract No.: GA 87600J
I.D. No.: 415-89-3765
Date of Service: April 28, 20–
Date Claim Submitted: May 1, 20–

A claim for the above patient was submitted on May 1, 20–, and we have not yet received payment. Will you please determine the status of the claim and let me know immediately whether there is a problem and, if not, when payment will be mailed.

A copy of the original claim form is enclosed. We will appreciate your prompt response to this inquiry.

Sincerely,

Casey Husted
Accounts Manager

FIGURE 13–15 Inquiry letter to insurance company

Salem Randall, M.D.
82-B Medical Building
Ambler, PA 19002

June 20, 20–

Medicare
Pennsylvania Blue Shield
Box 65, Blue Shield Building
Camp Hill, PA 17011

Ladies and Gentlemen:

Patient Name: Mary Ann Thomasini
Patient Address: 678 Penn Pike
                         Malvern, PA 19832
Medicare No.: 483-2878-32a

A claim form documenting Dr. Salem Randall's treatment of Mrs. Mary Ann Tomasini on April 3, 20– was filed with your office on April 6, 20–, and we have no response to the claim.

A copy of the original claim is enclosed. Please check your files and notify us on the status of this claim as soon as possible.

Sincerely,

Casey Husted
Accounts Manager

FIGURE 13–16 Inquiry to Medicare administrator regarding patient's claim

Salem Randall, M.D.
82-B Medical Building
Ambler, PA 19002

June 20, 20–

Ms. Barbara Hopewell
Personnel Supervisor
Markson Services
86 Hudson Lane
Ambler, PA 19002

Dear. Ms. Hopewell:

Employee: Randall Palmer
Date of Service: May 2, 20–

The claim submitted on behalf of
Mr. Randall Palmer to Aetna Life and
Casualty has not been paid. Please
contact the carrier and inquire about
the status of this claim; then inform us
immediately of your findings.

When insurance companies fail to make
payment for a medical claim within
eight weeks, the policy of this office
is to bill the patient. If you have a
question, please call me at 555-7823.

Sincerely,

Casey Husted
Accounts Manager

FIGURE 13–17 Letter to employer regarding workers' compensation claim

Telephone Collections

Patients who do not respond to collection letters cannot ignore a ringing telephone. Therefore, when a practice has received no payment after mailing several collection letters, a telephone call is in order to inquire about the past due balance. In medical offices where collections are handled internally, you as a medical assistant will assume the responsibility for telephone collections (Figure 13–18).

Telephone inquiries about unpaid bills are awkward, and you must use your best human relations skills to put the patient at ease while at the same time establishing control of the conversation. The purpose of a telephone inquiry is fourfold:

1. To inquire if there is a problem, error, or misunderstanding about the bill
2. To remind the patient of the bill
3. To stimulate the person to pay
4. To help find a way for the person to pay

Telephone collection calls can be made at the end of the collection series or at any point during the collection process. Several Do's and Don'ts for telephone collection are listed in Figure 13–19.

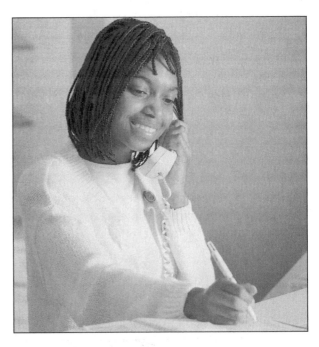

FIGURE 13–18 When collection letters receive no response, the medical assistant needs to call the patient to inquire about the past due balance.

Do	Don't
• Organize your thoughts before calling.	• Speak to anyone unfamiliar with the account.
• Identify the person to whom you are speaking. Ask for the person responsible for the account.	• Act harsh, belligerent, or threatening.
• Display a cooperative attitude.	• Use insurance "legalese" language.
• Speak on patient's level.	• Interrupt patients in an unkind or tactless manner.
• Listen respectfully to the person.	• Threaten or argue.
• Help the person think of multiple ways of solving the payment problem.	• Dive right into a conversation without thinking.
• Review the patient's past payment history.	• Put the patient in the position of correcting your information.
• Ask for a specific payment date.	• Leave the payment date unclear.
• Ask for partial payment when full payment cannot be paid.	• Make an impossible ultimatum.
• Refer the person to the physician if treatment is questioned.	• Discuss the value of medical treatment the patient received.
• Prompt answers by asking questions about the payment problem.	• Allow the individual to flounder for excuses.
• Wait for the patient to answer.	• Help the patient with excuses about why payment has not been made.
• Record results of the call in the patient's file.	• Try to remember everything the patient said.
• Tabulate results of all such calls to create an overdue account profile for the practice.	

FIGURE 13–19 Do's and Don't for telephone collection

Telephone collection is an effective method when handled properly. On the other hand, this task can be unpleasant if it is perceived negatively. Remember, each person who charges a product or service is morally, ethically, and legally bound to pay. Although some people are slow to pay, they should not be allowed to overlook the account. Although the medical assistant's patience may be tested at times, telephone collections are valuable in reaching people who ignore letters. Think of telephone collection as a method for the practice and the patient mutually to find a way for the bill to be paid.

TRUTH-IN-LENDING

Health insurance does not always cover the cost of a physician's service, and not all patients are covered by health insurance. Therefore, physicians occasionally find it necessary to extend credit, or "carry" an account over a period of time, allowing the patient to make several small, scheduled payments. For the privilege of receiving credit, patients must pay finance charges on the unpaid balance, just like an interest charge on a credit card. This substitutes for interest the practice could earn if fees were paid at the time of service and placed in an interest-bearing account. In other words, when a practice is willing to offer payment alternatives, it should not lose money doing so.

The Consumer Credit Protection Act of 1968, commonly called the Truth-in-Lending Act, requires providers of installment credit to state the charges in writing clearly and to express the interest as an annual rate. This law applies to medical practices as well as to other lenders; therefore, each time an account is to be paid "on time" a truth-in-lending letter should be written to the responsible person outlining the terms of the credit and the annual rate of interest. A cover letter and a truth-in-lending disclosure are shown in Figures 13–20 and 13–21.

Salem Randall, M.D.
82-B Medical Building
Ambler, PA 19002

June 15, 20–

Mr. Chamois Reilly
42 Jennings Drive
Ambler, PA 19002

Dear Mr. Reilly:

As you and Dr. Randall agreed in the office last week, your balance of $736 will be paid on an installment plan over the next six months. Two copies of a truth-in-lending disclosure statement showing the amount of money financed and the annual finance charge are enclosed. Please read the statement carefully, sign on the line called "Guarantor's Signature," and return one copy of the form to me.

If you have any questions, Mr. Reilly, please call me at 555-7823. Your first payment is due August 1, 20–.

Sincerely,

Casey Husted
Accounts Manager

FIGURE 13–20 Cover letter for truth-in-lending statement

Salem Randall, M.D.
82-B Medical Building
Ambler, PA 19002

Truth-in-Lending

This Truth-in-Lending Disclosure is made in compliance with the Consumer Credit Protection Act.

Chamois Reilly	Chamois Reilly
Patient's Name	Guarantor's Name

605	42 Jennings Drive Ambler, PA 19002
Patient Number	Address

1. Cash Price Medical Fee	$886
2. Less Cash Down Payment	150
3. Unpaid Balance of Cash Service	736
4. Amount Financed	736
5. Finance Charge	73.60
6. Total of Payment (4 plus 5)	809.60
7. Deferred Payment Price	809.60
8. Annual Percentage Rate	10%

The total of $809.60 is payable to Dr. Salem Randall at the address shown above in six (6) installments of $134.70 beginning August 1, 20– and due on the first day of each month thereafter through January 1, 20–.

_____   _____
Date   Guarantor's Signature

FIGURE 13–21 Truth-in-lending disclosure statement

IN YOUR OPINION

1. What might the result be from improperly aging accounts?
2. As a medical assistant, what could you do to make collection calls easier for both the patient and yourself?
3. What protections do truth-in-lending letters offer to both the patient and the practice?

INTERNET ACTIVITY

Log on to the Internet and locate an article on collections from customers. Use the keywords "Medical collections, collections, collecting payment, and others. Summarize what you learn.

STUDENT STUDY CHECKLIST

Workbook

1. Complete Chapter 13 exercises in the workbook.
2. Complete Chapter 13 simulations in the workbook that access the CD-ROM in the back of the book.

Administrative Skills CD-ROM

1. Go to the Library on the CD-ROM and play interactive games for Chapter 13.
2. Click on the Billings and Collections area of the office and select the Receipts folder. Complete the practice receipt exercises.

REFERENCES

Humphrey, Doris D. *Pediatric Associates, P.C.* Cincinnati, OH: South-Western, 1998.

Lindh, Wilburta Q., Marilyn S. Pooler, and Carol D. Tamparo. *Administrative Medical Assisting*, 2nd ed. Clifton Park, NY: Delmar Learning, 2002.

Money Line Lending Web site at moneylinelending.com, 2002.

CHAPTER ACTIVITIES

PERFORMANCE-BASED ACTIVITIES

1. Assume that you have been hired to handle collections at a private practice with three physicians. Collections have not been made since the last collection manager left six months ago. Most of the patients are covered by private or group insurance and a few patients are covered by Medicare. Write your recommendations for starting the collections process again, giving your reasons for each recommendation.

Recommended Steps for Collection

Type of Account	*Steps*	*Why*
1. Private Insurance	1. _____	1. _____
	2. _____	2. _____
	3. _____	3. _____
	4. _____	4. _____
	5. _____	5. _____
2. Group Insurance	1. _____	1. _____
	2. _____	2. _____
	3. _____	3. _____
	4. _____	4. _____
	5. _____	5. _____
3. Medicare	1. _____	1. _____
	2. _____	2. _____
	3. _____	3. _____
	4. _____	4. _____
	5. _____	5. _____
4. Other	1. _____	1. _____
	2. _____	2. _____
	3. _____	3. _____
	4. _____	4. _____
	5. _____	5. _____

2. Write a series of four form collection letters to mail to private insurers who do not pay claims promptly. Use the heading provided.

Garibaldi Medical Center
314 Walnut Street
San Francisco, CA 94122
415-555-1213

---

3. Write the dialogue for three conversations you would have with a patient who refuses to pay her account. Assume you call the first time when the account is three months overdue, the second time when the account is four months overdue, and the third time when the account is five months overdue. List in the chart below the key points to make and the patient's likely questions and objections. Role play your situations with a member of your class.

Key Points   *Patient Questions*   *Patient Objections*

Conversation 1.

Conversation 2.

Conversation 3.

EXPANDING YOUR THINKING

1. Compare the advantages and disadvantages of internal and external collection. Come to a conclusion about which method you would prefer.

Internal Collection

Advantages and Benefits   *Disadvantages*

1.

2.

3.

4.

5.

6.

7.

8.

External Collection

Advantages and Benefits	Disadvantages
1.	
2.	
3.	
4.	
5.	
6.	
7.	
8.	

2. Add your personal suggestions on the form below to the list of Do's and Don'ts for telephone collection listed in Figure 13–19.

Tone of Voice

Words to Use or Avoid

Helpful Questions

Making Sure You Gain Commitment to Pay the Bill

CHAPTER 14

Health Insurance and Coding

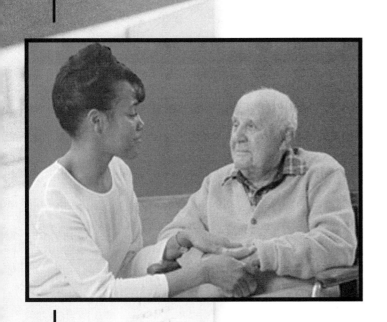

HUNTSVILLE, ALABAMA

At the risk of sounding a bit arrogant, I'd have to say that without my attention to insurance claims, this medical office would disappear. We serve a large elderly and below-poverty level groups of patients in the inner city, mixed with a few business people who use us because we're close to their offices.

Our elderly patients are covered by Medicare, and our pregnant moms without income and other poor patients are covered by Medicaid. I complete all the insurance claims forms for these patients, track them for payment, and follow up with the insurance companies when we aren't paid on time or correctly.

A big part of my job is making sure CMS forms are completed correctly. I check and recheck every detail, making sure all forms are dated, the CPT and ICD codes match the treatments and diagnosis, and the doctor's signature is present. The last thing I want is for a claim to get hung up in the bureaucracy of an insurance company because I didn't catch a mistake.

It's very rewarding to work for a practice that cares so much about treating the underprivileged. My job is to keep the cash flow on target by doing my job quickly and accurately.

John Christiansen
Medical Assistant/Claims Specialist

PERFORMANCE-BASED COMPETENCIES

After completing this chapter, you should be able to:
1. Use CPT-5 and ICD coding.
2. Analyze and use current third-party guidelines for reimbursement.
3. Discuss the different types of managed health care insurance.
4. Complete a CMS-1500 (formerly HCFA-1500) form.
5. Set up an audit trail for health insurance claims.

VOCABULARY

Basic insurance   Insurance benefits that cover physicians' fees, hospital expenses, and surgical fees as determined by the plan contract, usually after payment of a deductible by the patient.

Blue Cross and Blue Shield   Nonprofit insurers organized under the laws of individual states; generally, Blue Shield pays for physicians' services and Blue Cross covers hospital costs.

Capitation   A managed health concept whereby the physician is paid a certain amount per patient, no matter how much or how little service the patient receives.

Claim form   The documentation required by an insurance company before payment will be made for medical services.

Co-insurance   An insurance company and a patient share the cost of medical care, usually on an 80/20 split.

Commercial insurance   For-profit companies offering individual or group health insurance.

Comprehensive insurance   Combination of basic and major medical insurance.

Coordination of benefits   A policy requirement that insurance companies will share the cost of treatment when a patient is covered by more than one policy.

Co-payment   Percent of medical expenses for which the patient is responsible beyond the deductible.

Deductible   Amount paid by a patient prior to initiation of insurance benefits.

Diagnosis-related group (DRG)   Method of classifying patients into categories based on the primary diagnosis.

Exclusion   Illnesses or injuries not covered under an insurance policy.

Group insurance   Coverage of a group of people based on a common characteristic, such as employment at a company.

Major medical insurance   Insurance designed to offset potentially catastrophic expenses from a lengthy illness or accident.

Medicaid   Government health insurance program that protects the poor.

Medicare   Government health insurance program that protects the elderly.

Preexisting condition   A medical condition that existed before an insurance policy was approved.

Prospective payment   Term describing a method of flat fee pricing.

Usual and customary care   The fee that is usually charged for a specific service, one that is customary of the usual range and fees and is reasonable for the geographic area.

Waiting period   The time between when an insurance policy is approved and the patient is covered for benefits, often called the elimination.

Waiver   An attachment to a policy that excludes specific preexisting conditions.

Workers' compensation insurance   Employer-paid insurance that provides health care and income to employees and their dependents when employees suffer work-related injuries or illness.

Few families can afford to pay the expenses of a catastrophic illness or even the routine medical expenses of a family; therefore most Americans purchase insurance protection individually or through an organization. The federal government's Medicare and the states' Medicaid programs cover health care for the elderly and the poor.

Health insurance enables people to prepare financially for the high cost of an unexpected illness or injury by purchasing protection for an annual premium.

In response to the need for insurance, several financing plans besides the traditional private office, fee-for-service physician arrangement have evolved.

As a medical assistant, you will learn the differences among the plans under which patients are covered. Frequently, you will interpret benefits for patients to collect the practice's fees properly. Although patients are ultimately responsible for paying their accounts, they usually pay only a small portion of the costs of illnesses or accidents themselves, and some form of insurance pays for the remainder. Because the livelihoods of the physician and staff of a medical facility depend on income from insurance sources, managing insurance payments will be a fundamental part of your duties as a medical assistant.

TYPES OF HEALTH INSURANCE COVERAGE

In general, health insurance can be categorized in three ways: traditional coverage, managed care, and government or other program. The amount of premium a subscriber or purchaser pays determines the degree of protection a policy offers.

Traditional Coverage

Traditional insurance policies vary, but their basic characteristic is coverage on a fee-for-service basis. The insurance carrier generally pays 80% of the fee, and the patient pays a deductible 20%. Some companies require a waiting period after a policy is approved and before benefits begin. If during the waiting period a patient becomes ill or is injured, the insurance company will not pay. Insurance companies protect themselves further by excluding certain noncovered illnesses or disabilities and including waivers for preexisting conditions. Many traditional policies require patients to coordinate all their medical care with a primary care physician who refers the patients to specialists when needed.

A coordination of benefits statement, included in most policies, requires a sharing of the medical expenses by another insurance company when a patient is covered by more than one policy, for example, when both a father and mother receive insurance benefits for their children through insurance at work. After the health insurance claim form is received and reviewed by the insurance company, payment is made directly to the patient.

Basic Insurance

The physician's fee, hospital expenses, and surgical fees up to a maximum amount written in the contract are generally covered by basic insurance. Payment may be based on a "usual and customary fee," or the content may specify a stated amount. Usual and customary fee refers to the usual fee the physician charges most patients (usual), the midrange fee for this type of service (reasonable), and the average charge for the procedure by all physicians practicing the same specialty in the same geographic area (customary).

Many policies require a deductible or copayment from the patient with the patient typically paying the first $100, $200, or more of annual medical costs in addition to 20% of the remaining charges. For example, the patient whose medical expenses amount to $500 during one year might be required to a pay a $200 deductible and an additional $60 ($500 − $200 × 20%). The insurance company would reimburse the patient $240.

Hospital benefits for basic insurance may pay a certain dollar amount for a specified number of days, or they may pay full charges for a specific type of room, usually semiprivate (two patients per room), for a specified number of days. Inpatient services such as laboratory tests, x-rays, operating room, anesthesia, surgical dressings, and some outpatient services, though not all, are usually included (Figure 14–1). Some plans cover

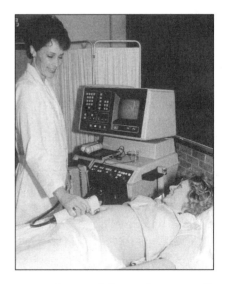

FIGURE 14–1 Ultrasound diagnostics are usually covered by basic insurance.

extended care at a skilled nursing facility after a patient's release from a hospital. A basic policy usually covers all or a portion of maternity care.

Major Medical Insurance

Major medical, or catastrophic, insurance takes up where basic insurance leaves off and is designed to help offset huge medical expenses that result from a lengthy illness or serious accident. Most major medical policies include a deductible provision that calls for a co-insurance, usually 20%, to be paid by the patient. Benefits, which usually range from $10,000 to unlimited coverage, determine the amount of the premium. Policies cover health services and supplies beyond those available in basic policies, including the services of special nurses, rental of medical equipment, prosthetic devices, and related items (Figure 14–2).

Comprehensive Major Medical Insurance

Comprehensive major medical insurance combines the benefits of basic medical and major medical protection. Coverage usually includes a small deductible and provides broad medical treatment under one contract.

Blue Cross and Blue Shield

Blue Cross and Blue Shield are nonprofit insurers organized under the laws of the individual states

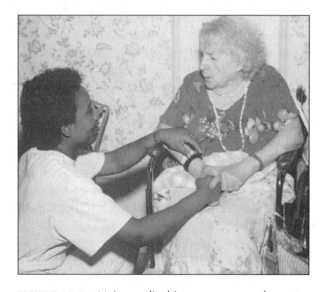

FIGURE 14–2 Major medical insurance covers the cost of items related to health care.

and regulated by boards of directors made up of public representatives, physicians, and other health care providers. Generally, Blue Shield plans pay for the services of physicians and other providers, and Blue Cross plans pay for hospital services. A patient may subscribe to either plan or to a combined plan. Each Blue Cross/Blue Shield plan develops and administers its own benefits package, although both plans usually cover groups of people with a common characteristic, for example, all the employees of a single company. In addition to the traditional Blue Cross and Blue Shield plans, health maintenance organization (HMO) plans are available.

Commercial Insurance Companies

Prudential Insurance, Nationwide Insurance, The Travelers Companies, and other similar companies are for-profit organizations that offer individual or group basic health and major medical insurance for an annual premium. In addition to health coverage, most sell other forms of insurance such as fire, theft, life, and casualty insurance.

Managed Health Care

Managed care is a belief that a health care system should work to keep people healthy and should ensure the right treatment in the right setting by the right person when they are sick or injured. Managed care exists in different forms, with different benefit structures, financing mechanics, and provider groups. It is still evolving and is very much a work in progress. Some managed health companies require that policyholders use medical services only from preferred providers.

Managed care plans are prepaid. Patients pay monthly premiums through their employer or individually. The physician provides service to the patient, and the patient either does not make any additional payment or makes co-payments and deductible payments required by the plan.

Health Maintenance Organizations (HMOs)

Millions of people belong to health maintenance organizations (HMOs). For a monthly pay-in-advance membership or annual prepayment paid through the employer or individually, each insured person is guaranteed physician and hospital services for little or no additional charge. Patients are attracted to HMOs because they guarantee no unexpected medical costs. Under an HMO plan, certain medical services are performed by participating physicians to a group of enrolled people. The physician is paid a per capita amount for each patient without considering the actual amount of service provided to each patient.

HMOs sometimes operate their own clinics with a salaried staff of physicians, or they may contract with groups of private physicians to provide service to members. In general, HMO members receive full medical services only if they use the physician groups and hospitals who participate in the plan, although under some plans emergency care will be covered outside the service area. When members are ill, they go to HMO clinics to see physicians who are salaried employees; if they need hospitalization, they are admitted to HMO-approved hospitals. The bill is sent to the HMO, and the members spend little or no money beyond the monthly or annual membership fee. When fees are charged, they are called co-payments. They range from $5 to $25 usually and are due at the time of the treatment. Prescriptions are usually covered also, with a small amount, usually $5 to $10, paid by the patient. A $100 prescription, which the patient has refilled monthly, might cost the patient only $5 per month, depending on the plan, a savings of $1,140 each year. In essence, a patient's choice of care is limited in exchange for a prepaid, preset price.

HMOs differ in the services they provide. An HMO may cover the entire cost of a medical or hospital service or may require a small charge for each visit or service. Because HMOs operate within a fixed budget based on prepayment, the HMO has a financial incentive to reduce the use of hospital facilities and emergency care, thus emphasizing "wellness" and "wellness checks" as a method of reducing expenses.

Two factors contribute to an HMO's ability to promise no unexpected costs:

1. Paperwork expenses are less for HMOs because there are no insurance forms to fill out. By eliminating time-consuming paper-

work activity, the HMO requires fewer employees.
2. With no profit incentive for ordering additional tests and procedures, HMO physicians are less likely to duplicate laboratory procedures or ask for secondary tests. Studies have shown that fee-for-service physicians order 50% more chest x-rays and ECGs than do HMO physicians.

Health maintenance organizations are controversial. Although HMOs appear to limit expenses, physicians and hospitals argue that they also limit care. When an extra x-ray reads negative for the average patient, it becomes an unnecessary expense; however, a second x-ray that finds a formerly undetected carcinoma may save the patient's life.

Exclusive Provider Organizations (EPOs)

In this approach to managed care, exclusive providers agree not to take work for any other managed care organization. Subscribers receive benefits for obtaining services from a network of providers who contract with a managed care plan, but they receive no benefits if they choose a provider who is not associated with the EPO.

Preferred Provider Organizations

A preferred provider organization (PPO) provides medical services at preset, usually lower, fees in return for a large number of referrals, such as a major corporation or a union who agrees to send all employee members of the group to physicians or hospitals affiliated with the PPO in return for volume discounts. Unlike some HMO physicians, PPO physicians are not employees of the treating organization; therefore, they can continue to provide service under the traditional fee-for-service arrangement. Usually, PPOs do not have contracts for laboratory or pharmacy services, but they do offer reduced rates at specific hospitals. Although the PPO member fee is usually lower than an HMO fee, co-payments are usually higher.

Integrated Delivery System (IDS)

Under this approach to managed care, groups of physicians and ambulatory centers affiliate to provide joining health care services to subscribers.

By subscribing to the plan, patients can choose their provider depending on the circumstance at the time.

Point-of-Service Plan (POS)

Subscribers to this type of plan have not only the option of going to a physician or facility that is part of the plan, but they also are free to "self-refer" to a non-HMO provider. When subscribers self-refer, they usually must pay a significant deductible fee — as high as $250 — and co-insurance charges as high as 25%.

Triple Option Plan (Cafeteria Plan)

Named because of the choices available to subscribers, Triple Option Plans, or cafeteria plans, offer traditional insurance, the HMO approach, or preferred provider services, as well as extra coverage options.

Medicare, Medicaid, and Other Government Programs

The fastest growing segment of the U.S. population is the group over 100 years old. The second fastest growing population group is 85 to 100 years old.

As might be expected and research confirms, the elderly are the biggest users of health care services in this country. The largest expenditures occur during the last year of life.

Because older people usually do not work and may depend on Social Security benefits, they cannot afford expensive health care. To address this problem, the U.S. government developed Medicare in 1965 to protect older citizens from the costs of illnesses (Figure 14–3). Medicaid, a similar program, was created to provide health services for the poor. This makes the U.S. government the largest purchaser in the country of health care services.

An aging population means continued increase in the rate of growth for Medicare spending. From 1993 to 2030, new entrants into the labor force are expected to increase by 20% while the numbers of people over the age of 65 are expected to double, or increase by 100%.

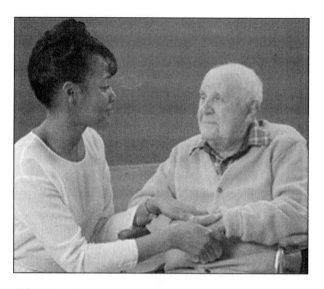

FIGURE 14–3 Americans over 65 are protected by Medicare.

Medicare

Medicare protects Americans aged 65 and over and citizens with disabilities under age 65. The coverage consists of two parts: A, hospital insurance; and B, medical insurance. Medicare hospital insurance pays for most but not all of a patient's hospital treatment and related expenses, and Medicare medical insurance pays 80% of reasonable physician's fees and related medical charges minus a deductible amount. Medicare is administered by the Centers for Medicare & Medicaid Services (CMS). Before 2001, this agency was known as the Health Care Financing Administration (HCFA, pronounced Hick-fa). In each state, an administering agency, often a large insurance company such as Equitable Life Assurance Society or Nationwide Insurance, is named to process Medicare claims. Because claims may be handled in a slightly different manner by the administering agency in each state, each state should be contacted for specific instructions. The local Medicare office in each area can provide the name of the administrator. Also, Parts A and B may be administered by two different contractors.

Medicare recipients are issued cards showing whether they have hospital benefits or a combination of hospital and medical benefits. The card also shows the Medicare identification number, which is needed for reporting Medicare claims. When a new Medicare patient registers with the medical office, the medical assistant should photocopy the Medicare card and store the photocopy in the patient's medical record.

When a physician agrees to accept Medicare assignment of benefits, he or she agrees to accept Medicare's predetermined payment in full for the services performed. Medicare pays 80% of the amount, and the patient pays 20%. The difference between what Medicare allows and what the physician normally charges is written off.

- **Part A** — Medicare, Part A, provides hospital benefits for the aged, disabled, or blind. Benefits begin the day a patient enters the hospital and ends when the patient has not been in a bed in any hospital for 60 consecutive days. Funds for Part A come from the employers and employees and the self-employed.

- **Part B** — Medicare, Part B, provides supplementary coverage for outpatient services for the aged, disabled, or blind. Premiums are deducted monthly from Social Security checks.

The five major classifications of Medicare Part A benefits are listed in Table 14–1, and Part B benefits are listed in Table 14–2.

TABLE 14–1
Five Major Classifications of Medicare Part A Benefits

Services	Benefit	Medicare Pays	Patient Pays
HOSPITALIZATION Semiprivate room and board, general nursing and miscellaneous hospital services and supplies. (Medicare payments based on benefit periods.)	First 60 days	All but $760	$760
	61st to 90th day	All but $190 a day	$190 a day
	91st to 150th day[1]	All but $380 a day	$380 a day
	Beyond 150 days	Nothing	All costs
SKILLED NURSING FACILITY CARE Patient must have been in a hospital for at least 3 days and enter a Medicare-approved facility generally within 30 days after hospital discharge.[2] (Medicare payments based on benefit periods.)	First 20 days	100% of app'd amount	Nothing
	Additional 80 days	All but $95 a day	Up to $95 a day
	Beyond 100 days	Nothing	All costs
HOME HEALTH CARE Part-time or intermittent skilled care, home health aide services, durable medical equipment and supplies, and other services.	Unlimited as long as Medicare conditions are met.	100% of approved amount; 80% of approved amount for durable medical equipment.	Nothing for services; 20% of approved amount for durable equipment.
HOSPICE CARE Pain relief, symptom management, and support services for the terminally ill.	If patient elects the hospice option and as long as doctor certifies need.	All but limited costs for outpatient drugs and inpatient respite care.	Limited cost sharing for outpatient drugs and inpatient respite care.
BLOOD	Unlimited if medically necessary.	All but first 3 pints per calendar year.	For first 3 pints.[3]

[1]This 60-reserve-days benefit may be used only once in a lifetime.

[2]Neither Medicare nor private Medigap insurance will pay for most nursing home care.

[3]To the extent the blood deductible is met under Part B of Medicare during the calendar year, it does not have to be met under Part A.

(Modified from *Your Medicare Handbook for Railroad Retirement Beneficiaries.* U.S. Government Printing Office, 1997.)

TABLE 14–2
Five Major Classifications of Medicare Part B Benefits

Services	Benefit	Medicare Pays	Patient Pays
MEDICAL EXPENSES Physicians' services, inpatient and out-patient medical and surgical services and supplies, physical and speech therapy, ambulance, diagnostic tests, and other services.	Unlimited if med-ically necessary.	80% of approved amount (after $100 deductible). Reduced to 50% for most outpatient mental health services.	$100 deductible, 20% of approved amount and limited charged above approved amount.
CLINICAL LABORATORY SERVICES Blood tests, urinalysis, and more.	Unlimited if med-ically necessary.	100% of approved amount.	Nothing for services.
HOME HEALTH CARE Part-time or intermittent skilled care, home health aide services, durable medical equipment and supplies, and other services.	Unlimited as long as patient meets conditions for benefits.	100% of approved amount; 80% of approved amount for durable medical equipment.	Nothing for services. 20% of approved amount for durable medical equipment.
OUTPATIENT HOSPITAL TREATMENT Services for the diagnosis or treatment of illness or injury.	Unlimited if medically necessary.	Medicare payment to hospital based on hospital cost.	$100 deductible, 20% of whatever the hospital charges.
BLOOD	Unlimited if medically necessary.	80% of approved amount (after $100 deductible and starting with 4th pint).	First 3 pints plus 20% approved amount for additional pints (after $100 deductible).
AMBULATORY SURGICAL SERVICES	Unlimited if medically necessary.	80% of predeter-mined amount (after $100 deductible).	$100 deductible plus 20% of predetermined amount.

[1]Once the patient has had $100 of expenses for covered services in the year, the Part B deductible does not apply to any further services received for the rest of the year.

[2]To the extent the blood deductible is met under Part A of Medicare during the calendar year, it does not have to be met under Part B.

(Modified from *Your Medicare Handbook for Railroad Retirement Beneficiaries.* U.S. Government Printing Office, 1997.)

Medicaid

Medicaid is a financial assistance program developed jointly by the federal government and the states to provide health care for the poor. Benefits offered are similar to other insurance programs, although they differ in amount from state to state. Medicaid generally pays the deductible amount charged under Medicare and the 20% not covered by Medicare medical insurance.

Again, the local Medicaid office should be called to determined what Medicaid benefits are paid in a specific state.

Medicaid claim forms are filed with the state administering agency, which determines whether the claim will be paid. Time limits for filing claims vary from state to state, and late claims may be rejected by the administrator. Individuals should contact their local agencies for information regarding filing deadlines and procedures. A Medicaid patient is issued an identifying card and number. The medical assistant should photocopy the card when a Medicaid patient registers and place the copy in the patient's medical record.

Health Insurance Portability and Accounting Act

The original intention of the Health Insurance and Portability and Accounting Act (HIPAA) of 1996 was to see to it that people who lost or switched jobs would be able to continue their health insurance coverage. Additionally, along the way, words were added to protect patient privacy in a health care setting. This grew out of the wish by Congress to assist the health care industry to realize the benefits of standardizing the computer/Internet transmission of information such as claims insurance verification and referrals. It was in the context of increased use of the Internet that the patient privacy issue was raised during passage of the legislation.

HIPAA gives patients statutory rights to determine the use of personal and medical information about them. Under the law, individually identifiable patient information is limited to three areas: patient treatment, payment collections, and provider operations.

The underlying philosophy is that patient information should be shared only on a need-to-know basis, and limited to only the information needed to perform a specific task. Along with the establishment of patients' rights with regard to information about them, the law provides for penalties for the improper use or disclosure of information. The final rules of privacy went into effect in 2003.

A medical provider or physician group must comply with HIPAA if it deals electronically with patient information in the form of "HIPAA transaction sets"— standardized, electronically formatted data blocks designed by the federal government with input from the insurance, provider, and consumer sectors. On the other hand, if the provider or group uses only paper, fax, or the telephone to store or send information, there is no requirement to comply with HIPAA patient privacy standards.

The protection extends to information stored in any form or hard copy. So, if a group practice,

for instance, exchanges patient information by using a HIPAA transaction set, it is required to comply with patient privacy rights under the law, and this compliance extends to paper records it maintains containing patient information.

As an additional mechanism to encourage providers to involve themselves in the electronic exchange of patient information, beginning October 2003, all physicians and other providers who have more than 10 employees were required to file Medicare claims electronically.

The HIPAA's privacy standards and transmissions sets are relatively new. Over time, the HIPAA will revolutionize the efficiency with which medical offices deal with patient information in the insurance context. Just as important, perhaps, is the increased privacy that patients will have with regard to the distribution of information about their medical condition. For the medical assistant, it will mean additional forms to learn, understanding of transmission sets, and a greater sensitivity to the privacy of patient information.

Other Government Programs

Military personnel and civilian employees of the federal government are covered under special insurance programs. Because the number of patient's covered under one of these plans in the average medical office is small, only a brief overview is provided here. When a patient enrolled in one of the programs comes under the care of the physician, the medical assistant should ask the patient for a brochure or other documentation that explains the benefits before making an insurance claim. Some restrictions exist for use of medical services off-base; therefore, this documentation should be carefully reviewed.

CHAMPUS **CHAMPUS** refers to the Civilian Health and Medical Program of the Uniformed Services (Army, Navy, Air Force, Marines, and Coast Guard). This program covers medical care not directly related to military service (for example, viral infection) for uniformed service personnel and their families. Although most uniformed services families obtain their medical care from government facilities, they are paid CHAMPUS benefits if they are referred to a private physician. The provider must be authorized by CHAMPUS.

Military dependents who prefer to be treated by a civilian medical facility can receive treatment by providing the office with a nonavailability statement or authorization issued by the commander of the military hospital. This statement should be attached to the CHAMPUS claim reporting form.

CHAMPVA **CHAMPVA** refers to the Civilian Health and Medical Program of the Veterans Administration and is similar to CHAMPUS. Those covered are (1) dependents of totally disabled veterans whose disabilities are service related, and (2) surviving dependents of veterans who have died from service-related disabilities.

FEHB Active and retired civilian employees of the federal government and their dependents may enroll in the Federal Employees' Health Benefits Program, which is administered by the Civil Service Commission through private insurers. The program is voluntary and offers similar benefits to the basic coverage and major medical coverage of other programs.

TRICARE This government sponsored managed care plan covers people in, affiliated, or retired from the uniformed services, the Public Health Service, and the North Atlantic Treaty Organization (NATO). TRICARE also provides coverage for their families and survivors. It covers medical care not directly related to military service (a viral infection, as contrasted with a shrapnel wound received in combat).

- TRICARE Prime: each enrollee is assigned a primary care manager; services are provided by military treatment facilities
- TRICARE Extra: a preferred provider option
- TRICARE Standard: a basic fee-for-service approach

Workers' Compensation Insurance

Workers' compensation insurance laws in each state require employers to purchase insurance that provides health care and income to employees and their dependents when the employee suffers or dies from a work-related injury or illness (Figure 14–4). The employer pays all premiums for workers' compensation insurance to a private carrier in return for protection from financial liability. Excluded from the workers' com-

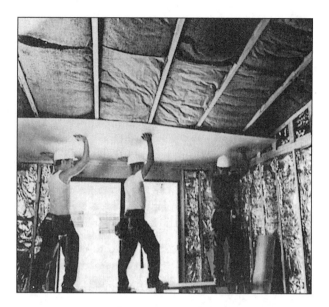

FIGURE 14–4 Workers' compensation insurance provides health care and income when an employee suffers a work-related injury, illness, or death.

pensation laws in some states are domestic workers, farmers, and employees of small companies. Federal workers' compensation laws have been enacted to provide benefits for people employed by the federal government.

The purpose of workers' compensation insurance is to return the employee to work. This includes providing medical treatment, hospital care, surgery, and therapy from the time of injury or diagnosis of an illness until recovery. In the case of total or partial disability, income benefits are paid to the injured or ill worker. If an employee is killed on the job or dies from a job-related disease or disability, a moderate funeral expense and living expenses are provided for the dependents. Benefits vary from state to state, so the Bureau of Workers' Compensation in each state must be contacted for an explanation of that state's law.

Claims for workers' compensation insurance are made with the Bureau of Workers' Compensation in each state. Because the claim forms for the states differ, the medical assistant should contact the patient's employer for a copy of the proper form. The attending physician is required to make a report before an employee may collect benefits under a claim. A workers' compensation insurance form from one state is shown in Figure 14–5.

1. Type answers to All questions and file original with the Workers' Compensation Commission within 72 hours after first treatment.
2. DO NOT FAIL to forward to the Workers' Compensation Commission PROGRESS REPORTS and FINAL REPORT upon discharge of patient.

WORKERS' COMPENSATION COMMISSION

DO NOT WRITE IN THIS SPACE

WCC CLAIM #

EMPLOYER'S REPORT Yes ☐ No ☐

This is First Report ☐   Progress Report ☐   Final Report ☐

EVERY QUESTION MUST BE ANSWERED AND FORM SIGNED

1. Name of Injured Person: Maureen A. Santega	Soc. Sec. No. 610-98-7432	D.O.B. 7/19/69	Sex M ☐ F ☑

2. Address: (No. and Street) 905 Raymond Lane   (City or Town) Atlanta   (State) GA   (Zip Code) 30385-8893

3. Name and Address of Employer: Majors Concrete Company, 238 Leaf Lane, Atlanta, GA 30342-3329

4. Date of Accident or Onset of Disease: 4/9/—   Hour: A.M. ☑   P.M. ☐   5. Date Disability Began: 4/9/—

6. Patient's Description of Accident or Cause of Disease: Concrete truck struck and backed over patient's foot while she was pouring concrete at job site

7. Medical description of Injury or Disease: massive bruising to left foot, no broken bones, great deal of pain associated with bruises

8. Will Injury result in: (a) Permanent defect? Yes ☐ No ☑ If so, what?   (b) Disfigurement Yes ☐ No ☑

9. Causes, other than injury, contributing to patients condition: None

10. Is patient suffering from any disease of the heart, lungs, brain, kidneys, blood, vascular system or any other disabling condition not due to this accident? Give particulars: No

11. Is there any history or evidence present of previous accident or disease? Give particulars: No

12. Has normal recovery been delayed for any reason? Give particulars: No

13. Date of first treatment: 4/10/—   Who engaged your services? patient

14. Describe treatment given by you: Darvon, 100 mg q4h prn for pain

15. Were X-Rays taken: Yes ☑ No ☐   By whom? — (Name and Address) Edwin Gordon, M.D. 802 Manor Lane, Atlanta 30303   Date 4/10/—

16. X-Ray Diagnosis: No broken bones

17. Was patient treated by anyone else? Yes ☐ No ☑   By whom? — (Name and Address)   Date

18. Was patient hospitalized? Yes ☐ No ☑   Name and Address of Hospital   Date of Admission: Date of Discharge:

19. Is further treatment needed? Yes ☐ No ☑   For how long?   20. Patient was ☑ will be ☐ able to resume regular work on: 4/14   Patient was ☐ will be ☐ able to resume light work on:

21. If death ensued give date: 22. Remarks: (Give any information of value not included above)

23. I am a qualified specialist in: orthopedics   I am a duly licensed Physician in the State of: Maryland   I was graduated from Medical School (Name) Johns Hopkins   Year 1967

Date of this report: 6/21/—   (Signed) *John N. Sparks, M.D.*

(This report must be signed PERSONALLY by Physician)

Address: 8504 Capricorn Drive Atlanta GA 30312   Phone: (404) 544-0078

FIGURE 14–5   Sample workers' compensation claim form

PROSPECTIVE PAYMENT SYSTEM

Diagnosis-related group is a term that describes a method of prospective pricing in which a hospital is paid a flat fee for medical service for Medicare patients based on an average cost of service, not on the actual cost per patient. The prospective pricing, or prospective payment, system was enacted in 1983 for hospitalized Medicare patients in an effort to reduce the cost of hospital care for the elderly.

As originally set up in 1965, Medicare payments were "passed along"; that is, hospitals assigned whatever cost they wished for medical care and passed the bill along to the government. Physicians, too, who treated Medicare patients could decide what fees were "customary" and pass along their bills to Medicare, which paid, usually without question. There was virtually no control over fee setting for either physicians or hospitals, and health care costs for the elderly skyrocketed. Predictably, those in control of financing government programs began to look for ways to contain expenses.

Diagnosis-Related Groups

The Health Care Financing Administration (HCFA), now known as the Centers for Medicare & Medicaid Services (CMS), which manages Medicare and Medicaid, adopted a plan developed at Yale University in the late 1960s in an effort to set a standard for hospital costs for Medicare patients. With minor changes, the plan, called diagnosis-related groups, was written into law in the Social Security Amendments Act in 1983.

A diagnosis-related group (DRG) is a method of classifying patients into categories based on the primary diagnosis. Hospitals are paid a flat fee for Medicare patients according to the category of illness. The fee is based on an average cost of service, not the actual cost. Every hospitalized Medicare patient must be placed in a category. The categories are derived from all of the possible diagnoses identified in *International Classification of Diseases, Clinical Modification* (ICD-9). Diseases are classified into forty-seven major diagnostic categories based on organ systems. All patients in the same DRG can be expected to

respond in a clinically similar manner, which, if averaged statistically, will result in about equal use of the hospital's facilities and resources, according to *DRGs and the Prospective Payment System*.

Five pieces of information are needed to place a patient in a DRG:

1. The patient's principal diagnosis and up to four complications
2. The treatment procedures performed
3. The patient's age
4. The patient's sex
5. The patient's status at discharge

The DRG program works in the following manner. After a patient is diagnosed, the hospital sends diagnostic information to the administering agency and receives a fixed fee based on the average cost of treating the patient's condition. If the patient's condition is corrected at less than average cost, the hospital makes money. However, if the patient's problem is more severe than average and takes more hospital days, physician time, and hospital resources than average, the hospital loses money. As an example, a Medicare patient diagnosed by a physician as suffering heart failure and shock would be classified in DRG 157, and the hospital would be reimbursed the amount allowed for that particular classification. In severe cases where expenses become catastrophic, an additional sum called an "outlier" is paid to offset the hospital's huge losses. The DRG system rewards efficiency in providing care, and a hospital that treats patients for less than the DRG payment receives a built-in bonus.

Significance of DRGs

Diagnosis-related groups caused a dramatic change in the way hospitals treat Medicare patients, and both hospitals and physicians argue that patients may not receive the treatment they need because of cost-cutting measures to stay within DRG limits. However, proponents of the system point out that physicians should not order duplicate procedures and services.

In an effort to maintain financial stability, hospitals have formed boards of physicians and other providers to set standards for what tests, procedures, and services are necessary to treat patients assigned to each DRG. Because physicians are responsible for diagnosing the condition that places a patient in a DRG, hospitals exert great pressure on them to make realistic diagnoses and to treat within the DRG payment system. Extra tests, procedures, and services are not allowed except in unusual cases.

The concept of DRGs and prospective payment is highly controversial because, based on Medicare's success in reducing costs, private insurance companies are now drawing plans for establishing their own standards. The time when hospitals and physicians can establish costs without outside review has passed.

IN YOUR OPINION

1. From the medical assistant's viewpoint, what are the advantages and disadvantages of the variety of health care financing plans available to patients?
2. What do you believe are the advantages and disadvantage of managed health care plans?
3. Since DRGs were developed to standardize hospital charges only, why are they important to private practice medical assistants?

FILING AN INSURANCE CLAIM

Payments by insurance companies, or third-party carriers, represent a large portion of a medical practice's income. Therefore, as a medical assistant, it is extremely important for you to understand the claims process if you file insurance claims or help patients file their own claims.

Following the Route of a Claim

Patients with insurance coverage must file claims with their carriers explaining the services received and the associated costs. Although patients are responsible for filing their own claims, some medical offices have found that their collection rate is better if they complete the forms for patients. Patients often are uncertain about how the form should be filled in, or they delay mailing the form, which delays the physician's payment.

Physicians have reduced this problem somewhat by requiring patients to pay at the time of their visit, then to collect reimbursement from their insurance carriers. Computers have also contributed to more efficient claim filing, because many software systems automatically print an insurance claim form at the end of each patient's visit. Some medical offices use modems for quick electronic filing of a claim with an insurance company.

Once a claim form has been properly completed using information obtained from the patient information sheet supplied at the first visit and signed by the physician and patient, it is mailed to the carrier's claim department or, in the case of a government agency, to the agency's administrator. The claims examiner evaluates the form and determines whether the patient's benefits cover the services provided. If the claim form is improperly filled out, incomplete, unsigned by either the patient or the physician, or in any way questionable, the form will be returned and the claim will not be paid. The form can be resubmitted; however, because payment often takes several weeks from the time a form is received in the claims department, resubmissions reduce a practice's cash flow and should be avoided whenever possible. When the insurance examiner is satisfied that all conditions of coverage have been satisfactorily met, the claims department mails a check for the covered services, minus the deductible or co-payment, to the patient or the physician.

Assignment of Payment

A physician may elect to accept assignment of the patient's benefits under Medicare and other government insurance programs. This means that the physician agrees to accept an amount predetermined by the third-party carrier instead of charging usual and customary fees. Many physicians will not accept assignment of benefits. In this case, patients should be informed prior to receiving services.

Insurance Coding Systems

Two types of codes are used to standardize information for insurance claim forms. They are CPT for identifying procedures, treatments, and services, and ICD-9-CM for identifying diagnoses.

CPT-5

CPT-5 codes, developed by the american Medical Association (AMA) are listed in the book *Current Procedural Terminology*, Fifth Edition, which identifies individual medical procedures, treatments, and services for all specialties by a five-digit code. The book lists all the procedures, treatments, and service for each specialty and identifies each with its own code. Most insurance companies require the use of CPT-5 codes on claim forms. CPT has been embraced by the federal government and incorporated into the Common Procedure Coding System used by the Centers for Medicare & Medicaid Services (CMS). It is required in filings of Medicaid Part B services, in reports to Medicaid agencies, and for outpatient surgical procedures.

Selecting a code to represent the level of service for a patient visit depends on seven components: history, examination, medical decision making, nature of the problem, counseling, coordination of care, and time required. A medical assistant should take a course in CPT-5 coding for in-depth understanding.

Fundamentally, under CPT all medical procedures have been broken down and coded into the following six categories (the reason that the first-listed category, Evaluation and Management, is out of numerical sequence is because the functions listed are common to all medical service facilities, no matter what their medical specialty. The remaining five categories are each specialties):

- Evaluation and Management   99201–99499
- Anesthesia   00100–01999
- Surgery   10040–69990
- Radiology   70010–79999
- Pathology and Laboratory   80049–89399
- Medicine   90281–99199

Physicians mark on the charge slip the service they performed, so the medical assistant will not be called on to make all the decisions regarding how service should be coded. A medical assistant who has a question about the level or type of service performed should check with the physician before filing a claim form. A compre-

hensive charge slip that lists most of the treatments, procedures, and services performed by specialty practice and matches them with a CPT code is an excellent time saver. This enables the physician to identify clearly the CPT designation simply by marking the service.

Successful coding depends on proper documentation. Each code must be supported by evidence of treatment, procedures, or service, or the practice will not be reimbursed for the amounts submitted. Inaccurate or incomplete documentation of claims can put a practice at legal risk.

Several sample procedures and treatments and their codes are listed below, on the charge slip in Figure 14–6 and on the CMS-1500 form in Figure 14–7. A hypothetical fee is listed for each service. Refer to Figure 14–6 and analyze the manner in which the CPT codes, ICD codes, and fees are used to document services.

1. Look at the section of the charge slip called Office Visits. This established patient was charged $72 for an Intermediate Office visit during which the physician performed an examination to help arrive at a diagnosis. The CPT code range for established patients is 99211 to 99215, depending on the duration and complexity of the visit. The range for new patients, is 99201 to 99205. All doctors do not list all levels on the charge slip. The level of service is determined by the length of time the physician spends with the patient and the complexity of the problem. When assigning levels of service, the physician considers three key components:

   - The amount of history taking necessary to clearly understand the problem
   - The level of physical examination necessary to adequately evaluate the patient
   - The complexity of the problem and the amount of medical decision-making necessary to determine an adequate treatment plan

   When assigning higher levels of service, the physician also determines the mortality risk associated with the patient's condition.

2. Look at the section of the charge slip called Laboratory Services. These laboratory services,

FIGURE 14–6 Charge slip used with CMS-1500 claim form

APPROVED OMB-0938-0008

CARRIER

| | PICA | | **HEALTH INSURANCE CLAIM FORM** | PICA | | |

| 1. MEDICARE | MEDICAID | CHAMPUS | CHAMPVA | GROUP HEALTH PLAN (SSN or ID) | FECA BLK LUNG (SSN) | OTHER | 1a. INSURED'S I.D. NUMBER | (FOR PROGRAM IN ITEM 1) |
| (Medicare #) | (Medicaid #) | (Sponsor's SSN) | (VA File #) | | | ☒ (ID) | 283-58-6871 | |

2. PATIENT'S NAME (Last Name, First Name, Middle Initial)
Shields, Nancy V.

3. PATIENT'S BIRTH DATE MM DD YY
08 15 41   M☐ F☒ SEX

4. INSURED'S NAME (Last Name, First Name, Middle Initial)
SAME

5. PATIENT'S ADDRESS (No., Street)
5168 Oak Terrace

6. PATIENT RELATIONSHIP TO INSURED
Self ☒ Spouse ☐ Child ☐ Other ☐

7. INSURED'S ADDRESS (No., Street)
5168 Oak Terrace

CITY Decatur   STATE GA

8. PATIENT STATUS
Single ☐   Married ☒   Other ☐

CITY Decatur   STATE GA

ZIP CODE 30033-8823   TELEPHONE (Include Area Code) (404) 721-9001

Employed ☒   Full-Time Student ☐   Part-Time Student ☐

ZIP CODE 30033-8823   TELEPHONE (INCLUDE AREA CODE) (555) 721-9001

9. OTHER INSURED'S NAME (Last Name, First Name, Middle Initial)
Shields, John H.

10. IS PATIENT'S CONDITION RELATED TO:

11. INSURED'S POLICY GROUP OR FECA NUMBER
TN 75281

a. OTHER INSURED'S POLICY OR GROUP NUMBER
US 8123976

a. EMPLOYMENT? (CURRENT OR PREVIOUS)
☐ YES ☒ NO

a. INSURED'S DATE OF BIRTH MM DD YY
08 15 41   M☐ F☒ SEX

b. OTHER INSURED'S DATE OF BIRTH MM DD YY
02 10 40   M☒ F☐ SEX

b. AUTO ACCIDENT?   PLACE (State)
☐ YES ☒ NO

b. EMPLOYER'S NAME OR SCHOOL NAME
Marshall Industries

c. EMPLOYER'S NAME OR SCHOOL NAME
United Surgical

c. OTHER ACCIDENT?
☐ YES ☒ NO

c. INSURANCE PLAN NAME OR PROGRAM NAME
MarshInd Plan

d. INSURANCE PLAN NAME OR PROGRAM NAME
United Surgical Plan

10d. RESERVED FOR LOCAL USE

d. IS THERE ANOTHER HEALTH BENEFIT PLAN?
☒ YES ☐ NO   *If yes*, return to and complete item 9 a-d.

READ BACK OF FORM BEFORE COMPLETING & SIGNING THIS FORM.
12. PATIENT'S OR AUTHORIZED PERSON'S SIGNATURE I authorize the release of any medical or other information necessary to process this claim. I also request payment of government benefits either to myself or to the party who accepts assignment below.

SIGNED *Nancy Shields*   DATE 4/20/—

13. INSURED'S OR AUTHORIZED PERSON'S SIGNATURE I authorize payment of medical benefits to the undersigned physician or supplier for services described below.

SIGNED *Nancy Shields*

14. DATE OF CURRENT: MM DD YY
02 25 —
ILLNESS (First symptom) OR INJURY (Accident) OR PREGNANCY(LMP)

15. IF PATIENT HAS HAD SAME OR SIMILAR ILLNESS. GIVE FIRST DATE MM DD YY

16. DATES PATIENT UNABLE TO WORK IN CURRENT OCCUPATION
FROM MM DD YY   TO MM DD YY

17. NAME OF REFERRING PHYSICIAN OR OTHER SOURCE
Dr. Frances Morgan

17a. I.D. NUMBER OF REFERRING PHYSICIAN
8439-71-10

18. HOSPITALIZATION DATES RELATED TO CURRENT SERVICES
FROM MM DD YY   TO MM DD YY

19. RESERVED FOR LOCAL USE

20. OUTSIDE LAB? $ CHARGES
☐ YES ☒ NO

21. DIAGNOSIS OR NATURE OF ILLNESS OR INJURY. (RELATE ITEMS 1,2,3 OR 4 TO ITEM 24E BY LINE)
1. 402.00 Hypertension with heart involvement
2. 413.9 Angina
3. |___.___
4. |___.___

22. MEDICAID RESUBMISSION CODE   ORIGINAL REF. NO.

23. PRIOR AUTHORIZATION NUMBER

24. A DATE(S) OF SERVICE						B Place of Service	C Type of Service	D PROCEDURES, SERVICES, OR SUPPLIES (Explain Unusual Circumstances) CPT/HCPCS MODIFIER	E DIAGNOSIS CODE	F $ CHARGES	G DAYS OR UNITS	H EPSDT Family Plan	I EMG	J COB	K RESERVED FOR LOCAL USE
From MM	DD	YY	To MM	DD	YY										
04	14	—				3		99214	1 and 2	79 00	1				
04	14	—				3		71010	1 and 2	50 00	1				
04	14	—				3		93000	1 and 2	50 00	1				
04	14	—				3		80003	1 and 2	35 00	2				

25. FEDERAL TAX I.D. NUMBER   SSN☐ EIN☐

26. PATIENT'S ACCOUNT NO.
839

27. ACCEPT ASSIGNMENT? (For govt. claims, see back)
☐ YES ☒ NO

28. TOTAL CHARGE
$ 214 00

29. AMOUNT PAID
$ 0

30. BALANCE DUE
$ 214 00

31. SIGNATURE OF PHYSICIAN OR SUPPLIER INCLUDING DEGREES OR CREDENTIALS
(I certify that the statements on the reverse apply to this bill and are made a part thereof.)

Signature on file

SIGNED   DATE

32. NAME AND ADDRESS OF FACILITY WHERE SERVICES WERE RENDERED (If other than home or office)

33. PHYSICIAN'S, SUPPLIER'S BILLING NAME, ADDRESS, ZIP CODE & PHONE #
John H. Sparks, M.D.
8504 Capricorn Drive
Atlanta GA 30033-7775
(404) 555-6078
PIN#   GRP#

(APPROVED BY AMA COUNCIL ON MEDICAL SERVICE 8/88)   **PLEASE PRINT OR TYPE**   FORM CMS-1500 (U2) (12-90) FORM OWCP-1500   FORM RRB-1500

PATIENT AND INSURED INFORMATION

PHYSICIAN OR SUPPLIER INFORMATION

FIGURE 14–7 Completed CMS-1500 claim form

which are identified with a CPT code, were performed to help the physician arrive at a diagnosis.

Chest x-ray	CPT code 71010	Fee $95.00
EKG	CPT code 93000	Fee $80.00
Electrolytes	CPT code 80003	Fee $75.00

Several CPT codes are shown in the following list.

99213	Level III Office visit, Established Patient	58.00
99214	Level IV Office Visit, Established Patient	98.00
99215	Level V Visit, Established Patient	175.00
99222	Level II Initial Hospital Care	215.00
99231	Subsequent Hospital Care	85.00
99238	Hospital Discharge	95.00
85007	Complete Blood Count	25.00
87060	Throat Culture	35.00
87086	Urine Culture	40.00
81000	Urinalysis	25.00

3. Look at the Diagnosis section of the charge slip immediately under the words Attending Physician's Statement. The diagnosis code 402.00 for hypertension with heart involvement is marked. In addition, the physician diagnosed angina, ICD-9 413.9, and spontaneous hypoglycemia ICD-9 251.2. The hypoglycemia was added in the Other diagnosis line. These diagnoses were reached through a combination of the physician's examination and the laboratory results.

ICD-9-CM

Standard nomenclature for diagnoses is contained in the *International Classification of Diseases, Ninth Edition, Clinical Modification*, which is available from the AMA. The tenth revision of the *International Classification of Diseases* (ICD), and its clinical modification, is expected to replace the ICD-9-CM Index to Diseases and Tabular List in 2005. Diagnosis codes are made up of three digits, followed by a decimal point and one or two additional digits. Claims submitted with a three- or four-digit code where a four- or five-level code is available will be returned for proper coding. The first three numbers identify the primary diagnosis and the extra digits differentiate within the diagnosis area. Several diag-

nosis codes are shown in the following list and on the CMS-1500 form in Figure 14–7.

244	Acquired hypothyroidism
250.9	Diabetes
251.2	Spontaneous hypoglycemia
401.0	Hypertension
402.00	Hypertension with heart involvement (fifth digit must be included)
413.9	Angina
414.0	Unstable arteriosclerotic heart disease
490	Bronchitis
493.9	Asthma

ICD coding is a complex issue and many times, physician's office personnel code conditions incorrectly. Incorrect codes often appear on charge slips because a single code cannot represent all aspects of one condition. A good example is hypertension, which is coded differently depending on associated problems. Because a general code for hypertension often appears on the charge slip, this condition can be easily miscoded. Several hypertension related ICD codes are shown below.

401.0	Malignant hypertension
401.1	Benign hypertension
402.00	Hypertension with heart involvement
403.00	Hypertension with renal involvement
405.09	Hypertension due to brain tumor

The Healthcare Common Procedure Coding System

The Healthcare Common Procedure Coding System (HCPCS, pronounced: hickpicks) is used to document the furnishing of medical equipment, procedures, services, and supplies and is based on CPT coding. It was developed by HCFA in the early 1980s to eliminate confusion arising from myriad, differing claims forms being submitted for Medicare payment. HCPCS is the common language that emerged. It is used by most state Medicaid programs.

HCPCS is organized into two levels:

• Level I is the same as CPT.
• Level II codes are also called National codes. They cover medical services and supplies not included in CPT (Level I), including services supplied by physicians and nonphysicians, such as nurse practitioners and physical therapists,

as well as transportation and durable medical equipment and orthotic supplies (wheelchairs, canes), and medications.

Charge Slip as Documentation

Most charge slips provide a complete list of procedures and treatments and their accompanying codes; many also list diagnoses and diagnosis codes. Space is given for writing the charge for each service and for the physician to write a diagnosis. Formerly, a charge slip could be submitted in place of a completed CMS-1500 form. At present, the trend is away from this practice. Medicare and many other insurers will no longer accept the charge slip. This practice varies by insurance carrier because many companies are using computer scanners on the claims.

COMPLETING A UNIVERSAL HEALTH INSURANCE CLAIM FORM

A Universal Health Insurance claim form (CMS-1500, formerly HCFA-1500), developed by the AMA, has been adopted for use by most group and individual insurance claim organizations, HMOs, PPOs, and government health programs. some carriers, however, require their own special form for reporting claims.

The CMS-1500 form is divided into two sections: patient and insured information and physician or supplier information. The patient and insured section contains eleven spaces for information and two spaces for signatures; the physician or supplier information section consists of nineteen spaces for information, and one space for the physician's signature. For Blue Shield claims, refer to the local plan. An illustration of how to complete a CMS form for Nancy Shields is shown in Figure 14–7.

Establishing an Audit Trail

An audit trail should be established to determine the status of all insurance claims at all times. This is especially important for medical offices that file a large number of insurance claims for patients. When a carrier fails to make a timely reimbursement, the medical assistant must call or write the company, determine the problem, and assist in rectifying the situation. An alert medical assistant should be able to give an up-to-date status report on a claim at any time if the physician or patient inquires. Two simple methods of tracing claims are discussed in the next section.

Claims Register

A claims register is a continuing log that lists the following information about each claim submitted to an insurance carrier: (1) the claim number, (2) the patient's name, (3) the carrier, (4) the date the claim was submitted, (5) the amount of the claim, (6) dates of follow-up requests, and (7) final disposition of the claim, including (a) the date the claim was made, (b) the amount paid, and (c) any difference between the amount of the claims and the amount paid.

For greatest efficiency, complete the claims register when an insurance claim form is mailed to the carrier, or keep all claims in a stack to be registered at the end of each day. Depending on the number of forms submitted, one sheet from the claims register can be used for several days. When the sheet is full, continue listing claims on a new page.

The follow-up date refers to a future date when an inquiry should be made if the carrier has not responded. Because most claims require two to six weeks for processing, a date six weeks away is realistic. People who work with the various carriers learn how long a claim takes for processing, and can adjust the follow-up dates accordingly. A claims register is shown in Figure 14–8.

Tickler File

A ticker file is a dated file that holds a copy of each claim form until it is paid. In a tickler file, primary dividers are labeled with the name of each month, and two sets of folders list the numbers 1–31. One set of folders is placed behind the divider for the current month, and the second set is placed behind the divider for the upcoming month. follow the procedures below for using a tickler file (Figure 14–9).

1. When the claim form is submitted to the insurance carrier, place a copy of the form in the proper folder behind a date approximately

INSURANCE CLAIMS REGISTER

Claim No.	Patient	Carrier	Claim Submitted Date	Claim Submitted Amount	Follow-up Date	Claim Paid Date	Claim Paid Amount	Difference (Submitted - Paid)	
1	601	Clara Vinings	Liberty Mutual	5/17	62.00	6/30	6/2	54.00	8.00	1
2	602	Jason Martin	Blue Shield	5/17	26.00	6/30	6/15	20.00	6.00	2
3	603	Anthony Garcia	Nationwide	5/18	78.00	6/30				3
4	604	Barbara Cosby	Aetna Life + Casualty	5/18	26.00	6/30	6/4	26.00	—	4
5	605	Serand Jackson	Blue Shield	5/23	84.00	7/7				5
6										6
7										7
8										8
9										9
10										10
11										11
12										12
13										13
14										14
15										15

FIGURE 14–8 Claims register

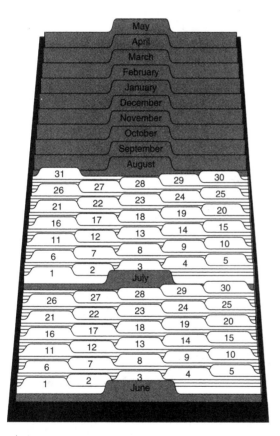

FIGURE 14–9 Tickler file

six weeks in advance. (For example, for a claim submitted on June 1, file the copy of the claim form in the folder for July 15.)

2. When a claim is paid, record the payment on the patient's ledger card, then remove the copy of the claim form from the tickler file.

(Destroy this copy, because another copy should already be filed in the patient's medical record.)

3. At the end of each billing period, review all claim forms in the tickler file to determine which claims are more than six weeks old. Begin the follow-up procedure described in the next section.

Follow-Up Procedure

When payment has not been received from a carrier at the end of six weeks (or the next billing period after six weeks), write a follow-up letter asking for payment and enclose a copy of the claim form. Enter the date of the letter in the claim register and record a new follow-up date two to six weeks away. Or, attach a copy of the letter to the file copy of the claim form in the tickler file and return it to the tickler file in a folder dated before the next billing period. Continue with the collection process discussed in Chapter 13 until the claim is paid.

Computerizing the Claims Process

Computers have revolutionized the processing of claims. With a few simple commands, the medical assistant can instruct the computer to print insurance forms daily, weekly, or monthly and to submit them electronically to the insurance carrier. The computer can also track the forms on a standard schedule, thus providing an up-to-date analysis of each form's location in the insurance cycle.

Most medical software is capable of automatically printing the CMS-1500 form, and the instruction to bill the insurance company for patient charges is coded when the information is entered on the patient's first visit. When the medical assistant instructs the program to print an insurance form, it searches through the transactions previously posted to the account from the charge slip and prints complete details about each office visit, procedure, or service.

Most computer systems can print individually or in bulk on a daily, weekly, or monthly basis at the rate of two to four forms a minute, depending on the printer. The computer will even print two forms automatically if the patient has two insurance policies. In medical offices that do not prepare insurance forms for patients, the program can generate a detailed charge slip for the patient to attach to the insurance form.

Look at the computer-completed CMS-1500 form in Figure 14–10. A computer program enters the correct information for each patient onto the form as it is fed into the computer, providing a detailed description of the services provided. This form provides the insurer with all the information needed to quickly process the insurance claim. The computer program eliminates the tedious task of handwriting the information onto the form and greatly reduces errors. Some government agencies do not accept the CMS-1500 form. It is possible to program most computer systems to accept various other formats for claims forms. An example is the Workers' Compensation First Report of Injury form shown in Figure 14–4. The computer can also be programmed to produce the Attending Physician's Report and other relevant forms.

IN YOUR OPINION

1. Is it preferable for the patient or the medical assistant to complete insurance claims forms? Explain your thinking.
2. What are the advantages and disadvantages to the health practitioner of traditional insurance and managed health care insurance?
3. What advice would you give a new medical assistant whose job is to complete insurance forms for patients?

INTERNET ACTIVITY

Log on to the Web site www.pohly.com. Scroll down the page and click on Glossary of Managed Care Terminology. Choose twenty words and their definitions to add to the vocabulary at the front of this chapter.

STUDENT STUDY CHECKLIST

Workbook

1. Complete Chapter 14 exercises in the workbook.
2. Complete Chapter 14 simulations in the workbook that access the CD-ROM in the back of the book.

Administrative Skills CD-ROM

1. Go to the Library on the CD-ROM and play interactive games for Chapter 13.
2. Click on the Insurance area of the office and review the information and complete three of the exercises provided, using the CMS-1500 claim form presented on screen. Begin by clicking on the computer in the office. Why is medical insurance data so detailed and complicated? Can you justify this to someone not familiar with the practice of medicine?

REFERENCES

Binder, Darren T., J D, "Determining Who is Covered by HIPAA Privacy Regulation," *Managed Care Law Strategist*, November, 2001.

Fordney, Marilyn T. and Joan J. Follis. *Administrative Medical Assisting*, 4th ed. Clifton Park, NY: Delmar Learning, 1998.

HIPAA Online at http://cms.hhs.gov/hipaa

Humphrey, Doris D. *Pediatric Associates*, P.C. Cincinnati, OH: South-Western, 1998.

Integrated Healthcare Association Web site at http://www.iha.org/evolve.htm, Walnut Creek, CA: 2002.

Lindh, Wilburta Q., Marilyn S. Pooler, and Carol D. Tamparo. *Administrative Medical Assisting*, 2nd ed. Clifton Park, NY: Delmar Learning, 2002.

Porkorney, Joseph, "HIPAA Raises Patient Privacy Issues," *Information Systems*, November 15, 2000.

Rowell, JoAnn C. and Michelle A. Green. *Understanding Health Insurance*, 6th ed. Clifton Park, NY: Delmar Learning, 2002.

Epsilon Life & Casualty
P.O. Box 189
Macon, GA 31298

APPROVED OMB-0938-0008

HEALTH INSURANCE CLAIM FORM

PICA			PICA

| 1. MEDICARE (Medicare #) | MEDICAID (Medicaid #) | CHAMPUS (Sponsor's SSN) | CHAMPVA (VA File #) | GROUP HEALTH PLAN (SSN or ID) | FECA BLK LUNG (SSN) | OTHER ☒ (ID) | 1a. INSURED'S I.D. NUMBER (FOR PROGRAM IN ITEM 1) 756575675 |

| 2. PATIENT'S NAME (Last Name, First Name, Middle Initial) Evans   Patricia | 3. PATIENT'S BIRTH DATE MM DD YY 12 13 40 M☐ F☒ SEX | 4. INSURED'S NAME (Last Name, First Name, Middle Initial) Evans   Patricia G |

| 5. PATIENT'S ADDRESS (No., Street) 8907 Harbor Drive | 6. PATIENT RELATIONSHIP TO INSURED Self ☒ Spouse ☐ Child ☐ Other ☐ | 7. INSURED'S ADDRESS (No., Street) 8907 Harbor Drive |

| CITY Madison | STATE CA | 8. PATIENT STATUS Single ☐ Married ☐ Other ☐ | CITY Madison | STATE CA |

| ZIP CODE 95653 | TELEPHONE (Include Area Code) ( ) | Employed ☐ Full-Time Student ☐ Part-Time Student ☐ | ZIP CODE 95653 | TELEPHONE (INCLUDE AREA CODE) ( ) |

| 9. OTHER INSURED'S NAME (Last Name, First Name, Middle Initial) | 10. IS PATIENT'S CONDITION RELATED TO: | 11. INSURED'S POLICY GROUP OR FECA NUMBER |

| a. OTHER INSURED'S POLICY OR GROUP NUMBER | a. EMPLOYMENT? (CURRENT OR PREVIOUS) ☐ YES ☒ NO | a. INSURED'S DATE OF BIRTH MM DD YY   M☐ F☐ SEX |

| b. OTHER INSURED'S DATE OF BIRTH MM DD YY   M☐ F☐ SEX | b. AUTO ACCIDENT? ☐ YES ☐ NO   PLACE (State) | b. EMPLOYER'S NAME OR SCHOOL NAME |

| c. EMPLOYER'S NAME OR SCHOOL NAME | c. OTHER ACCIDENT? ☐ YES ☐ NO | c. INSURANCE PLAN NAME OR PROGRAM NAME |

| d. INSURANCE PLAN NAME OR PROGRAM NAME | 10d. RESERVED FOR LOCAL USE | d. IS THERE ANOTHER HEALTH BENEFIT PLAN? ☐ YES ☐ NO   If yes, return to and complete item 9 a-d. |

READ BACK OF FORM BEFORE COMPLETING & SIGNING THIS FORM.

12. PATIENT'S OR AUTHORIZED PERSON'S SIGNATURE I authorize the release of any medical or other information necessary to process this claim. I also request payment of government benefits either to myself or to the party who accepts assignment below.

SIGNED   Signature on File   DATE 02/03/—

13. INSURED'S OR AUTHORIZED PERSON'S SIGNATURE I authorize payment of medical benefits to the undersigned physician or supplier for services described below.

SIGNED   Signature on File

| 14. DATE OF CURRENT: ILLNESS (First symptom) OR INJURY (Accident) OR PREGNANCY(LMP) MM DD YY 12 30 | 15. IF PATIENT HAS HAD SAME OR SIMILAR ILLNESS. GIVE FIRST DATE MM DD YY 01 10 | 16. DATES PATIENT UNABLE TO WORK IN CURRENT OCCUPATION MM DD YY   FROM   TO   MM DD YY |

| 17. NAME OF REFERRING PHYSICIAN OR OTHER SOURCE Leland W Groves, M.D. | 17a. I.D. NUMBER OF REFERRING PHYSICIAN | 18. HOSPITALIZATION DATES RELATED TO CURRENT SERVICES MM DD YY FROM 01 26 — TO 01 31 — |

| 19. RESERVED FOR LOCAL USE | 20. OUTSIDE LAB? ☐ YES ☐ NO $ CHARGES |

21. DIAGNOSIS OR NATURE OF ILLNESS OR INJURY. (RELATE ITEMS 1,2,3 OR 4 TO ITEM 24E BY LINE)

1. 174.9
2. ____.__
3. ____.__
4. ____.__

| 22. MEDICAID RESUBMISSION CODE   ORIGINAL REF. NO. |
| 23. PRIOR AUTHORIZATION NUMBER |

24. A DATE(S) OF SERVICE						B Place of Service	C Type of Service	D PROCEDURES, SERVICES, OR SUPPLIES (Explain Unusual Circumstances) CPT/HCPCS | MODIFIER	E DIAGNOSIS CODE	F $ CHARGES	G DAYS OR UNITS	H EPSDT Family Plan	I EMG	J COB	K RESERVED FOR LOCAL USE
From MM	DD	YY	To MM	DD	YY										
01	10	—				3		99214	174.9	50 00	1				
01	10	—				3		76088	174.9	125 00	1				
01	10	—				3		71020	174.9	58 00	1				
01	26	—				3		99223	174.9	180 00	1				
01	31	—				3		99238	174.9	38 00	1				
01	27	—	01	31	—	3		99232	174.9	208 00	1				

| 25. FEDERAL TAX I.D. NUMBER   SSN ☐ EIN ☐ | 26. PATIENT'S ACCOUNT NO. | 27. ACCEPT ASSIGNMENT? (For govt. claims, see back) ☒ YES ☐ NO | 28. TOTAL CHARGE $ 659 00 | 29. AMOUNT PAID $ 00 | 30. BALANCE DUE $ 659 00 |

| 31. SIGNATURE OF PHYSICIAN OR SUPPLIER INCLUDING DEGREES OR CREDENTIALS (I certify that the statements on the reverse apply to this bill and are made a part thereof.) Signature on File SIGNED   DATE | 32. NAME AND ADDRESS OF FACILITY WHERE SERVICES WERE RENDERED (If other than home or office) | 33. PHYSICIAN'S, SUPPLIER'S BILLING NAME, ADDRESS, ZIP CODE & PHONE # 9169876543 Sydney Carrington & Assoc. 34 Sycamore St. Suite 300 Madison, CA 94303 PIN#   GRP# |

(APPROVED BY AMA COUNCIL ON MEDICAL SERVICE 8/88)   **PLEASE PRINT OR TYPE**

FORM CMS-1500 (U2) (12-90)
FORM OWCP-1500   FORM RRB-1500

790-0115(12/90) (OCR) 1 pt.

FIGURE 14–10 Computerized insurance form

CHAPTER ACTIVITIES

PERFORMANCE-BASED ACTIVITIES

1. Contact the administrative office of an HMO and a PPO in your area. Ask for the information shown in the chart. Compare the two types of plans.

   a. What benefits do the plans offer?

   b. What are the provisions of the physician's contract?

   c. Who pays for the plan and when is it paid?

   d. What are the advantages for the insured person and the physician?

   Comparison of HMO and PPO Plans

	HMO Plan	*PPO Plan*
Covered Benefits	_____	_____
Physician's Contract Provisions	_____	_____
Who Pays the Plan?	_____	_____
When Is the Plan Paid?	_____	_____
Advantages for the Patient	_____	_____
Advantages for the Physician	_____	_____

2. Review the procedures and codes on page 301 and the charge slip on page 299. List the correct CPT-4 codes, ICD-9 codes, and fees for patients with the services and diagnoses listed below:

BARBARA GONZALES	*CPT CODE*	*ICD CODE*	*FEE*
SERVICE			
Level III			
Established Patient	_____		_____
CBC	_____		_____
Urinalysis	_____		_____
DIAGNOSIS			
Goiter		_____	
Hyperthyroidism		_____	

FRED CHEN	*CPT CODE*	*ICD CODE*	*FEE*
SERVICE			
Intermediate Visit			
Established Patient	_____		_____
Throat Culture	_____		_____
CBC	_____		_____
DIAGNOSIS			
Bronchitis		_____	

JUANITA DAVIS	CPT CODE	ICD CODE	FEE
SERVICE			
Level IV			
Established Patient	_____		_____
Chest X-ray	_____		_____
EKG	_____		_____
CBC	_____		_____
Urinalysis	_____		_____
Electrolytes	_____		_____
DIAGNOSIS			
Cardiac Arrhythmia		_____	

3. What is the medical assistant's responsibility at each step in the health insurance claim process? Fill out the chart below.

Step   *Medical Assistant's Responsibility*

   1. Completing Form

   2. Form Signatures

   3. Form Mailing

   4. Claim Examination

   5. Form Return (if incomplete)

   6. Form Resubmission
     (if original was incomplete)

   7. Check Sent to Patient or Physician

   8. Account Credited

1. Contact the claims department of a major insurance company and inquire about the types of problems it encounters.

Problems with Claim Forms   *Conclusion*

_____   _____

_____   _____

_____   _____

_____   _____

_____   _____

_____   _____

_____   _____

_____   _____

_____   _____

_____   _____

_____   _____

_____   _____

_____   _____

_____

_____

_____

_____

2. Log on to the Internet and review information from a Web site about CPT-5 and ICD-9-CM coding. Make a list of ten procedures or treatments you recognize and ten diagnoses you have heard about.

Medical Diagnoses   *Diagnosis Code*

_____   _____

_____   _____

_____   _____

_____   _____

_____   _____

_____   _____

_____   _____

_____   _____

_____   _____

_____   _____

PART V

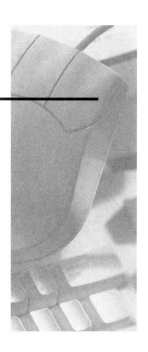

Becoming a Career Medical Assistant

Whether you are about to begin your first job now or in a few months, expectations for your performance will be high from the first day. You will receive training in the medical office, and you may have worked in a medical assisting internship before, but probably you will get less training than you think you need and almost certainly not as much as you want. Whether your training is for a few days, or longer, you will be expected to deliver value right from the start. You will be evaluated on how much you deliver to the practice and how hard you work. You will be expected to demonstrate commitment to your job and to the practice.

Your challenge is to find ways to show why the practice made a good decision in hiring you. This is hard when you are brand new, do not know the ropes, and are afraid of making a mistake. A good way to start is to complete all work on time and then take on any small tasks that will add to the practice's efficiency.

You may find yourself helping other staffers, serving in a secondary role, or taking work that is dull and boring. If that is the case, smile, tough it out, and ask for more work. Show that you are willing to follow through on every task, no matter how small or insignificant it may seem. Your attitude will impress the doctors, the staff, and the patients. That attitude, your professional attitude, as you show it, as you live it, is what gets you a job and what keeps it for you. It is a way of behaving — of being — that makes for success, whatever you do.

CHAPTER 15

Seeking Employment

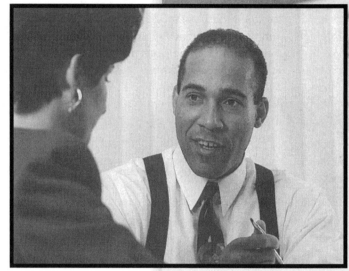

WASHINGTON, DC

In this big city, you would think it would be easy to get a medical assisting job. From experience, I've learned that it's harder than it seems. The process I had to go through seemed endless, though I actually got the job I wanted within two weeks. It took a lot of work, though.

I started by reading newspaper classified ads, but I soon learned that what sounded good in the paper might not be so good, once I went to the interview. Eventually, I got over my resistance to asking my friends and acquaintances to recommend me for jobs. My luck changed when I went to a meeting of the local chapter of the AAMA and got to know some of the CMAs who attended. They took me under their wing and started introducing me to other medical assistants whose practices were looking for employees.

Networking was never one of my strong characteristics, but I've learned it's an invaluable way to get your foot into the door of a first job. When someone who works in a medical office recommends you, the interviewer pays more attention.

Cassie Longfelter
Medical Assistant

PERFORMANCE-BASED COMPETENCIES

After completing this chapter, you should be able to:
1. Identify the skills and characteristics needed to be a successful employee.
2. Formulate a career objective.
3. Prioritize the sources available for learning about medical assisting jobs.
4. Develop a resume and application letter.

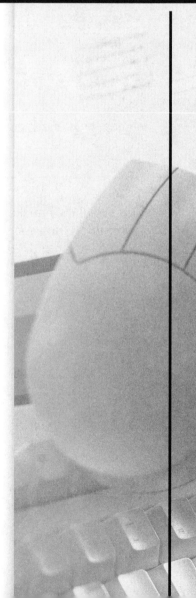

Application letter   The letter that accompanies the resume. It highlights the most important information from the resume.

Credentialing   Verifying that an individual has met certain industry standards.

Employment agencies   Companies that charge a fee to connect employers and job applicants.

Employment application   A standard form for providing personal information and employment history, an identification of places where an applicant has worked, and the types of responsibilities.

Expectations   Standards of performance set by an individual or an employer.

Networking   Interacting with a circle of acquaintances.

Recredentialing   Renewing a previously awarded recognition of industry standards.

Resume   A formatted document listing an applicant's personal and employment information.

Employers say that "being ready to work" is far more important than having training as a medical assistant. In fact, they say that a medical background is secondary when it comes to getting and keeping a job. You may find this surprising since most of your training focuses on the clinical or administrative aspects of being a medical assistant.

Doctors often describe a good medical assistant as someone who "cares about the work." What they are referring to is a professional attitude, and they make the distinction between *being able* to do a job well and *wanting* to do the job well (Figure 15–1). These labels can also

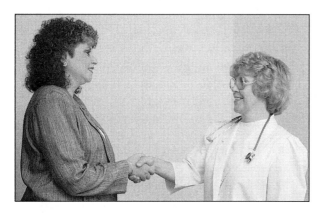

FIGURE 15–1   When first meeting the medical staff, greet each person and show a friendly manner.

apply to the differences between having a job and having a career. The person whose preference is for a career will possess an intense desire to go beyond the minimum requirements of the job.

FINDING AND KEEPING A JOB

Doctors have a well-defined understanding of the characteristics they want in new hires and long-time employees. Here are a few traits doctors say they look for in staff members:

- *Cheerful.* You have a pleasant, happy, energy about you. You take things in stride. Your manner helps to ease the way of people with medical difficulties. It also helps your coworkers as they go about their responsibilities. Cheerful does not mean an automatic smile and a mechanically happy greeting. It means not complaining, not being negative, and — even if you are distressed about something—not behaving in a way that calls attention to your distress.

- *Considerate.* You consider, and respect, the differences in others — those with whom you work and those you serve. You are aware of the possible implications of your actions on others and you manage your behavior so as not to cause them distress. This does not mean that you will always get along with everyone. What it does mean is that when you express your differences, you will stick to the subject and not act in a disrespectful way of others.

- *Dependable.* You are a person of your word. You do what needs to be done without having to be asked. You are on time. You are someone that people turn to for help when things go wrong, because they know that you will find a way to be supportive. Another word that works here is reliable. You are someone whom others can rely on. You are always "there" for others.

- *Detail-oriented.* You understand the phrase, "the devil is in the details." You understand that the little things can make a huge difference. Accurately writing down what patients say, correctly noting instrument readings, and preparing injections carefully, for instance, make a huge difference. Another phrase says,

"If you pay attention to the details, the large problems take care of themselves."

- *Discreet.* You honor the privacy of patients, and the confidentiality with which information about them should be treated. When you communicate information about a patient to someone else in the office, it is on a need-to-know basis, and it is done out of the earshot of others. You make sure that you have written permission from a patient before giving out information about them in writing, electronically, or over the phone.

- *Energetic.* You have a way of doing things, whatever they are, with zeal, communicating a sense of enthusiasm with the task at hand. You help to keep things moving, rather than being a brake on activity. Your personal energy helps to move the enterprise.

- *Flexible.* You are easy to get along with. If work schedules change, or you have to take on duties you had not expected, you are able to go with the flow.

- *Friendly.* You deal with coworkers and patients as people you truly are concerned about and care for. This means referring to patients by their name preceded by Mr., Mrs., and Ms., and actually talking with them rather than voicing instructions. You can put yourself in the role of advisor or concerned other without walking over the patient—employee line.

- *Knowledgeable.* You are intelligent, or you would not be working in this field. But you realize that one of the keys to success is using your intelligence to keep on learning. Staying current about new pharmaceuticals, computer systems, patient privacy requirements — the list can go on — and being able to respond and contribute in the office setting is a key factor for success. Be informed and stay informed. Keep learning.

- *On time.* You understand that being at work when work is due to begin says worlds about your attitude, your self-discipline, your personal organizational ability, and the perception that coworkers and superiors have of you. You realize that the person who is consistently late gets a label, and not a good one. You realize that the person who arrives on time, even if there is little to be done that day, is the person who commands respect.

- *Persistent.* You press on, even at the end of the work day, when there are still many tasks to be accomplished. You have an attitude of not giving up, not quitting, not leaving your post. Your persistence may take the form of enlisting others to assist you, but your primary focus is to get the job done.

- *Polite.* You understand that the formalities of please and thank you, excuse me, and hello and good by are accepted and used by people as a way of showing respect and courtesy. True politeness comes from the heart, even though it is uttered from the mouth. By being polite and considerate, you will do much to make your workplace experience a positive one.

- *Self-starter.* You see things in the office that need to be done and you tackle them, without waiting for someone to ask or instruct you. Of course, being a self-starter does not extend to responsibilities out of your area of expertise, nor does it extend to actions that would be perceived by others as encroaching on their territory. But basically, you do not avoid work by using the excuse that you were not told to work.

- *Sensitive.* You are aware of the subtleties of tone of voice and body language to help you work with patients and coworkers. Most importantly, you use this awareness to treat others in a positive and useful way, reaching out to them in time of worry or anxiety to give them support. You know that just because someone does not ask for help does not mean that they are not wishing for help. Using your sensitivity, your awareness of others and the situation can help you go a long way toward being the kind of medical assistant practices and groups want to hold on to.

- *Tactful.* You are able to find a way of expressing a fact or opinion in a difficult situation, without hurting, attacking, or insulting the person you are speaking to. An example of a tactless remark might be, "Well, that's just stupid," even if, in fact, it is stupid. A more tactful way of expressing yourself might be to say, "Well, I have some concerns about that." The latter statement gives you room to expand on your reservations without upsetting the other person.

RESEARCHING EMPLOYMENT OPPORTUNITIES

After spending many years in school preparing for a productive career, you are ready to go to work now. You know you want to be a medical assistant, and you have been told that many positions exist, but how do you locate a job?

Finding employment in a personally and financially rewarding position takes time, patience, perseverance, and confidence. In addition, locating the right job requires an understanding of (1) your skills and abilities, (2) the types of positions available in your area, and (3) your goals for the future.

Opportunities abound in many different types of medical offices, both large and small. You may choose to work for a private solo or group practice, a hospital, an outpatient clinic, an emergency center, a research center, a teaching center, or in some other medical setting. Whatever your ambitions, the decisions you make now will influence the rest of your life. Make your basic decisions only after thoughtful study of the job market and after considering the implications for your career. Talk over your questions and concerns with someone you trust, preferably someone who is knowledgeable about the medical assisting field and who has several years of experience. Because your future happiness may depend on selecting a good first job, do not take any position unless it feel right to you.

The time you spend now investigating the medical assisting job market will yield dividends later in saved time, reduced frustration, and fatigue. It will also give you a good understanding of what positions are available. Begin your research while you are still in school and have access to both your instructors and the Internet. By beginning early, you will be able to discuss your questions and concerns with instructors who can provide assistance and objectivity about prospective employers. Your best sources for job information are (1) your school placement office, (2) newspaper classified advertisements, (3) professional organizations, (4) professional organizations, (4) acquaintances, (5) employment agencies, (6) instructors at your school, (7) medical societies, (8) the Internet, and (9) the yellow pages directory.

School Employment Offices

Colleges, universities, trade schools, and other educational institutions keep a list of employers who are actively recruiting. Be sure to visit the employment office of your school and review the job listings. Sometimes students fail to take advantage of this excellent source.

Newspaper Classified Advertisements

Medical practices often advertise positions in the classified section of the newspaper because they recognize that this is a fast way of reaching a large number of prospective employees. The Sunday edition's classified advertisements are an especially rich source of opportunities. Do not set your expectations for finding a job through the newspaper too high, however. One study showed that only 11% of jobs are advertised in newspapers.

Advertisements for medical assistants may be found under many headings, including (1) medical assistant, (2) phlebotomist, (3) medical secretary, (4) secretary, (5) ECG technician, (6) receptionist, (7) nurse assistant, (8) bookkeeper, (9) billing clerk, (10) administrative assistant, (11) medical office manager, (12) insurance clerk, or (13) transcriptionist. Do not overlook an advertisement just because it does not have "medical" in the title. The "medical" reference may be buried in the body of the copy or it may be identifiable only from the company or institution named. For example, an advertisement for an "administrative assistant in a psychiatric clinic" clearly would be worth investigating even though the word "medical" is not used. Many large city newspapers print a special section called "Health Care Opportunities" or some similar label. Be sure also to review this section thoroughly (Figure 15–2).

Do not dismiss an ad just because the position does not sound exactly like the one you are seeking. After all, it is very difficult for a personnel manager to describe fully the features of a job in only a few lines.

Professional Organizations

Members of the local chapters of the AAMA and other organizations are employees in medical institutions. Sometimes they also do hiring. By

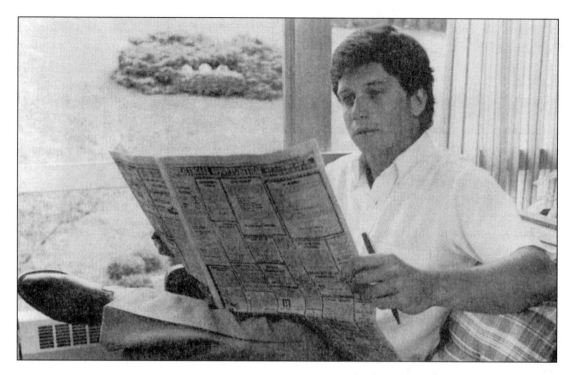

FIGURE 15–2 Be sure to carefully review the classified sections of newspapers when researching medical assisting employment opportunities. Not all job titles list the word "medical."

becoming acquainted with members of a local organization, you may hear of positions in your area. If you do not personally know any members, determine the name of the organization's president through the local AAMA chapter and give that person a call. Usually, they are very willing to help new employees get started in the field.

Acquaintances

Friends and acquaintances may know about potential openings before an announcement is made in the newspaper. Word-of-mouth is a valuable source of information. Networking is considered one of the best sources for finding employment.

Employment Agencies

Employment agencies match medical assistants with physicians, medical companies, and other institutions. The agency provides pre-employment screening for the physician. When the agency is satisfied that an applicant meets the qualifications specified, it makes a referral to the medical office.

Employment agencies charge a fee, usually a percentage of the medical assistant's beginning salary. The amount can become quite large when the beginning salary is large. Some practices pay the agency's fee, because they think the best-qualified applicants have many employment opportunities and will not take a job for which they must pay. Fortunately, in the last few years, more and more agencies are advertising "fee-paid" jobs. The fee is an important consideration that you should discuss with an employment agency before registering for its service (Figure 15–3).

When using a private employment agency, you will probably be asked to sign a legally binding contract that holds you to certain requirements. Do not sign a contract unless you have read it carefully and are fully satisfied with its terms. A typical binding clause states that you cannot tell other people about the position. If you do and someone else takes the job, you may be held responsible for paying the agency fee. The contract may also state that you are not allowed to take the job at a later date to avoid paying the agency's fee.

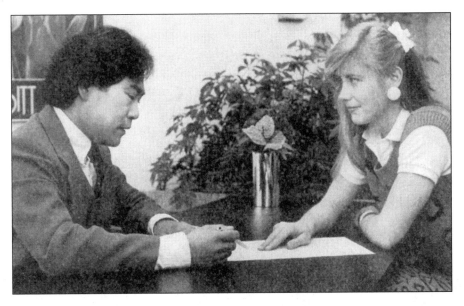

FIGURE 15–3 Before signing a contract with a private employment agency, read the document and study its terms carefully.

Internet

If you want a job as a medical assistant anywhere in the world, you are likely to be able to find it on the Internet. Enter keywords "medical assistant employment, employment, jobs, job search, careers" or other words to start your search. Most listings are by job title and many, though not all, list the potential salary. Skills and personal characteristics are also listed. A good first place to check is the AAMA Web site (http://www.aama-ntl.org), which features an employment opportunity link on its homepage.

Yellow Pages

Medical assistants have a distinct advantage over many other job-seekers because physicians, hospitals, and other medical facilities have specialized listings in the yellow pages. Although going through the yellow pages and dropping a resume in person to each physician or facility is not recommended as a first source of employment, this method could be used with selected physicians. This type of contact also has word-of-mouth potential, and you may learn of prospects in other medical offices when you make random calls. Most medical office managers are willing to talk with potential applicants.

THE JOB APPLICATION PROCESS

The process of applying for a job requires several steps. The person who methodically and confidently works through each step will likely find worthwhile employment, whereas those who attempt to shortcut the process will undermine their own efforts.

The Resume

The most important document you will prepare for an interview is a resume, which is a thorough, yet concise, summary of your background, education, and abilities. A resume is an advertisement of you. Just as companies spend time and effort ensuring that their advertisements deliver the right message to the people they want to reach, your resume should deliver the right message about you. Before you distribute a resume, you should rewrite, edit, and proofread it several times.

Preparing a Resume

Just as the packaging for a product should be attractive, neat, and visually appealing, so should your resume. Use good quality buff or off-white bond paper, a business-like typeface, and an attractive format. Write objective, brief sentences that clearly describe your background; then ask a friend or a relative to proofread the resume for you. Grammatical or typographical mistakes, careless corrections, misspelled words, wrinkled or poor-quality paper, smudges, and awkward placement leave a poor impression. A resume should be limited to one page.

Personal Information List your full name, address, and telephone number as the heading for a resume. Discrimination laws prohibit employers from requiring some personal information such as age, height, weight, sex, and marital status.

Career Objective State your career objectively concisely. Rewrite the objective to fit the position for which are interviewing. For example, if you are applying with a private practice, the following objective would be appropriate:

Career Objective: To provide my strong medical assisting skills in a private practice that serves diverse patients.

If you are applying with a nursing home, your objective might be similar to the one below:

Career Objective: To apply my medical assisting skills as a member of a team serving elderly patients.

Special Strengths Compile a list of what makes you special to an employer. Be honest and list only the items that you are sure you possess.

Work Experience Experience in a former job is a

yardstick against which prospective employers measure an applicant's abilities. The breadth and depth of your background and the type of work you did in former jobs is a big factor in landing a job. The practice's interviewer will look at how long you stayed with the previous employer and at the type of duties you performed, whether administrative, clinical, or both.

On your resume, you should list the dates of all employment, beginning with the most recent, and give a brief description of your responsibilities for each job. Include details about any previous jobs, even though they might not relate directly to medical assisting.

Students are so busy attending school that they often do not have a broad employment background. Although experience in a related job is very helpful, all job experience is valuable and should be listed, including employment at fast food restaurants, babysitting, lifeguarding, volunteer work, or camp-related employment. Physicians want to see a pattern of responsibility and professional growth.

Education List your college, university, business school, or other postsecondary education. If you have attended more than one school, give the most recent first, even if you did not graduate, and list other institutions and dates of attendance in reverse chronological order. Include the dates of graduation and a list of any degrees, licenses, or applicable certification. Emphasize your clinical training and externship.

Honors and Awards If you have received honors and awards that demonstrate resourcefulness, hard work, or a good attitude, you should list them, especially if they relate to the job for which you are applying.

Extracurricular Activities Many students participate in valuable extracurricular activities because they represent commitment and responsibility. You might include in this portion of a resume some of these extracurricular activities: president of a club, band or chorus member, stage crew member for a class play, member of a sports team, or editor of the school newspaper or yearbook.

References References are names of people who know your work habits and skills. Previous employers or supervisors are the best references, followed by teachers or club advisors. Never use a parent or other relative, a minister, or a friend as a reference. These personal references cannot evaluate your abilities objectively and using them leaves an impression that you do not know about appropriate business practices.

Some applicants do not list names of references on their resume; instead, they use the phrase, "References Upon Request." Unless you have a specific reason not to name a reference, it is a good practice to list the names directly on the resume and relieve the employer of the annoyance of having to call you for the names. If you wish to keep your employment search confidential, you will want to be selective in listing references. Figure 15–4 shows a sample form for collecting the information needed for a resume. Figure 15–5 shows an example of a completed resume.

---

1. Your name, address, and telephone number(s).

2. Employment objective — your career goal.

3. Special skills — what makes you unique.

4. Work experience — list the name of the job, description of duties, and dates of employment.

Employer	Job Title	Job Duties	Dates of Employment

5. Education — list the type of diploma, major, and schools attended with dates. You need go no further back than high school. List courses and project-related to the job you want, especially those that have to do with your clinical experience.

School	Major	Dates Attended	Special Projects

6. Certificates and licenses related to the job.

7. Awards and honors.

8. References — list three references.

Name	Phone	How Known

FIGURE 15–4 Resume data collection form

Karen Beyer
78 Justine Lane
Nashville, TN 19087
615-555-2836

CAREER OBJECTIVE: A medical assistant position that allows me to use my clinical and administrative skills.

EDUCATION: Volunteer Community College, Nashville, TN.
Associate Degree in Medical Assisting, June 2002.

Major Courses:

Medical Terminology	Machine Transcription
Anatomy and Physiology	Medical Word Processing
Medical Law and Ethics	Computer Applications
Business English	Medical Office Procedures
Business Communication	Human Relations

Internship Program: Participated in a one-year, half-day internship program as a medical assistant trainee for Adele R. Matz, M.D.

WORK EXPERIENCE:

2001–02   Adele R. Matz, M.D., 804 Oakdale Drive, Lebanon, TN 37087 615-555-7432. Internship Employer. Transcribed case histories, answered telephone, substituted at reception desk during lunch hour and other special times.

1999–2000   McDonald's, 1801 Main Street, Lebanon, TN 37087 615-555-2945. Part-time work during summer and after school. Waited on customers.

HONORS AND AWARDS:

Outstanding Office Administration Student, Volunteer Community College, 2002.

EXTRACURRICULAR ACTIVITIES:

Representative, Radnor High School Student Council, 1999.

Member, Future Business Leaders of America, 1998.

REFERENCES:

Adele R. Matz, M.D., 804 Oakdale Drive, Lebanon, TN 37087 615-555-7432

Mr. Ralph Gallagher, Office Manager,
Adele R. Matz, M.D., 804 Oakdale Drive, Lebanon, TN 37087

Ms. Rachel Sellers, Supervisor, McDonald's, 1801 Main Street, Lebanon, TN 37087 615-555-2945

FIGURE 15–5   Completed resume example

Writing an Application Letter

Always write an application letter to accompany your resume. It provides an opportunity to emphasize important parts of your background and offers one more way to sell yourself to a prospective employer. To be effective, it must be well written, visually attractive, error free, and relatively short. The letter should not review all the information provided in your resume, but it should explain why you are interested in the job and why your background has prepared you for the particular position. Mention both front office and back office skills that qualify you for the position.

Although you may copy a resume and use it to apply for several different positions, each application letter should be an original document written for the specific position. The letter should be easy to read and unique without being clever or cute. Above all, it should be interesting, because a dull application letter may discourage an employer from thoroughly reviewing a resume. Refer to Figure 15–6 for a sample cover letter. Use the following procedures for writing your application letter.

Procedures for Writing an Application Letter

1. Send the letter to a specific person, using the person's title. If you do not know the name or title, call the office, and ask the person who answers the telephone for the information you need. ("Hello, this is Alison Rivers. I wish to write a letter to your office manager, but I don't have a name. Will you please tell me the name of the office manager?")
2. Use the "You" viewpoint. Do not overuse "I."
3. Begin with a brief first paragraph describing how you heard of the job and why you are interested. Explain the reasons that you would be good for the job, not the reasons that job would be good for you. Refer to the resume for brief details about your background.
4. Summarize pertinent information about your education or background and employment history that have prepared you for the job. This is the "selling" section of your let-

ter, so include important details that distinguish you from other applicants. Use two paragraphs if you have enough to say that is different, but do not repeat everything already stated in the resume.
5. Request a personal interview so that you can discuss how your background and the employer's needs match. Make the situation easy by offering to call the employer within a few days to set an appointment; then follow through on the call.
6. Make a copy of the letter for your file. See Figure 15–7.

Completing an Application Form

As a matter of policy, and for legal purposes, most practices require all applicants to complete an application form in addition to submitting an application letter and resume. Transferring information from your resume to an application form is a relatively simple matter, but remembering all the dates of employment and years of education can be difficult if you do not have a resume handy. Therefore, it is a good idea to take a copy of your resume with you to every interview. Answer each question on the application form fully; do not skip any questions. If a question does not apply to you, write "N/A" for "not applicable." Write your answers neatly.

Providing Documentation

Some practices may require you to submit an official school transcript as documentation of your education. Since obtaining a transcript may be a lengthy process at some schools, you should begin this step immediately after graduation. Ask for one official copy of your transcript as soon as you are allowed and then make several additional copies that you can give to employers. You will not want to postpone employment because of bureaucratic delays.

If you have been employed previously, you may have achieved special recognition or professional certification. You should have any important professional certifications or supporting documents available in case an employer asks for them. For example, the Certified Medical Assistant, Certified Professional Secretary, Registered

78 Justine Lane
Nashville, TN 19087

June 16, 20–

Ms. Anna Capodici, CMA
Office Manager
Orthopedic Associates, P.C.
20-A Medical Arts Building
Nashville, TN 19087

Dear Ms. Capodici:

Your advertisement for a medical assistant in the June 15 *Nashville Tennessean* seeks an employee with the skills and abilities I possess, and I would like to be considered for the position. The enclosed resume describes thoroughly my education and work background that prepare me for employment in your medical office.

At Volunteer Community College, I majored in Medical Assisting. The curriculum focused on medical terminology, office technology, and human relations in the medical office. As a high B student, I was able to participate in the college's Internship Program, attending school half-time each day and working in the medical office of Dr. Adele Matz the other half.

Dr. Matz and her office manager, Ralph Gallagher, made certain that I received a thorough orientation to medical office work. Initially, my job was to transcribe case histories and other dictation; however, by the end of my internship year, I had gained broad experience in all areas of medical office work. Frequently, I was asked to fill in for other employees during their lunch hour or absence from work. Dr. Matz and Mr. Gallagher both encouraged me to use their names as references.

May I come to your office for an interview, so we can further discuss how my background and your needs for a skilled employee are similar? You may call me at 555-2836; however, because I am sometimes difficult to reach, I will call your office next Tuesday morning. I look forward to discussing your position further.

Sincerely,

Karen Beyer

Enclosure

FIGURE 15–6 Sample cover letter

```
Your Address

Date


Name of Person
Title
Company Name
Street Address
City, State, Zip Code

Dear _____:

Opening Paragraph:
     Your purpose in writing the letter.

Middle Paragraph:
     Why this employer should consider
     you for this job.

Closing Paragraph:
     Thanks, and plan for your future
     contact with this employer.

Sincerely,



Your Name
```

FIGURE 15–7 Cover letter form

Medical Assistant, and other similar certifications are valuable recognitions of your extensive background that an employer may wish to include in your file.

IN YOUR OPINION

1. How can you convince an employer that you would make a good medical assistant when you do not yet have broad work experience?
2. How can you write a letter accompanying a resume and use the "You" viewpoint?
3. What initial steps can you take while still in school to prepare for interviewing?

INTERVIEWING FOR A POSITION

A personal interview is the most important part of the employment process because both the practice interviewer and prospective medical assistant get a chance to evaluate one another. Personal "chemistry," or the way the interviewer and applicant relate to each other, plays a subtle, yet crucial, role in any interview. Although the interviewer is responsible for helping the applicant relax, the medical assistant must be at his or her best. The employer will dismiss an impressive resume and a wonderfully written application letter if the interview does not go well.

Appearance

When a prospective medical assistant walks through the door, an interviewer immediately evaluates the person's appearance. Any negative reactions will subconsciously affect the interviewer's opinion and the outcome of the interview. You should look rested, alert, comfortable, and business-like. Dress conservatively and neatly. If you own a tailored suit, this is the time to wear it; if not, wear a jacket over tailored clothes. Wear a white or light-colored blouse or shirt, a tie if you are a man, and clean, polished shoes. You should eliminate clothes that are too tight, too baggy, too faddish, or "too" anything from your business wardrobe.

Style your hair in a conservative, becoming manner. Long, flowing, or unkempt hair will project a casual, nonbusiness-like image. Use makeup and jewelry sparingly. Any makeup or jewelry should enhance your general appearance and not stand out as gaudy or heavy. Very trendy or provocative styles announce that you are unsophisticated in the ways of professional dress. Dress in a way that reinforces the message that you would be a valuable addition to the practice staff (Figure 15–8).

To add a measure of polish to your image, carry an 8½" by 11" portfolio. The folder holds extra copies of your resume, provides paper for taking notes, gives you something to do with your hands, and projects a business-like feeling. Taking a briefcase to an interview, however, is

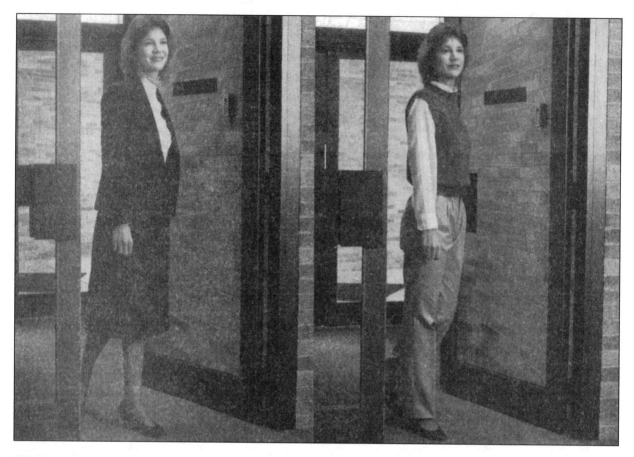

FIGURE 15–8 A neat, conservative, businesslike appearance (left) is preferable for an interview. Sport or casual clothes (right) are too informal.

not recommended because it may appear pretentious. For women, matching your purse, shoes, and portfolio color in black, navy, brown, or burgundy will give you an especially polished, pulled-together appearance.

Conduct

An interviewer will pay close attention to your behavior during an interview because it shows how you react under pressure. Showing a confident, natural manner will help reduce any anxiety you feel. Be honest, and answer all questions thoroughly, but refrain from talking too much or speaking too loudly. Shake hands when you meet the interviewer and make confident eye contact without appearing bold. Your facial expression should be pleasant and attentive.

An applicant who appears nervous, aloof, inattentive, or arrogant during an interview will spoil any positive impressions that the resume generated. Although a certain amount of ner-

vousness may provide the edge that makes for a strong interview, try to control your nervousness instead of letting it control you. Be mindful of nervous habits like running your fingers through your hair, biting your nails, fiddling with jewelry, or swinging your foot. These nervous reactions are unconscious, and they may be annoying to the interviewer. They will certainly show that you are ill at ease and not in control.

You should sit so that you face the interviewer squarely, with your arms in a relaxed, "open" posture. Hands should rest in your lap or on the arms of the chair (Figure 15–9).

Knowledge of the Employer

Before going for an interview, obtain as much information as possible about the practice and about the position for which you are being interviewed. A good place to seek information about a practice is from your medical assisting instructors. They may know the physicians or someone

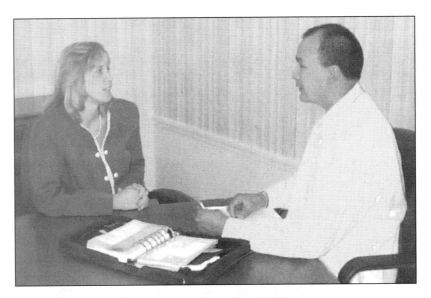

FIGURE 15–9 The interviewer will pay close attention to the applicant's conduct during their meeting. An honest, natural manner is most effective.

on the staff. If not, they may be able to direct you to another person who can share information about the practice. You may also call the Physician Licensing Department in your state for routine information, such as the year the physician started the practice and number of years at the current address, and related information. Another source of information is your local chapter of the AAMA. Obtain the name of the president or another officer from a local hospital personnel office, or contact the national office of the AAMA at http://www.aama.com and ask for the name of the president of your local chapter.

Use the officers as resource people to answer questions you may have about a particular practice or position. Most professionals are pleased to be able to help one another find employment. You will quickly build a network of acquaintances through these valuable sources. Here are several questions that need answers before you attend an interview:

- What is the physician/practice's specialty?
- How large is the practice?
- How many staff members does the practice employ?
- What hospitals does the physician(s) serve as staff member (if applicable), or at which hospital(s) does the physician(s) have privileges?
- What medical product or service does the company make or sell (if appropriate)?
- How long has the company or practice been operating?
- What is the "style" of the office; family-like or professional? Hectic or relaxed?

Asking the Right Questions

The purpose of an interview is to provide information that both you and the employer can use to make a sound decision about employment. The employer should cover basic facts, such as responsibilities of the position, office hours, benefits, and salary. You are expected to have additional questions and to ask them with confidence. However, you should be careful not to appear overly concerned about a high salary, the number of days off, coffee breaks, and other matters that are too "me-oriented."

If an employer asks you how much you want to be paid, it is best not to give an exact number. A good answer to this question is, "I expect to be compensated according to my background and experience."

The interviewer will most likely address the list of questions given in the next section; if not, you may tactfully ask the questions that are appropriate to the size of the practice. Review the list and add questions of your own that you would like answered before agreeing to assume a new position.

- What are the responsibilities of the position?
- To whom will you report?
- What is the potential for career growth?
- Does the office promote from within?
- Is the practice growing?
- What does the employer envision for the practice in five years?
- What is the "style" or culture of the office?
- What is the salary range? Are increases automatic or based on merit?
- What are the benefits? Are continuing education units (CEUs) paid for, and is membership in AAMA included?
- Are health and/or dental insurance offered? Who pays?
- What is the sick leave policy?
- How much vacation time is allowed each year?
- How is vacation time accrued?
- Are there any education benefits? Will the company reimburse for college courses? Will the cost of textbooks be included?
- How many days of released time to attend professional conferences per year are given?
- Who pays for registration and travel expenses?

Illegal Questions

Prospective employers are prohibited by law from asking certain questions. As an interviewee, you should know (1) which questions are illegal, and (2) how to handle the situation gracefully if you are asked an illegal question.

Religion Employers cannot ask your religious faith. They can, however, ask if your faith will interfere with your ability to execute the duties of the job for which you are interviewing. If asked your religion, respond this way, "If you are asking me if my faith will prevent me from being able to do this job, let me assure you that it will not." If, in fact, your religion prohibits you from working on certain days or from carrying out any duties in the job description, you should discuss this with your employer. "My faith prohibits me from working on a Saturday. Would this present a problem?" The discussion should be about the job requirements, not about your personal beliefs.

Marital Status An employer cannot ask if you are married, if you have children, or if you plan to have children. The employer may ask a question similar to the one on religion; "Will your obliga-

tions prevent you from being able to execute the duties of this job?"

If asked if you have small children or plan to become pregnant soon, you could answer, "I have no family commitments that will interfere with this job as described." If you do have a responsibility that compels you to leave work promptly, for example, to pick up a child at day care, do not give personal details. Say, "I will need to leave work at 5:00 PM unless we arrange an alternative schedule that allows me to meet family responsibilities."

Arrests Employers can ask if you have been *convicted* of a crime, but cannot ask if you have been *arrested*. This is unlikely to be asked on an interview, but a question about conviction will almost certainly be included on a written application.

Drug Testing An employer is allowed to, and often does, ask for drug testing as a part of a pre-employment physical exam.

In general, if a question seems too personal or seems unrelated to the job for which you are interviewing, it is perfectly correct to ask, "Can I ask you how this would affect the job we are discussing?"

Writing a Follow-Up Letter

If you are interested in a position after the interview, write a courteous follow-up letter to the interviewer. The letter should thank the person for the interview, express your interest in the position, and further sell your abilities. Because many people do not write follow-up letters, yours will remind the interviewer of you and perhaps give you an advantage over other applicants. Figure 15–10 shows a sample follow-up letter.

IN YOUR OPINION

1. If two applicants appear to be equally qualified for a job, what factors might influence the physician in favor of one applicant?
2. How can a medical assistant ask the right questions about a position without appearing too aggressive?
3. How can a medical assistant ask the right questions about a position without appearing overanxious?

June 25, 20–

Ms. Anna Capodici, CMA
Office Manager
Orthopedic Associates, P.C.
20-A Medical Arts Building
Nashville, TN 19087

Dear Ms. Capodici:

Thank you for discussing your opening for a medical assistant with me. As a result of our conversation, I am convinced that my experience as a medical transcriptionist and as an internship student has prepared me well for your position. I hope we have the opportunity to work together and look forward to hearing from you soon.

Sincerely,

Karen Beyer

FIGURE 15–10 Sample follow-up letter

CONTINUING THE EDUCATION PROCESS

College was traditionally viewed as the end of formal education and the beginning of a career. Graduates happily received their diplomas and then went about their business of being employees. Those days are gone for the medical assistant and others in the allied health professions. Advances in technology, changes in the health care delivery system, and other trends create modifications, new procedures, and increased paperwork almost daily.

Several resources exist for continuing education — from formal college and university courses leading to a degree to informal courses, seminars, and workshops conducted by vendors, professional organizations, employers, and medical institutions and the AAMA's "Quest for Excellence" series of home study courses for continuing education credit. Courses may be taken for a variety of reasons including (1) intrinsic value and the satisfaction they offer, (2) advancement potential and salary increase, (3) necessity to keep current with the field, (4) certification, and (5) recertification.

Although certification is voluntary for practicing, the AAMA strongly encourages medical assistants to take the certification examination. The exam measures professional competency at the entry level and successful completion earns the designation of certified medical assistant (CMA). This credentialing is prestigious and sets the CMA apart from noncredentialed medical staff. In some areas of the United States, practices and other medical employers hire only CMAs. The examination is offered twice yearly at more than 200 test sites across the United States. The logo of the AAMA is shown in Figure 15–11.

Certification by professional organizations offers several advantages:

1. It affirms to employers that you are a skilled professional who has gained recognition through formal procedures conducted by a professional organization.
2. It offers prestige among your contemporaries in the field.
3. It often leads to a higher salary.
4. It provides personal satisfaction for achieving a professional standard.

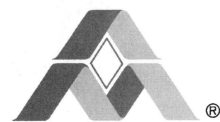

AFFILIATE OF THE
AMERICAN ASSOCIATION
OF MEDICAL ASSISTANTS

CERTIFIED MEDICAL ASSISTANTS:
HEALTHCARE'S MOST VERSATILE PROFESSIONALS

FIGURE 15–11 Logo of the AAMA (Courtesy of the American Association of Medical Assistants.)

Do not underestimate the importance of certification. If you were a potential employer choosing between a certified medical assistant and a noncertified medical assistant, which candidate would you select? As you begin your career as a medical assistant, check with the local chapter of your professional organization about dates and procedures for testing.

Re-Certification

Within five years of the date of certification, a CMA must become re-certified. This can occur in two ways:

- By accumulating approved continuing education hours
- By retaking the examination

Re-certification attests to a medical assistant's or other health practitioner's continued competency and commitment. Because the CMA certification examination of the AAMA is based on entry-level competency and is not a measure of continued competency, the Certifying Board of the AAMA developed a revalidation program based on continuing education. For this program, the certified medical assistant is required to obtain a given number of continuing education credits in specified subject areas.

Registered Medical Assistant

The American Medical Technologists (AMT) registers health professionals in a variety of fields, including medical assisting. Successful completion of the exam leads to the designation of registered medical assistant (RMA). The RMA certification examination is given yearly in June and November at schools that have been accredited by the Accrediting Bureau of Health Education Schools (ABHES). Those who take the examination must have graduated from a medical assisting program accredited by ABHES or meet designated experience requirements. The logos of the RMA and AMT are shown in Figure 15–12.

OFFICE MANAGEMENT

Chances are that at some point in your career you will aspire to become a medical office manager. In the Health and Medicine career pathway, management is a natural step in the progression of your career. Management responsibilities are different from medical assisting tasks; for one thing, you will probably work less with patients and more with staff, coordinating the work of others. Some people like this, whereas others prefer the day-to-day involvement with patients.

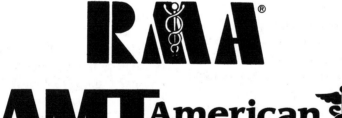

FIGURE 15–12   (A) Logo of the Registered Medical Assistant, representing a credential awarded by the American Medical Technologists. (B) Logo of the American Medical Technologists (AMT). (Reprinted with permission from American Medical Technologists)

An office manager juggles many priorities — from organizing the work schedule so the office is always covered, to seeing that accounts get paid and patients get billed, to observing how well the office and medical assisting staff are performing their responsibilities, and, always, to making sure that the patients are well served and the physicians are properly assisted. A discussion of typical medical office management responsibilities will help you understand what you can expect if you choose to become a manager.

Personnel

Hiring, evaluating, and firing personnel requires excellent people skills, good judgment, and outstanding communication skills. Although the final decision for hiring and firing may come from the physician, the office manager does the bulk of the background investigations that lead to the decisions. A few important guidelines will help you with your personnel responsibilities:

- Gather complete background information about applicants, including references, and analyze the information carefully before making a hiring recommendation.
- Treat all applicants and staff courteously and fairly.
- Make sure personal feelings do not enter into your personnel decisions.
- Do a careful evaluation of all employees under your supervision at least once a year, evaluating new employees more often.
- Arrange a meeting with each person who was evaluated and share your comments about both their best work and about areas that need improvement.
- Prepare and distribute a policy manual that includes accepted dress, behaviors, time off and pay policies, and insurance and other benefit information.
- Prepare a procedure manual that describes how the office functions, including everything from methods for dealing with emergencies, to scheduling, to postal procedures. (You can develop a short procedures manual by selecting and summarizing key topics from this book).

Fringe Benefits

Employee benefits will need your attention, because benefits are as important to some workers as the base salary. Benefits vary from one medical office to another.

- *Vacation.* Two weeks with pay after one full year of employment.
- *Holiday.* New Year's, Memorial Day, Fourth of July, Labor Day, Thanksgiving, and Christmas, plus others the practice may designate.
- *Sick time.* Three to five sick days with pay per year; however, one popular concept allows a designated number or days per year — say 15 — and allows an employee to use them for vacation, sick days, appointments, bereavement, or other reasons. After 15 days, pay is deducted.
- *Insurance.* Health, life, and disability insurance, sometimes for the employee only and sometimes for the employee's family also.
- *401K or profit sharing.* A percentage is set aside by the practice to go into a fund that the employee can collect after working a specific number of years and on leaving the employment of the practice.
- *Complimentary health care.* Often, this benefit is for the employee only, but may also extend to the employee's immediate family.

Patient Flow

The success of the practice will depend, to some extent, on how quickly patients are seen; therefore, patient flow is something you will want to monitor often. If patients have long waiting periods before being called to the examining room, or, once there, if they have to wait indefinitely for the physician, something is probably wrong with the scheduling sequence. Ask these questions to determine the reason for a patient flow problem and to find a solution. Conducting a small investigation will give you the information you need before addressing the issue with the physician.

- Is the scheduling strategy effective? For instance, if the practice uses the wave scheduling method, should it use another method?
- Is the staff well trained? Should training sessions be scheduled?

- Is the office understaffed? Is additional staff needed to handle the traffic?
- Does the staff come to work every day, on time, and do staff members work efficiently?
- Does the staff refrain from lengthy, nonhealth-related conversations with patients or other staff?
- Are enough doctors available to handle the number of patients served by the practice?
- Are patients encouraged to be on time and tactfully reminded when they are late?

Facilities, Equipment, and Supplies Responsibilities

To operate at top efficiency, a medical office needs up-to-date equipment and adequate supplies. The equipment needs to be serviceable at all times, and a replacement plan needs to be in place. Supplies should be ordered routinely and in the correct quantities. As office manager, it will be your job to make sure that everyone on the staff has the equipment and supplies to do the job. Here are a few guidelines.

- Maintain an inventory of equipment, showing the date purchased and the replacement date. Make sure replacement dates are met.
- Purchase maintenance agreements for new equipment and make sure the maintenance company services the equipment on time.
- Clean and maintain the equipment on a daily basis as recommended by the equipment manufacturer.
- Order essential supplies before the inventory becomes dangerously low.
- Contract with a cleaning service to ensure sanitary and attractive facilities.
- Keep files of contracts for all space, furniture, and equipment and call on the landlord or rental/leasing company when a problem occurs.
- Develop a plan for waste management.

Financial Matters

Although you will not be expected to handle all financial matters personally, you will be responsible for coordinating all the details, such as working with the accountant, analyzing practice management software for usefulness, and recommending benefit plans for the staff. Your knowledge needs to be broad but not deep, that is, you must know the right questions to ask and the proper sources to use, and you should be able to analyze materials that are prepared for you by individuals who handle the finances. Here are a few of the financial areas you will oversee:

- Accounts receivable and accounts payable
- Payroll
- Quarterly tax reports prepared by the accountant
- Third-party payer procedures
- Employee benefit packages

IN YOUR OPINION

1. Why does a medical office manager need to know about many different areas, when not required to do the actual work in those areas?
2. What do you believe are the top three priorities for medical office managers?
3. Name several benefits you believe staff members would prefer.

INTERNET ACTIVITY

1. Go to the Web site http://www.salaries.com and compare medical office assistant salaries in five cities where you might like to live. What is the salary range across these five cities?
2. Go to the Web site http://www.keirsey.com and use the Keirsey Temperament Sorter to identify your personality characteristics. Write an opinion regarding how your characteristics match the characteristics needed by medical assistants. Could any of your personality features be detrimental to your career if not adjusted? If yes, what can you do to overcome them?

STUDENT STUDY CHECKLIST

Workbook

1. Complete Chapter 15 exercises in the workbook.
2. Complete Chapter 15 simulations in the workbook that access the CD-ROM in the back of the book.

Administrative Skills CD-ROM

1. Go to the Library on the CD-ROM and play interactive games for Chapter 15.
2. Click on the Employment Strategies tab at the upper right of the opening screen of the CD-ROM and complete the exercises presented.
3. What do you think are the advantages of keeping the master copy of your resume in a computer?

REFERENCES

Career Solutions Training Group. *The Quick Skills Series: Advancing Your Career.* Cincinnati, OH: South-Western, 2001.

Career Solutions Training Group. *How to Find and Apply for a Job,* Cincinnati, OH: South-Western , 2001.

Career Solutions Training Group. *What Your Employer Expects.* Cincinnati, OH: South-Western, 2000.

Kier, Lucille, Barbara A. Wise, and Connie Krebs. *Medical Assisting: Administrative and Clinical Competencies,* 5th ed. Clifton Park, NY: Delmar Learning, 2003.

Lindh, Wilburta Q., Marilyn S. Pooler, and Carol D. Tamparo. *Administrative Medical Assisting,* 2nd ed. Clifton Park, NY: Delmar Learning, 2002.

CHAPTER ACTIVITIES

PERFORMANCE-BASED ACTIVITIES

1. Following the example shown on page 320, prepare and key your resume. Include all sections that relate to your background. Make sure your document is perfect with no typographical mistakes, messy corrections, bad grammar, or misspelled words. Begin by completing the information sheet below, then transfer the information to the resume form and key and print the completed resume.

RESUME DATA COLLECTION FORM

(1) Your name, address, and telephone number(s).

(2) Employment objective — your career goal. Make it clear and short.

(3) Special skills — characteristics and skills that make you special and that will be valuable to an employer.

(4) Work experience — any jobs you have done, including work at home and volunteer work or community projects. List the name of the job, description of duties, and dates of employment. List your clinical externship.

	Employer	Job Title	Job Duties	Dates of Employment
1.				
2.				
3.				
4.				

(5) Education — type of diploma, major, all schools attended with dates of attendance and graduation. List courses and projects related to the job you want, especially those that have to do with your clinical experience.

School	Major	Dates Attended	Special Projects

(6) Certificates and licenses related to the job

(7) Awards and honors

(8) References — include full names, phone numbers, and how you know the person. List at least three references.

	Name	Phone	How Known
1.	_____	_____	_____
2.	_____	_____	_____
3.	_____	_____	_____

2. Find a position that appeals to you in the classified advertisements of your local newspaper or on the Internet. Write a cover letter applying for the position. Use the format below to compose your letter, then key and print a final copy.

COVER LETTER FORM

Your Address
Date

Name of Person
Title
Company Name
Street Address
City, State, ZIP Code

Dear _____:

Opening Paragraph:
   (Your ad in the Sunday *Inquirer* for the position of medical assistant interests . . .)

Middle Paragraph:
   (Your practice is known for its good rapport with patients. I have experience in . . .)

Closing Paragraph:
   May I come for an interview? I will call your office . . .)

Sincerely,

Your Name

3. Using the advertisement from No. 2 above, develop a list of questions you think the interviewer might ask an applicant. Prepare answers to the questions based on your background.

4. Select a classmate to serve as interviewer in a mock interview with you. Give your classmate the advertisement from No. 2 above and the list of questions you developed for No. 3. Ask the classmate to add other questions and keep them secret. Conduct a mock interview for the class. Dress appropriately for the interview. At the conclusion, ask for a critique of the interview from other class members.

INTERVIEW CRITIQUE FORM

(1) Did each person sit straight and face the other person?

(2) Did each speak clearly?

(3) Did the the interviewee make good eye contact?

(4) Did the interviewer listen and pay attention?

(5) What kind of impression did the interviewee make?

(6) Did either person seem to be uncomfortable? Why?

(7) Did the interviewer ask good questions and were they appropriate to the job?

(8) Did the interviewee give good answers? What made them good?

(9) Did the interviewer ask any illegal questions? If so, how well did the interviewee handle them?

(10) What suggestions would you make to help each person improve?

5. Analyze the Sunday advertisements in your local newspaper and compare the skills and abilities required for five medical office positions. Using the following chart as an example, develop a list of the requirements for each position. Tally the number of positions, naming each individual skill or ability. Make a priority list of skills needed based on your tally.

Skills and Abilities Required for Medical Office Employment

	Title of Position	*Skills and Abilities Needed*
Job No. 1	_____	_____
Job No. 2	_____	_____
Job No. 3	_____	_____

EXPANDING YOUR THINKING

1. Assume that you are ready to begin a job search. Compile your "network" of friends and acquaintances who might help you learn of available positions. Include family members, current and former employers, teachers, classmates, your friends' parents, and people you know through civic organizations, sports, church, scouts, or clubs.

Networking Data Collection Form

Name of Person	How Known	Questions to Ask, or Information to Seek	Follow-up or Referral
1.			
2.			
3.			
4.			
5.			
6.			
7.			
8.			
9.			
10.			
11.			
12.			
13.			
14.			
15.			
16.			
17.			
18.			
19.			
20.			
21.			
22.			
23.			
24.			
25.			

2. Identify several of your habits that might be distracting or annoying to an interviewer. What can you do to break these habits?

Distracting Behaviors

Related to Speech

1. _____
2. _____
3. _____
4. _____
5. _____

Related to Eye Contact

1. _____
2. _____
3. _____
4. _____
5. _____

Related to Posture and Movement

1. _____
2. _____
3. _____
4. _____
5. _____

Other

1. _____
2. _____
3. _____
4. _____
5. _____

3. Create a list of information you should have about employers before attending an interview. Add other information you might want to learn about a prospective employer.

Information About Job Duties

1. _____
2. _____
3. _____
4. _____
5. _____

Information About Working Conditions, Hours, and Overtime

1. _____
2. _____
3. _____
4. _____
5. _____

Information About Computers and Software

1. _____
2. _____
3. _____
4. _____
5. _____

Information About Career Planning and Continuing Education

1. _____
2. _____
3. _____
4. _____
5. _____

Information About Practice Type and Specialty

1. _____
2. _____

APPENDICES

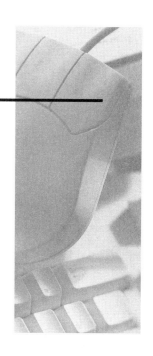

Appendix A

AAMA MEDICAL ASSISTANT ROLE DELINEATION CHART

AAMA Role Delineation Study

Occupational Analysis of the Medical Assisting Profession

Administrative
Administrative Procedures
Practice Finances

Clinical
Fundamental Principles
Diagnostic Orders
Patient Care

General
Professionalism
Communication Skills
Legal Concepts
Instruction
Operational Functions

Update on the medical assisting profession

The health care delivery system is dynamic and changing. Medical assistants, who work in ambulatory health care settings and assist physicians in meeting the clinical and administrative demands of the medical office, must adapt with these changes. For this reason, the American Association of Medical Assistants (AAMA) publishes updates to its *Role Delineation Study* to provide a current analysis of the profession.

Last published in 1996, the update to the Role Delineation Chart is based on a survey conducted by an outside research firm. In April 2002, the survey was sent to a random sampling of 15,268 current CMAs, including AAMA members, nonmembers and former members. A total of 4,004 responses were received. This extraordinary response rate (26%) allowed for a 99% confidence level, with a reliability factor of plus or minus 1.7%.

The survey included a real-world component of what medical assistants are actually performing in the workplace and a forward-looking component of what the respondents thought medical assistants might be doing during the next five years. The survey results

indicated an increasing percentage of respondents (as compared to past surveys) are spending a greater portion of their time performing clinical tasks. Respondents also listed the tasks they think medical assistants will be delegated more frequently during the next five years. The top tasks included assisting in clinical or patient care procedures, patient education, management and supervisory tasks, coding and billing, intravenous procedures, and medical records.

The chart illustrates the areas of competence required for an entry-level medical assistant. Potential uses of the chart include the following:

Description of the field of medical assisting for other health care professionals

Identification of the entry-level areas of competence for medical assistants

Framework for the development of continuing education programs

Framework for self-assessment by practitioners

Acknowledgments
The AAMA Board of Trustees formed an ad hoc committee to analyze the results of the survey. The committee consisted of the chair, two CMA practitioners, one CMA educator, and the chairs of the Certifying Board, Curriculum Review Board, Continuing Education Board and Physician Liaison Board. The AAMA president, vice president and executive director served ex officio.

Committee members
Kathryn Panagiotacos, CMA, Chair
Boni Bruntz, CMA-A
Mary Dey, CMA-AC
Kristina Frye, CMA
Lisa Gibbons, CMA
Rebecca Newsome, PhD, CMA, MT(ASCP)
Deborah Rossi, MA, CMA
Catharine Tabb, MD

Ex officio
Julianna Drumheller, CMA, 2001–02 President
Luella Wetherbee, CMA, CPC, 2001–02 Vice President
Donald A. Balasa, JD, MBA, Executive Director

A PUBLICATION OF

AMERICAN ASSOCIATION OF MEDICAL ASSISTANTS
20 N. WACKER DR., STE. 1575
CHICAGO, ILLINOIS 60606

web site: www.aama-ntl.org   800.228.2262

Copyright 2003 by the American Association of Medical Assistants, Inc. For more information or additional copies, contact the AAMA.

1/03

Reprinted with permission from the American Association of Medical Assistants.

Medical Assistant Role Delineation Chart

Administrative

ADMINISTRATIVE PROCEDURES

- Perform basic administrative medical assisting functions
- Schedule, coordinate and monitor appointments
- Schedule inpatient/outpatient admissions and procedures
- Understand and apply third-party guidelines
- Obtain reimbursement through accurate claims submission
- Monitor third-party reimbursement
- Understand and adhere to managed care policies and procedures
- *Negotiate managed care contracts*

PRACTICE FINANCES

- Perform procedural and diagnostic coding
- Apply bookkeeping principles
- Manage accounts receivable
- *Manage accounts payable*
- *Process payroll*
- Document and maintain accounting and banking records
- *Develop and maintain fee schedules*
- *Manage renewals of business and professional insurance policies*
- *Manage personnel benefits and maintain records*
- *Perform marketing, financial, and strategic planning*

Clinical

FUNDAMENTAL PRINCIPLES

- Apply principles of aseptic technique and infection control
- Comply with quality assurance practices
- Screen and follow up patient test results

DIAGNOSTIC ORDERS

- Collect and process specimens
- Perform diagnostic tests

PATIENT CARE

- Adhere to established patient screening procedures
- Obtain patient history and vital signs
- Prepare and maintain examination and treatment areas
- Prepare patient for examinations, procedures and treatments
- Assist with examinations, procedures and treatments
- Prepare and administer medications and immunizations
- Maintain medication and immunization records
- Recognize and respond to emergencies
- Coordinate patient care information with other health care providers
- Initiate IV and administer IV medications with appropriate training and as permitted by state law

General

PROFESSIONALISM

- Display a professional manner and image
- Demonstrate initiative and responsibility
- Work as a member of the health care team
- Prioritize and perform multiple tasks
- Adapt to change
- Promote the CMA credential
- Enhance skills through continuing education
- Treat all patients with compassion and empathy
- Promote the practice through positive public relations

COMMUNICATION SKILLS

- Recognize and respect cultural diversity
- Adapt communications to individual's ability to understand
- Use professional telephone technique
- Recognize and respond effectively to verbal, nonverbal, and written communications
- Use medical terminology appropriately
- Utilize electronic technology to receive, organize, prioritize and transmit information
- Serve as liaison

LEGAL CONCEPTS

- Perform within legal and ethical boundaries
- Prepare and maintain medical records
- Document accurately
- Follow employer's established policies dealing with the health care contract
- Implement and maintain federal and state health care legislation and regulations
- Comply with established risk management and safety procedures
- Recognize professional credentialing criteria
- *Develop and maintain personnel, policy and procedure manuals*

INSTRUCTION

- Instruct individuals according to their needs
- Explain office policies and procedures
- Teach methods of health promotion and disease prevention
- Locate community resources and disseminate information
- *Develop educational materials*
- *Conduct continuing education activities*

OPERATIONAL FUNCTIONS

- Perform inventory of supplies and equipment
- Perform routine maintenance of administrative and clinical equipment
- Apply computer techniques to support office operations
- *Perform personnel management functions*
- *Negotiate leases and prices for equipment and supply contracts*

* Denotes advanced skills.

Appendix B

CAAHEP STANDARDS

Content: To provide for student attainment of the Entry-Level Competencies for the Medical Assistant, the curriculum must include, but not necessarily be limited to:

a. **Anatomy and Physiology**
   (1) Anatomy and physiology of all the body systems
   (2) Common pathology/diseases
   (3) Diagnostic/treatment modalities

b. **Medical Terminology**
   (1) Basic structure of medical words
   (2) Word building and definitions
   (3) Application of medical terminology

c. **Medical Law and Ethics**
   (1) Legal guidelines/requirements for health care
   (2) Medical ethics and related issues
   (3) Risk management

d. **Psychology**
   (1) Basic principles
   (2) Developmental stages of the life cycle
   (3) Hereditary, cultural, and environmental influences on behavior
   (4) Mental health and applied psychology

e. **Communication**
   (1) Principles of verbal and nonverbal communication
   (2) Recognition and response to verbal and nonverbal communication
   (3) Adaptations for individualized needs
   (4) Applications of electronic technology
   (5) Fundamental writing skills

f. **Medical Assisting Administrative Procedures**
   (1) Basic medical office functions
   (2) Bookkeeping and basic accounting
   (3) Insurance and coding
   (4) Facility management

g. **Medical Assisting Clinical Procedures**
   (1) Asepsis and infection control
   (2) Specimen collection and processing
   (3) Diagnostic testing
   (4) Patient care
   (5) Pharmacology
   (6) Medical emergencies
   (7) Principles of radiology

h. **Professional Components**
   (1) Personal attributes
   (2) Job readiness
   (3) Workplace dynamics
   (4) Allied health professions and credentialing

i. **Externship**
   (1) A minimum of 160 contact hours
   (2) Placement in an ambulatory health care setting

Reprinted with permission of the Commission on Accreditation of Allied Health Education Programs.

Appendix C

ABHES COURSE CONTENT REQUIREMENTS FOR MEDICAL ASSISTANTS

1. **Orientation**
   a. Introduction and review of program
   b. Employment outlook
   c. General responsibilities

2. **Anatomy and Physiology**
   a. Anatomy and physiology
   b. Diet and nutrition
   c. Study of diseases and etiology

3. **Medical Terminology**
   a. Basic structure of medical words (roots, prefixes, suffixes, spelling, and definitions)
   b. Combining word elements to form medical words
   c. Medical specialties and short forms
   d. Medical abbreviations

4. **Medical Law and Ethics**
   a. Ethical decisions, medical jurisprudence, and confidentiality
   b. Legal terminology pertaining to office practice
   c. Medical/ethical issues in today's society

5. **Psychology of Human Relations**
   a. Dealing with difficult patients with normal/abnormal behavior
   b. Caring for patients with special and specific needs
   c. Caring for cancer and terminally ill patients
   d. Emotional crises, patients, and/or family
   e. Various treatment protocols

6. **Pharmacology**
   a. Occupational math and metric conversion (drug calculations)
   b. Use of Physician's Desk References (PDRs) and medication books
   c. Common abbreviations used in prescription writing
   d. Legal aspects of writing prescriptions
   e. FDC and state laws
   f. Medications prescribed for the treatment of illness and disease based on a systems method

7. **Medical Office Business Procedures/ Management**
   a. Manual and computerized records management
      1. Patient case histories (confidentiality)
      2. Filing
      3. Appointments and scheduling
      4. Inventory/control
   b. Financial management
      1. Basic bookkeeping
      2. Billing and collections
      3. Purchasing
      4. Banking and payroll
   c. Insurance (including Health Maintenance Organizations [HMOs], Preferred Provider Organizations [PPOs], co-pays, Current Procedural Terminology [CPT] coding, etc.)
   d. Equipment and supplies (including ordering, maintaining, storage, and inventory)
   e. Reception, public, and interpersonal relations
      1. Telephone techniques
      2. Professional conduct and appearance
      3. Professional office environment and safety
   f. Office safety and security

8. **Basic Keyboarding**
   a. Office machines, transcriptions, computerized systems, and medical data processing
   b. Transcribing medical correspondence and medical reports
   c. Medical terminology review

9. **Medical Office Clinical Procedures**
   a. Basic clinical skills (e.g., vital signs)
   b. Basic skills and procedures used in medical emergencies
   c. Patient examination
      1. Patient histories
      2. Patient preparation
      3. Physical exam
      4. Instruments
      5. Assisting the physician
      6. Housekeeping
   d. Medical equipment
      1. Electrocardiogram, centrifuge, etc.
      2. Physical therapy
      3. Radiography
         a) Safety
         b) Patient preparation
         c) Radiography of chest and extremities
   e. Medical asepsis/sterilization and minor office surgery
   f. Specialties
   g. First aid, cardiopulmonary resuscitation (CPR)
   h. Injections (dosage calculations)
      1. IM (intramuscular)
      2. Sub q (subcutaneous)
      3. ID (intradermal)
   i. Universal Precautions in the medical office

10. **Medical Laboratory Procedures**
    a. Orientation
       1. Laboratory equipment and maintenance
       2. Safety
       3. Storage of chemicals and supplies
       4. Fire safety
       5. Care of microscope (introduction)
    b. Urinalysis
       1. Specimen collection
       2. Physical exam

3. Chemical analysis
4. Microscopic exam
   c. Hematology
      1. Personal protective equipment
      2. Specimen collection
         a) Venipuncture
         b) Finger puncture
      3. Hemoglobin
      4. Hematocrit
      5. WBCs (white blood cells)
      6. RBCs (red blood cells)
      7. Slide preps
      8. Serology
         a) Blood typing
         b) Blood morphology
      9. Quality control
   d. Basic blood chemistries
   e. Human immunodeficiency virus (HIV)/acquired immunodeficiency syndrome (AIDS)
   f. OSHA (Occupational Safety and Health Administration) Compliance Rules and Regulations

11. **Career Development**
    a. Instruction regarding internship rules and regulations
    b. Job search, professional development, and success
    c. Goal setting, time management, and employment opportunities
    d. Resumé writing, interviewing techniques, and follow-up
    e. Dress for success
    f. Professionalism

12. **Guidelines for Acceptable Externship (160 Hours)**
    a. The externship should provide students practical experience in ambulatory health care facilities, including hospitals, physician's offices, or other health care facilities.
    b. Before assigning a student to an externship location, there must be a prior evaluation by the school that a viable externship site exists for an effective externship. In addition, the physician shall be provided with a written contract setting forth the conditions for the externship.

c. Visitation by a qualified member of the school staff should be made during the externship of a trainee if the locale is within a reasonable distance from the school. In any event, telephone follow-up should be made to determine that the experience is a valid and satisfactory one for the trainee.

d. The externship should include appropriately diversified learning experiences.

e. A documented report on student performance must be submitted by the physician and/or the supervisory person involved. The report must be kept at the school in the student's file.

Reprinted with permission from the Accrediting Bureau of Health Education Schools.

Appendix D

REGISTERED MEDICAL ASSISTANT (RMA [AMT]) CERTIFICATION COMPETENCY SUMMARY

I. GENERAL MEDICAL ASSISTING KNOWLEDGE
   A. Anatomy and Physiology
      1. Body systems
      2. Disorders of the body
   B. Medical Terminology
      1. Word parts
      2. Definitions
      3. Common abbreviations and symbols
      4. Spelling
   C. Medical Law
      1. Medical Law
      2. Licensure, certification, and registration
   D. Medical Ethics
      1. Principles of medical ethics
      2. Ethical conduct
   E. Human Relations
      1. Patient relations
      2. Other interpersonal relations
   F. Patient Education
      1. Patient instruction
      2. Patient resource materials

II. ADMINISTRATIVE MEDICAL ASSISTING
   A. Insurance
      1. Terminology
      2. Plans
      3. Claim forms
      4. Coding
      5. Financial aspects of medical insurance
   B. Financial Bookkeeping
      1. Terminology
      2. Patient billing
      3. Collections
      4. Fundamental medical office accounting procedures
      5. Banking
      6. Employee payroll
      7. Financial mathematics
   C. Medical Secretarial-Receptionist
      1. Terminology
      2. Reception
      3. Scheduling
      4. Oral and written communications
      5. Records management
      6. Charts
      7. Transcription and dictation
      8. Supplies and equipment management
      9. Computers for medical office applications
      10. Office safety

III. CLINICAL MEDICAL ASSISTING
   A. Asepsis
      1. Terminology
      2. Universal blood and body fluid precautions
      3. Medical asepsis
      4. Surgical asepsis
   B. Sterilization
      1. Terminology
      2. Sanitization
      3. Disinfection
      4. Sterilization
      5. Record keeping
   C. Instruments
      1. Identification
      2. Usage
      3. Care and handling
   D. Vital Signs
      1. Blood pressure
      2. Pulse
      3. Respiration
      4. Height and weight
      5. Temperature

E. Physical Examinations
  1. Problem-oriented records
  2. Positions
  3. Methods of examination
  4. Specialty examinations
  5. Visual acuity
  6. Allergy testing
F. Clinical Pharmacology
  1. Terminology
  2. Injections
  3. Prescriptions
  4. Drugs
G. Minor Surgery
  1. Surgical supplies
  2. Surgical procedures
H. Therapeutic Modalities
  1. Modalities
  2. Patient instruction

I. Laboratory Procedures
  1. Safety
  2. Quality control
  3. Laboratory equipment
  4. Urinalysis
  5. Blood
  6. Other specimens
  7. Specimen handling
  8. Records
  9. Microbiology
J. Electrocardiography
  1. Standard, 12-lead ECG (electrocardiogram)
  2. Mounting techniques
  3. Other ECG procedures
K. First Aid
  1. First aid procedures
  2. Legal responsibilities

Reprinted with permission of American Medical Technologists.

GLOSSARY

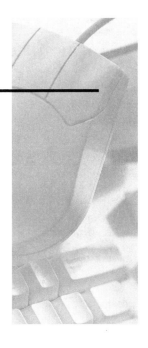

AAMA The American Association of Medical Assistants, a professional organization for all practicing medical assistants, certified and noncertified

account aging Method for reporting how long an account has been due

active listening Conscious attention to the speaker, asking open-ended questions that elicit additional information, and using verbal and nonverbal skills to provide feedback

advance directives Patient's wishes regarding future treatment if the patient is incapacitated

allocation Deciding how to divide available resources, such as time, among conflicting demands

ambulatory care centers Twenty-four-hour medical centers that treat patients with minor illnesses or injuries

answering service Twenty-four-hour service that answers phones for a fee

anxiety An intense feeling of dread or worry; fear of a situation or of the unknown

application letter The letter that accompanies the resume. It highlights the most important information from the resume

appointment book A daily record of each patient's name, telephone number, appointment time, and the reason for the medical visit

assignment of benefits Signing over benefits from an insurance payment to a third party

association Organization that advocates special interests through information or lobbying

balance Amount remaining owed on a patient's account or the amount of money in a checking account at any given moment

basic insurance Insurance benefits that cover physicians' fees, hospital expenses, and surgical fees as determined by the plan contract, usually after payment of a deductible by the patient

billing Reminding patients that money is owed to the practice

bioethics Branch of medical ethics concerned with moral issues resulting from high technology and sophisticated medical research. Social issues such as abortion, fetal research, artificial insemination, and euthanasia are important bioethical questions

block Letter format in which all lines begin at the left margin

blood tests Analysis of blood to determine whether infection is present, excessive urea is evident, or glucose or other substances are present in too high or too low a concentration

Blue Cross and Blue Shield Nonprofit insurers organized under the laws of individual states; generally, Blue Shield pays for physicians' services and Blue Cross covers hospital costs

burnout The physical and mental letdown that occurs after a period of stress, intensity, or overwork

business class Flight class that offers more amenities than coach, but fewer than first

CAAHEP Commission on Accreditation of Allied Health Education Programs, a group that accredits a school's medical assisting program. Medical assistants who wish to sit for the CMA examination should select a CAAHEP-approved school for their education

callback A message that requires a return call

capitation A managed health concept whereby the physician is paid a certain amount per patient, no matter how much or how little service the patient receives

case history Analysis of the patient's complaint, examination results, lab results, diagnosis, prescribed treatment, and family and personal history

cellular phone Portable telephone that operates by means of batteries, independent of any fixed location

Centers for Disease Control and Prevention Federal medical research center located in Atlanta, Georgia

central processing unit (CPU) The electronic circuitry that translates software instructions

charge slip Receipt listing the typical examinations, procedures, treatments, and services a patient might have during one visit

check register The record book in which all information about checks is recorded

civil law Rights and obligations that people have toward one another, usually concerned with a wrong or injury one person inflicts on another

claim form The documentation required by an insurance company before payment will be made for medical services

clearinghouse Centralized location where claims are received, reviewed, and distributed electronically to insurance companies

closed files Medical records of patients who are no longer under the physician's care because they have moved, changed doctors, or died

CMA Certified Medical Assistant, a credential earned by passing the comprehensive examination offered by the American Association of Medical Assistants

co-insurance An insurance company and a patient share the cost of medical care, usually on an 80/20 split

co-payment Percent of medical expenses for which the patient is responsible beyond the deductible

co-payment The amount the policyholder must pay for each visit or medical service received

collection Process for expediting overdue accounts

commercial insurance For-profit companies offering individual or group health insurance

comprehensive insurance Combination of basic and major medical insurance

computer scheduling Scheduling patient appointments with computer software

conference call A single call that allows several individuals — perhaps in different cities — to participate. Even the most inexpensive office telephone systems usually provide a feature that allows a medical office assistant to connect up to three or four individuals to one call

confidentiality Maintaining secrecy about all information regarding patients, including placing the fax machine in a secure location, storing patient files out of the view of everyone except the medical staff, and securing computer records so they are visible only to individuals with a pass code

coordination of benefits A policy requirement that insurance companies will share the cost of treatment when a patient is covered by more than one policy

CPT Current Procedural Terminology

credentialing Verifying that an individual has met certain industry standards

criminal law Rights and obligations people have toward society

culturally diverse Representing a variety of traditions, language, and customs

Current Procedural Terminology (CPT) Industry coding standard recognized by most insurance companies and widely used in medical offices to identify procedures and services performed

cycle billing Process for spreading billing over the whole month instead of sending all bills at the same time

daily list of appointments A list showing names of all patients who will be seen in one day

daily log The day's summary of patient transactions

database Software application for sorting and summarizing large amounts of data

DDD Direct Distance Dialing; placing long-distance calls directly, without intervention of an operator

deductible Amount paid by a patient prior to initiation of insurance benefits

dependents Individuals covered under a policyholder's insurance contract, including children and spouse

desktop publishing Creating professional quality brochures, flyers, and other printed communications pieces that incorporate words, charts, pictures, and clip art

diagnosis-related group (DRG) Method of classifying patients into categories based on the primary diagnosis

direct flight Flight that connects two cities without a plane change

disability An illness or injury that affects an individual's ability to continue in the job held previously

disabled Unable to participate at the normal level because of a physical or mental weakness or incapacitation

DNR Do Not Resuscitate order permits the patient to die without cardiopulmonary resuscitation. This order is commonly used in treating terminally ill or elderly patients

doctor's notes, or progress notes Doctor's comments that are added to the medical record each time the patient is treated

domestic mail services Mail services performed by the United States Postal Service

drug schedules Categories of drugs divided according to their potential for abuse

durable power of attorney Document that provides broad powers of medical authority to an individual often either a family member or an attorney, who is given legal power to decide what extraordinary measures should be taken with a patient when the patient is too sick to decide. A durable power of attorney usually accompanies a DNR in the patient's hospital record

E-mail Electronic mail routed through a computer network allows persons at different computer terminals around the world to write messages for others on the network

effective Achieving the mission of the practice in serving patients, whether or not resources are used efficiently

efficient Making good use of available resources

electrocardiogram Graphic illustration of the heart's activity

electronic fund transfer Using computer networks to move money from one bank account to another

elimination period Period of time after the onset of a disability for which no benefits are made

empathy Mentally putting oneself in another's situation

employment agencies Companies that charge a fee to connect employers and job applicants

employment application A standard form for providing personal information and employment history, an identification of places where an applicant has worked, and the types of responsibilities

exclusions Services that are not paid under the terms of an insurance contract

expectations Standards of performance set by an individual or an employer

explanation of benefits (EOB) A report from an insurance company that is sent with claim payments to provide details about the reimbursement

extended benefits Supplemental coverage to a basic hospital plan, sometimes includes diagnostic x-rays and laboratory examinations

fax Facsimile transmission of documents by telephone line from one location to another

fee-for-service Payment system in which the full bill is paid each time a patient visits the physician

feedback Responses that provide direction

FICA Federal Insurance Contribution Act; set up by the social security retirement system. Social Security deductions are called FICA deductions

Form W-2 The form sent by every employer to every employee, with copies to the IRS and state government, summarizing the year's gross income, tax deductions, and net income

Form W-4 The employee's withholding allowance certificate, filled out at the beginning of employment and whenever exemptions change, listing the exemptions from taxation that the employee is claiming

formatting Placement of the parts of a letter or medical document

gender bias Subtle form of verbal sex discrimination

gender neutral Language that is not biased toward either sex

genetic counseling Counseling related to gene disorders. Prospective parents often receive genetic counseling regarding the likelihood of bearing a child with genetic disorders

genetic engineering Advanced, complex, and often controversial means of isolating and replacing part or all of a "mutant" gene to reduce or eliminate the chances that a person will develop a particular disease

genetics Study of genes and their role in illness and disease. Gene therapy is an exciting, emerging field of medical study because it promises a cure for some illnesses now considered terminal

good Samaritan laws Laws that protect the physician and other health care professionals who assist people in unusual emergency situations

graphics Pictures or charts designed on a computer

group insurance Coverage of a group of people based on a common characteristic, such as employment at a company

hardware Machines in a computer system

hold Telephone function that allows a call to be kept waiting on the line

ICD codes Diagnosis codes from the International Classification of Diseases, Tenth Edition, used to identify the patient's medical problem

inactive files Medical records of patients who have not visited the physician for an extended period

informed consent Law that states a patient must be given medical information about risk before undergoing a procedure

Internet search Locating information through the Internet

interpersonal From one person to another

inventory Store of supplies

inventory issue Taking an item out of inventory to use it

inventory receipt Taking an item into inventory

invoice Statement of services

itinerary Schedule of travel, including departure and arrival times, flight numbers, lodging, and telephone numbers

keyboard Input device that allows the operator to key data into the computer

keywords Words that identify the information you want to locate through the Internet

laboratory request Test to be administered and the name of the attending physician

lead time Delay between placing a purchase order and receiving the item

ledger card Chronological listing of one family's financial activity with the practice

literature search Review of published sources at the library or by computer to find articles on a specified topic

living will Legal document, signed by an individual, that provides precise instructions about the amount of extraordinary care to be delivered in the event of a life-threatening medical situation

major medical insurance Insurance designed to offset potentially catastrophic expenses from a lengthy illness or accident

malfeasance Wrongful treatment of a patient

managed competition Medical care in which physicians and hospitals compete for patients

Medicaid Government health insurance program that protects the poor

medical ethics Term applied to the principles governing medical conduct. Medical ethics deals with the relationship of the physician to the patient, the patient's family, fellow physicians, and society

medical law Standards set by elected officials in the state and nation. An illegal act is always unethical according to the American Medical Association's Principles of Medical Ethics, but an unethical act may not be illegal

medical specialties Branches of medicine that concentrate on specific body systems

Medicare Government health insurance program that protects the elderly

misfeasance Lawful treatment performed in the wrong way

modem Hardware that connects your computer, via phone lines, to other computers and to the Internet

modified block Format in which the date and closing lines begin at center

monitor Television-like screen on which words, charts, letters, and other data appear

multiskilled medical assistant Medical assistant who is trained in both administrative and clinical duties

network The computer components that are connected to each other, resulting in a system that allows each component to communicate with the other pieces

networking Interacting with a circle of acquaintances

no show The term given to a patient who fails to keep an appointment

non-stop Flight that connects two cities without making intermediate stops

nonfeasance Failure to act when duty requires

nonverbal communication The signals humans send out without speaking, including facial expressions, gestures, posture, and appearance

objective The intent of the process

obsolete supplies Inventory items that are no longer used

OMA Ophthalmic Medical Assistant, a credential earned through the Joint Commission on Allied Health Personnel in Ophthalmology

on call Medical care in which physicians are available on an as-needed basis, no matter the time of day. Doctors in a single practice are always on call. Doctors in a group practice can rotate the responsibility

optimal Making the best use of a resource

orient To provide an informational overview

overbooking Scheduling more patients than the physician can see in the time available

overdraft A check written for an amount that exceeds the balance of the account the check is drawn on. When such a check is not honored — paid — by a bank, it is said to have bounced. A bounced check is an overdraft that comes back to the person who drafted it

pathology and cytopathology Field of laboratory testing that shows the results of studies of body tissue and body cells

patient health questionnaire Questions about the patient's previous health and surgical history and family history

patient information form Completed by a patient immediately on arriving at the medical office for the initial visit

Patient Self-Determination Act Federal law requiring all hospitals and nursing homes to explain in detail the extraordinary care their state permits. These facilities must alert patients of their right to execute living wills or appoint a health care proxy through a durable power of attorney

Patient's Bill of Rights Established by the American Hospital Association in 1972, the Patient's Bill of Rights provides basic guidelines for the care of hospitalized patients

payables Amount of money owed by a practice to those from whom it purchases goods and services

PC Personal computer

pegboard accounting Traditional method of maintaining accounts, named for the flat writing board on which accounting papers are prepared

physician extenders Paramedical staff trained to support the physician by performing some tasks previously performed only by the physician

practice analysis Overview of procedures and treatments provided and income derived during a specified period

preexisting condition A medical condition that existed before an insurance policy was approved

problem-oriented medical record Patient's complaints identified in list form

progress appointments Follow-up appointments that monitor the progress of treatment

proof of posting Verification of the calculation of columns in the daily log

proofread To examine a document for errors

prospective payment Term describing a method of flat fee pricing

RDC The Role Delineation Chart, developed by the Endowment of the American Association of Medical Assistants to define the basic competencies for an entry-level medical assistant professional

receivables Amount of money owed to a practice by those who purchase its services

reconciliation The monthly task of ascertaining that the practice's determination of the amount of its account balance agrees with the balance arrived at by the bank

recredentialing Renewing a previously awarded recognition of industry standards

redundancy Unnecessary repetition of words

referral Determination by a physician that a patient should see a specialist or subspecialist for a consultation

residency Three years of specialty training that occurs after a physician finishes medical school

resume A formatted document listing an applicant's personal and employment information

reversed charges Collect call

RMA Registered Medical Assistant, a credential earned by passing the comprehensive examination offered by the American Medical Technologists

root medical word Basic medical word used in combination with other words or prefixes and suffixes

scanner A machine that takes a snapshot of forms, pictures, graphs, and some written material and merges them with computer-created words or images

schedule The daily calendar of times when patients will be seen

screening Evaluation of a call for proper referral

shingling Method of filing small reports

SOAP Method of reporting patient's diagnosis and treatment plan: subjective examination (S), objective test results (O), doctor's assessment (A), and treatment plan (P)

software Programs or instructions that operate computers

source-oriented medical record Information grouped according to its source

spreadsheet Software application for rows and columns of numbers and their calculation

stored letter parts Standard paragraphs that are stored in the computer's memory

supply disposal Getting rid of out-of-date or obsolete items

tact Diplomacy in handling difficult situations

thesaurus Reference book or word processing feature containing synonyms and antonyms

third-party payers Insurance companies or others who will pay the patient's bill

third-party reimbursement A form of payment for medical services where someone other than the patient — a third party — pays the doctor or hospital. Third parties include insurance companies, health maintenance organizations, and Medicare and Medicaid. Under the fee-for-service payment system, fees can be paid directly by the patient, or by a third party; either way, it is considered a fee paid for a service received

time zone Geographic area identified by its time of day in relation to time in other parts of the country or world

tone Sound of letters; what is said and how the writer chooses to say it

transcription To write from one source to another

triage Screening calls, usually associated with emergencies, so as to prioritize the schedule, putting worst cases first

urinalysis Routine laboratory test of urine often requested by physicians

usual and customary care The fee that is usually charged for a specific service, one that is customary of the usual range and fees and is reasonable for the geographic area

vendor Supplier of products or services

videoconference A conference that connects participants in various locations through telephone lines, a video camera, and computer hookups. Videoconferences are often substituted for costly in-person conferences that would require participants to travel long distances

voice mail Voice messages that are left in an answering system when the office staff is not available to take a call personally

waiting period The time between when an insurance policy is approved and the patient is covered for benefits, often called the elimination

waiver An attachment to a policy that excludes specific preexisting conditions

wave scheduling Clustering appointments by time block; flow is maintained by rotating patients among needed procedures

word processing Processing of words to form narrative documents using a computer and software package instead of a typewriter

workers' compensation insurance Employer-paid insurance that provides health care and income to employees and their dependents when employees suffer work-related injuries or illness

x-rays, CAT scans, and ultrasound Diagnostic tests to determine whether any unusual medical condition, such as a tissue mass, is present in the body

"you" viewpoint Focusing the language of a written document on the best interests of the reader

INDEX

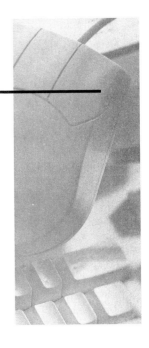

Entries followed by f *reference figures*
Entries followed by t *reference tables*

A

AAA. *See* American Automobile Association (AAA)
AAMA. *See* American Association of Medical Assistants (AAMA)
Abbreviations
   defined, 10
      used in recording patient care, 227–229t
ABHES. *See* Accrediting Bureau of Health Education Schools (ABHES)
Abortion, medical ethics and, 43
Abuse
   child, medical ethics and, 43
   drug, medical ethics and, 47–48
   elderly, medical ethics and, 43
   substance, medical ethics and, 47–48
Account aging, 269
Accounting procedures
   check entries, 247–248
   computerized account management, 252–253, 255–256
   daily deposits, 245
   ledger entries, 247
   payroll accounting procedures, 250, 252
   pegboard accounting, 241–245
      charge slip, 241–242
      daily log, 241–242, 244f
      ledger card, 241–242, 244f
Account management, computerized
   daily activities
      cash and check register, 256
      daily log, 255
      list of appointments, 253, 254
      patient charge slip, 255, 255f

patient ledger, 255, 256f
      patient registration form, 254f
      practice analysis, 257
   patient accounts, 252–253
Accounts receivable
   control, 244–245
   report, 270f
Accrediting Bureau of Health Education Schools (ABHES), 328
   course content requirements for medical assistants, 343–345
Active files, 230
Active listening, Medical Assistant and, 85
Active voice, letter writing and, 165, 166f
Adjusted Checkbook Balance, 248
Advance directives, 58
Advertisements
   misleading, 60
   newspaper classified, job search process and, 315
Aggressiveness *vs.* assertiveness, 28f
AIDS
   ethical concerns, 47
   health care costs and, 1
   research on, 7
Allergy and immunology, as specialty, 13f
Allocation, 126
Alphabetic card file, 233–234
Alphabetic filing guides and tabs, 233
Alphabetic indexing, 231–232
Alzheimer's disease, genetic engineering and, 46
AMA. *See* American Medical Association (AMA)
Ambulatory care centers, 20, 22–23
Ambulatory centers, 6
American Association of Medical Assistants (AAMA), 4, 20, 21, 22, 39, 41–42, 63
   Code of Ethics, 41–42
   role delineation study, 340

American Automobile Association (AAA), 201
American Board of Medical Specialties, 11
American Hospital Association, 38–39
American Medical Association (AMA), 20
  Code of Medical Ethics, 38
  position on computer security, 50
  principles of Medical Ethics, 37–38
Anesthesiology, as specialty, 13f
Annotating mail, 208–209
Answering services/machines, 104, 119–120
Antiabortion, 43
Anxiety, 85, 93
Appearance, job interview and, 323–324
Application form, job application process, 321
Application letters, job application process, 321, 322f
Appointment scheduling, 126–138
  the appointment book, 126, 129, 130f
    computer scheduling, 129–130
    overbooking (double tracking), 130–131
    procedures, 130
    rescheduling/canceling appointments, 131
      by computer, 131
  by computer, 129
  coordinating delays/unexpected appointments, 131–132
  emergency appointments, 131
  follow-up appointments, 137–138
  maintaining, 128–135
  nonpatient appointments, 133
  patient appointments, 128–129
  patients for outside facilities, 136–137
  patients for referral, 137
  patients for surgery, 136
  patients for the hospital, 136
  preparing a daily list, 135
  rescheduling missed appointments, 132–133
Arteriosclerosis, genetic engineering and, 46
Assertiveness, medical assistant and, 27–28
Assignment of benefits, defined, 214
ATM. See Automated teller machine (ATM)
Audit trail, establishing
  claims register, 302, 303f
  computerizing the claims process, 303–304, 305f
  follow-up procedure, 303
  ticker file, 302–303
Automated teller machine (ATM), 248, 249
Automobile travel, 201

B
Balance, defined, 248
Banking, medical office and, 245
  electronic, 248–250
Basic insurance, 287–288
Beepers, cellular telephone and, 120
Benefits
  assignment of, 214
  coordination of, 214
  extended, 214

fringe, 329
Betty Ford Drug Treatment Center, 9
Bibliography, business reports, 186
Billing patients. See also Billing
  cycle, 268
  external service, 268
  internal, 263–266
  monthly, 266–268
Bioethics, 36
Biological terrorism, health care costs and threat of, 1
Block letter, 174
  block/modified, 175f, 176f, 177f
Blood banking, as subspecialty, 13f
Blood tests, 214, 222
Blue Cross and Blue Shield, 286, 288
Body systems, 10
Burnout, defined, 85
Business analysis summary, daily log and, 245
Business associates, scheduling appointments for, 134
Business report formatting
  bibliography, 186
  footnotes, 186
  job instructions, 183
  margin guide, 183
  table of contents, 186
  title page, 186

C
CAAHEP. See Commission on Accreditation of Allied Health Education Programs (CAAHEP)
Cafeteria Plan. See Triple Option Plan (Cafeteria Plan)
Callback messages, 104, 111f
Cancer, genetic engineering and, 46
Capital punishment, medical ethics and, 43
Capitation, 214, 286
Cardiovascular medicine, as subspecialty, 13f
Case history, defined, 214
Cash and check register, computerized, 256
Cash control, daily log and, 245
Cash paid-outs , daily log and, 245
CDC. See Centers for Disease Control (CDC)
Cellular phones
  beepers and, 120
  defined, 104
Centers for Disease Control and Prevention (CDC), 4, 7, 8f
Centers for Medicare and Medicaid Services (CMS), 2, 290, 296
Central processing unit (CPU), 145, 147
Certification, 21–22
Certified Medical Assistant (CMA), 21, 327
CEUs. See Continuing education units (CEUs)
CHAMPUS. See Civilian Health and Medical Program of the Uniformed Services (CHAMPUS)
CHAMPVA. See Civilian Health and Medical Program of the Veterans Administration (CHAMPVA)
Charge slip or receipt, 241, 242–243
  as documentation, 302

Charitable organizations representatives, scheduling
    appointments for, 134
Check(s)
    entries, 247–248
    office management and, 245
    register, 246–247
Chemical pathology, as subspecialty, 13f
Child abuse, medical ethics and, 43
Circulatory system, 10
Civilian Health and Medical Program of the Uniformed
    Services (CHAMPUS), 293–294
Civilian Health and Medical Program of the Veterans
    Administration (CHAMPVA), 294
Civil law, 58, 60, 61
Claims
    insurance, 297
    Medicaid, 292–293
    Medicare, 290
    register, 302
    settlement of, 75
Clearinghouse, 214
Clinical investigation, medical ethics and, 43–44
Clinical supplies, 152–153
Clinics, 6
Closed files, 214, 230
Clustering appointments, 127
CMA. See Certified Medical Assistant (CMA)
CMS. See Centers for Medicare and Medicaid Services (CMS)
Code of Ethics
    American Association of Medical Assistants (AAMA),
        41–42
    American Medical Association (AMA), 38
Code of Hammurabi, 37
Coding systems, insurance, 297–298, 301
Co-insurance, 286
Collection process, 268–278
    aging accounts, 269
    collection letters, 271–276f
Colon and rectal-surgery, as specialty, 13f
Color coding the folder, 216–218
Commercial insurance
    companies, 288
    defined, 286
Commission on Accreditation of Allied Health Education
    Programs (CAAHEP), 20, 21
    standards, 342
Communication. See also Telecommunications
    feedback, 92
    interpersonal, 85–86
        concern for the patient, 86
        empathy, 87
        listening, 86-87
        patience, 88-89
        tact, 87-88
    nonverbal, 90–91
    verbal, 89–90
Complaint, legal, 77f
Comprehensive insurance, 286
Computer

confidentiality and, 49–50, 50–51f
    in the hospital, 15
    insurance claims forms, 303–304, 305
    mechanical failures of, 155
    Medical Assistant and, 23
    medical office and, 146f
    in private practice, 14
    and relationships with patients, 92–93
    rescheduling or canceling an appointment, 131
    scheduling an appointment, 126, 129
    system, 147
    troubleshooting, 155
Computerization of the office
    medical software applications, 147–150
    software applications
        graphics, 145, 149
        spreadsheet, 145, 148
        word processing, 173
Computerized billing statement, 265–266, 267f
Computerized practice lists
    developing, 150–152
    patient-related information, 152
    practiced management information, 152
Computer system, 147
    central processing unit (CPU), 145, 147
    keyboard, 145, 147
    modem, 104
    monitor, 162
    software, 145, 147
Conduct
    job interview and, 324
    unprofessional, 60
Conference call, 104
Confidentiality, 36
    agreements, 73, 74
    computers and, 49–50, 50–51f
    Fax transmissions and, 72
    patient information and, 52
    patient's rights to, 69–70
        exception to, 69
        and insurance companies, 70
    and telecommunications, 72–73
Consulting physician's report, 182f
Contents of the medical record. See Medical records
    management, contents of the medical record
Continuing education process, 327–328
Continuing education units (CEUs), 22
Controlled substances, physicians and, 78
Cooperation, medical assistant and, 26–27
Coordination of benefits, 214
Co-payment, defined, 214
Correspondence file, 234
Correspondence management, 230
Correspondence report formatting, 173–182
Cost of health care, medical ethics and, 48
Court papers, 75
CPT. See Current Procedural Terminology (CPT)
CPT-5 codes, 298, 301
CPU. See Central processing unit (CPU)

Creating text, 173
Credentialing, 20
  defined, 313
  medical records personnel, 25
Criminal law, 58, 60, 66
Critical care, surgical as subspecialty, 13f
Critical care medicine, as subspecialty, 13f
Cross-posting report, 257
Cross-referencing, 232
Culturally diverse, 85
Current Opinions of the Judicial Council of the American
    Medical Association, 43
Current Procedural Terminology (CPT), 2, 20, 241
Cycle billing, 268
Cystic fibrosis, genetic engineering and, 46

D
DACUM, 23
DACUM analysis, Medical Assistant, 23
Daily list of appointments, 126
Daily log
  computerized, 253, 255
  pegboard accounting, 241–242, 244f
Database, 145, 148–149
  partial
    of drug and drug codes, 151f
    of patients, 149f
DDD. *See* Direct Distance Dialing (DDD)
Defensive medicine, 60
Delineation Study Analysis, 23
Delivery services, 204–209
Dental specialties/subspecialties, 12
Dentists, licensure of, 59
Dependability, medical assistant and, 28
Dependents, defined, 214
Deposits, daily, 245–246
Deposit slips, preparing for, 245–246
Dermatology, as specialty, 13f
Desktop publishing, 145, 149–150
Developing A CUrriculuM. *See* DACUM
Diabetes, genetic engineering and, 46
Diagnosis-related group (DRG), 286, 296–297
Diagnostic laboratory immunology, as subspecialty, 13f
Diagnostic radiological physics, as subspecialty, 13f
Dictation, 170
  machine, 170
  voice-activated, 170
Digestive system, 10
Direct Distance Dialing (DDD), 104, 113–114
Directory assistance, 115
Disability, defined, 214
Disabled, 85
DNR (Do Not Resuscitate), 36, 47
Documents, procedures for formatting, 174
Domestic mail services, 204–205
Do Not Resuscitate. *See* DNR (Do Not Resuscitate)
Double booking, 127
Double tracking, 130

DRG. *See* Diagnosis-related group (DRG)
Drugs
  narcotic drug records, 78
  schedules, 79
  security, 78
Drug schedules, 58
Drugs/substance abuse, medical ethics and, 47–48
Dual-organ transplants, 44
Durable power of attorney, 36, 39

E
Editing text, 173
Elderly abuse, medical ethics and, 43
Electrocardiogram, 214, 222
Electronic banking, 248–250
Electronic deposits and payments, 249
Electronic fund transfers, 241, 248
Electronic mail (E-mail), 72–73, 104, 107
  writing, 167, 169
Elephant man's disease, genetic engineering and, 46
E-mail. *See* Electronic mail (E-mail)
Emergencies
  arranging for medical care, 99
  handling appointments for, 131
  handling patients in, 96–99
  reassuring family and waiting patients, 99
  recognizing, 96–97
  screening method for, 97–98
Emergency medicine, as specialty, 13f
Empathy, Medical Assistant and, 85, 87
Employee earnings records, 252
Employment
  agencies, 316
  finding, 313–314
  job titles/job sites for Medical Assistant, 23–24
  Medical Assistant, 22
  trends, 5
Employment application, defined, 313
Employment opportunities, researching
  acquaintances, 316
  employment agencies, 316
  Internet, 317
  newspaper classified advertisements, 315
  professional organizations, 315–316
  school employment offices, 315
  yellow pages, 317
Endocrine system, 11
Endocrinology, as subspecialty, 13f
Environment, medical, 1–2
EOB. *See* Explanation of benefits (EOB)
EPOs. *See* Exclusive Provider Organizations (EPOs)
Equipment
  inventories, 152, 153f
  as responsibility of the manager, 330
Ethical behavior, 38
Exclusive Provider Organizations (EPOs), 8f, 289
Explanation of benefits (EOB), 214
Extended benefits, 214

F

Facial expression, communication and, 91f
Facilities, as responsibility of the manager, 330
Family practice, as specialty, 13f
Fax machines, 72, 73f
FAX transmission, 120, 121f
Federal and state withholding taxes, 250
Federal Employees' Health Benefits Program (FFHB), 294
Feedback
    and communication, 92
    defined, 85
Fee for service, 4, 5
Fees, ethics and physician, 51–52
Fetal research, medical ethics and, 2, 45
FFHB. *See* Federal Employees' Health Benefits Program (FFHB)
FICA, 241
Files
    active, 230
    closed, 214, 230
    correspondence, 234
    inactive, 214, 230
    management, 230
    paper, 230
    research, 234
Filing
    alphabetic filing guides and tabs, 233
    cross-referencing, 232
    geographic, 234
    numeric, 233–234
    rules for, 231
    subject, 234
Finances
    discussing with patient, 95–96
    as responsibility of the manager, 330
Follow-up appointments, 137–138
Follow-up letter, job interview and, 326
Follow-up procedures, insurance claims, 303
Footnotes, business reports, 186
Forensic pathology, as subspecialty, 13f
Formatting, defined, 162
Form(s)
    standardization of, 216
    W-2, 241, 252, 253f
    W4, 241
    W-4, 251f
"Franchised" medicine, 6
Fraud/abuse, in the health care system, 48
Fringe benefits, 329

G

Gastroenterology, as subspecialty, 13f
Gender bias
    defined, 162
    letter writing and, 164–165
Gender neutral, defined, 162
General hospitals, 9
General surgery, as specialty, 13f

Genetic counseling, 36
Genetic engineering, 36, 37
    medical ethics and, 2, 45–46
Genetics, 36
Geographic filing, 234
Good Samaritan laws, 78
Government insurance programs, 293–294
Graphics, computer, 145, 149
    presentations as form of, 150
Greeting patients, 94
Group insurance, 286
Group practices, 5–6
Gynecologic oncology, as subspecialty, 13f

H

Hardware, computer, 145, 147
HCFA. *See* Health Care Financing Administration (HCFA)
HCPCS. *See* Healthcare Common Procedure Coding System (HCPCS)
Health care. *See also* Health insurance
    costs, 1–2
    types of delivery systems, 2
Healthcare Common Procedure Coding System (HCPCS), 301–302
Health Care Financing Administration (HCFA), 290, 296
Health care professionals, licensure of, 59
Health care system, fraud/abuse in, 48
Health insurance
    types of coverage
        managed health care, 288–290
        Medicare, Medicaid, and other government programs, 290–294
        traditional, 287–288
Health insurance claims
    CMS-1500 claim form, charge slip used with, 299f
    CMS-1500 claim form, completed, 300f
    establishing audit trail
        claims register, 302, 303f
        computerizing the claims process, 303–304, 305f
        follow-up procedure, 303
        ticker file, 302–303
    filing a claim
        coding systems
            CPT-5 codes, 298, 301
            ICD-9-CM, 301
Health Insurance Portability and Accountability Act (HIPAA), 2, 293
Health Maintenance Organizations (HMOs), 8f, 288–289
Health resources, allocation of, medical ethics and, 43–44
Heart disease, genetic engineering and, 46
Hematology, as subspecialty, 13f
HIPAA. *See* Health Insurance Portability and Accountability Act (HIPAA)
HIV. *See* Human Immunodeficiency virus (HIV)
HMOs. *See* Health Maintenance Organizations (HMOs)
Hold function etiquette, 105–106, 107f
Honesty, medical assistant and, 27

Hospitals, 8–9
  computers in, 15
  scheduling patients for, 136
Human Immunodeficiency virus (HIV), 47
  testing, medical ethics and, 47

I

ICD. *See* International Classification of Diseases (ICD)
ICD-9-CM, 301
ICD codes, 241
IDS. *See* Integrated Delivery System (IDS)
Illegal acts, by physicians, 66
Immunopathology. as subspecialty, 13f
Inactive files, 214, 230
Infectious diseases, as subspecialty, 13f
Informed consent, 58, 63
Input, sources of, 169–172
Institutions
  hospitals, 8–9
  laboratories, 7–8
  nursing homes, 8
  research centers, 6–7
  specialized care centers, 8
Instructions
  for new patients, 95
  patient, 197–198
Insurance
  coding systems, 297–298, 301
  filing an insurance claim, 297
  types of health insurance
    basic, 287–288
    Blue Cross and Blue Shield, 288
    coding systems, 297–298, 301
    Comprehensive Major Medical Insurance, 288
    Major Medical Insurance, 288
    major medical insurance, 288
    professional liability, 61
Insurance companies
  patient confidentiality and, 70
  payments by, 96
Integrated Delivery System (IDS), 8f, 289–290
Integumentary system, 11
Internal medicine, as specialty, 13f
International Classification of Diseases, Clinical Modification (ICD-9), 296, 301
International Classification of Diseases (ICD), 216
International Statistical Classification of Diseases and Related Health Problems (ICD), 2
International travel, 202
Internet, job search process and, 317
Internet searching, 194–195
Interpersonal communication, 85–89
Interviewing
  appearance, 323–324
  asking the right questions, 325–326
  conduct, 324
  follow-up letter, 326
  knowledge of the employer, 324–325

In utero gene testing, 45
Inventories
  categories of office, 154f
  clinical supplies, 152–153
  equipment, 152
  office supplies, 153–154
  purchasing, 154
Inventory issue, 162
In vitro fertilization, 43
Itinerary preparation, 202, 204f
"I" viewpoint, 163

J

Job application process
  the application form, 321
  the application letter, 321, 322f
  interviewing for a position
    appearance, 323–324
    asking the right questions, 325–326
    conduct, 324
    follow-up letter, 326
    knowledge of the employer, 324–325
  providing the documentation, 321
  the resume, 317–319, 320f
Job instructions, 183, 185f
Job titles/job sites
  of Medical Assistant, 23–24

K

Keyboard, 145, 147
Keywords, 194, 195

L

Laboratories, 7–8
Laboratory reports
  blood test, 222, 224f
  electrocardiogram, 222, 224f
  pathology/cytopathology report, 222–223, 226f
  radiology report, 222, 225f
  urinalysis, 222, 223f
Law
  medical ethics and, 36–37
  physicians and, 60
Ledger card, 241
  as billing statement, 264–265
  computerized, 255
  entries, 247
  pegboard accounting, 241–242, 244f
Legal complaint, 77f
Letter writing, 162–166
  active *vs.* passive voice, 165, 166f
  collection letters, 271–276f
  correct word choice, 164
  developing communications, 166–168
  developing tone, 162
  eliminate redundant words, 166

Letter writing, *continued*
   gender bias and, 164–165
   for the physician's signature, 167
   use of short sentences and paragraphs, 165–166
Licensed practical nurses (LPNs), 24
Licensure, 59
   renewal of license, 59
   revocation/suspension of license, 59–60
Listening, Medical Assistant and, 86–87
Literature search, defined, 194
Living will, 36, 39, 66
Logs, telephone, 116
Loyalty, medical assistant and, 29
LPNs. *See* Licensed practical nurses (LPNs)
LVN. *See* Licensed practical nurses (LPNs)

M
Machine dictation, 170
Magnetic resonance imaging (MRI), 2, 15
Mail. *See* Postal delivery services
Mailing, private, 204
Major medical insurance, 288
Malfeasance, 58, 62
Malpractice
   claims, 61–62
   complaint, 75–76, 77f
   by the physician's staff, 62–63
   preventing malpractice claims, 63
      advance directives, 64, 66
      informed consent, 63–64, 65f
      living wills, 66
      medical records, 64
      power of attorney, 66
   professional liability insurance for, 61
   summons to court, 75, 76f
Malpractice insurance, costs and, 1
Managed competition, 4
Managed competition organizations, 5, 8f
Managed health care, 288–290
Manic depression, genetic engineering and, 46
Margin guide, business reports, 183
Material risk, 63
Maternal-fetal medicine, as subspecialty, 13f
Medicaid, 1, 286, 292–293
Medical Assistant(s), 20–22
   Accrediting Bureau of Health Education Schools
      (ABHES) course content requirements for, 343–345
   Certified Medical Assistant, 19
   characteristics of, 26–29
   confidentiality and, 52
   do's and don'ts in using computers, 93
   employment
      opportunities, 2
      percent employed by type of practice, 5f
   job titles/job sites, 23–24
   professional activities, 194–198
   registered, 328
   responsibilities of, 23

   developing practice lists and reports, 150–152
   for patient confidentiality, 70, 72
   patient information and confidentiality, 52
   for reporting crimes, 69
   for reviewing equipment and software contracts, 148f
   role delineation chart, 23, 341
   role in ethical issues, 51–52
   role in record keeping, 235
   traits for, 313–314
   as witness, 78
   working with the medical professionals
      hospital staff, 29–30
      other outside professionals, 30
      physician and health care team, 26–29
Medical Associations
   ethics of, 37–38
Medical ethics, 36
   AMA principles of, 37–38
   Code of Hammurabi, 37
   computers and, 48
      confidentiality, 49–50
   Medical Assistant's role in, 51–52
   medical association statements, 37
Medical information, insurance form for release of, 71f
Medical law, 36
Medical microbiology, as subspecialty, 13f
Medical nuclear physics, as subspecialty, 13f
Medical office management, 328–330
Medical office management, banking, 245–250
Medical offices, high tech, 145–147
Medical oncology, as subspecialty, 13f
Medical Practice Acts, 58
Medical professionals
   roles of, 24–25, 26
   working with, 25–26
Medical records administrators, role of, 25
Medical records management. *See also* Filing
   color coding the folder, 216–218
   contents of the medical record
      laboratory reports
         blood test, 222
         electrocardiogram, 222
         pathology/cytolopathology, 222
         radiology, 222
         urinalysis, 222
      patient-completed forms, 218–219
      physician-completed forms, 219–222
         case history, 219, 220f, 221
         doctor's notes, 221
         laboratory request, 221–222
   discussion, 213–215
   medical assistant's role in record keeping, 235
   medical record defined, 214
   methods, trends, and issues in, 214–215
Medical records technicians, role of, 25
Medical report formatting, 179–180
Medical software applications, 147–150
Medical specialties, 4
Medical specialties/subspecialties, 11–14

Medical Technologists, role of, 24–25
Medical terminology, 165f
Medicare, 1, 286, 290–292
Memorandums, 179
Message taking, 110–111
 callback messages, 110, 111f
 computer message screen, 112f
 emergency calls, 111–113
 procedures for prescription refill requests, 110
 procedures for taking messages regarding an illness, 111
Microbiology, as subspecialty, 14F
Misfeasance, 58, 62
Modem, computer, 104, 145, 147
Modified block, defined, 162
Modified wave scheduling, 127–128
Monitor, computer, 162
Monthly billing, 266–268
Multi-skilled medical assistant, 20, 22–23
Muscular dystrophy, genetic engineering and, 46
Muscular system, 11

N
Narcotic drug records, 78
Negligence, concept of, 61–62
Nephrology, as subspecialty, 13f
Nervous system, 11
Network, 162
Neurofibromatosis, genetic engineering and, 46
Neurological surgery, as specialty, 13f
Neurology, 9–10
 as specialty, 13f
Neuropathology, as subspecialty, 13f
Newspaper classified advertisements, job search process
  and, 315
Nonfeasance, 58
Non-medical terminology, 165f
Nonverbal communication, 85, 90–91
Nuclear medicine, as specialty, 13f
Nuclear radiology, as subspecialty, 13f
Numeric filing, 233–234
Nurses
 licensure of, 59
 role of, 24
Nursing homes, 8

O
Oath of Hippocrates, 37
Obsolete supplies, 162
Obstetrics, as specialty, 13f
Office management, 328–330
Office supplies, inventory of, 153–154
OMA. See Ophthalmic Medical Assistant (OMA)
On call, 4, 6
Online research, 194–196
Open hours scheduling, 128
Opening mail, 208
Ophthalmic Medical Assistant (OMA), 20, 21

Ophthalmology, as specialty, 13f
Optimal, defined, 162
Oral and maxillofacial surgeon, 12
Oral pathologist, 12
Organ transplantation, medical ethics and, 43, 46
Orthodontist, 12
Orthopedics, 9–10
Orthopedic surgery, as specialty, 13f
Otolaryngology, as specialty, 13f
Outside facilities, scheduling appointments for,
  136–137
Overbooking patients, 126, 130–131
Overdraft, 241, 248

P
Packaging mail, 205, 207
Paper files, 230
Passive voice, letter writing and, 165, 166f
Passports, obtaining, 202
Pathology, as specialty, 14f
Pathology and cytopathology report, 222–223, 226f
Patience, Medical Assistant and, 88–89
Patient accounts, computerized, 252–256
Patient appointment. See Appointment scheduling
Patient billing
 collection process
  aging accounts, 269
  collection letters, 271–276f
  telephone collections
   dos and don'ts for, 277f
  truth-in-lending letters, 277, 278f
 cycle billing, 268
 external billing service, 268
 internal billing
  billing statement, 263–264
  charge slip as statement at time of service, 263
  computerized statement, 265–266
  ledger card as statement, 264–265
  monthly billing, 266–268
  special statement form, 265
 monthly billing, 266–268
 truth-in-lending letters, 277, 278f
Patient Care Partnership, 39, 40–41f
Patient charge slip, computerized, 255
Patient complaint, procedures to identify, 128–129
Patient confidentiality
 and insurance companies, 70
 Medical Assistants and, 69–70
 patient-physician privilege
  exception to, 69–70
Patient flow, 329–330
Patient information
 computerized lists and reports and, 152
 confidentiality and, 52
Patient instruction, 197–198
Patient medical record
 problem-oriented medical record (POMR), 223, 225
 source-oriented medical record (SOMR), 225

Patient-physician relationship, 69
Patient registration form, 254f
Patients
    abbreviation for care of, 227–229t
    computers and relationships with, 92–93
    discussing finances and billing with, 95–96
    established, 95
    greeting, 94
    managing activities of, 93–95
    new, 95
    reassuring family and waiting patients, 99
Patient's Bill of Rights, 36, 39
Patient Self-Determination Act, 36, 39
Payable, defined, 262
Payroll accounting procedures, 250–252
Payroll register, 250, 252
Pediatrics
    dentist, 12
    as specialty, 14f
    surgery, as subspecialty, 14f
Pegboard accounting, 241–245
Periodic appointments follow-up, 138
Periodontist, 12
Personal identification number (PIN), 249
Personnel, 329
Pharmacists, licensure of, 59
Physical medicine and rehabilitation, as specialty, 14f
Physical violence, medical ethics and, 43
Physician extenders, 20
    role of, 24
Physician(s)
    controlled substances and, 78
    as defendant, 73, 74
    ethics and fees of, 51–52
    Illegal acts by, 66
    law and, 60–66
    licensure of, 59–60
    and patient relationship, 69
    role of, 24
    as witness, 78
    working with, 26–29
Physician's Current Procedural Terminology (CPT), 2. See
        also Current Procedural Terminology
Physician-withdrawal letter, 64, 66f
PIN. See Personal identification number (PIN)
Plastic surgery, as specialty, 14f
Point-of-Service Plan (POS), 8f, 290
POMR. See Problem-oriented medical record (POMR)
POS. See Point-of-Service Plan (POS)
Postal delivery services, 204–209
    domestic, 204205
    processing incoming mail
        distributing, 209
        expediting, 209
        opening, 208
        packaging and sorting, 205–206
        reading, underlining, and annotating, 208–209
        sorting, 208
    recalling the mail, 207

special, 205
Posture, communication and, 91f
Power of attorney, 66
    health care declaration and, 67–68f
PPOs. See Preferred Provider Organizations (PPOs)
Practice analysis, 257
Practiced management information, 152
Practice management, 256–257
Practices, types of
    ambulatory centers, 6
    clinics, 6
    group, 5–6
    managed competition organizations, 6, 8f
    medical centers, 6
    Prefixes, 10
    Preventive medicine, as specialty, 14f
    solo-physician, 5
Preferred Provider Organizations (PPOs), 8f, 289
Presentations, as form of graphics, 150
Principles of Medical Ethics, 38
Problem-oriented medical record (POMR), 214, 223, 225
Pro-choice, 43
Professional activities, medical assistant, 194–198
Professional organizations
    as information sources, 195–196
    job search process and, 315–316
Progress appointment follow-up, 137–138
Progress appointments, 126, 137–138
Progress notes, 226
Pro-life, 43
Proofreading, 162, 186–187
    sample of, 171f
Prospective payment system, 296–297
Prosthodontist, 12
Psychiatry, as specialty, 14f
Public health dentist, 12
Pulmonary diseases, as subspecialty, 13f
Purchasing, medical office and, 154

Q
Quality of life, medical ethics and, 46–47

R
Radiological physics, as subspecialty, 14f
Radiology
    report, 222
    as specialty, 14f
    as subspecialty, 14f
Reading mail, 208–209
Recalling mail, 207
Receivable, defined, 262
Reception area/lobby, management of, 93–94
Re-certification, 328
Reconciliation
    defined, 248
    form, 249f
Recredentialing, defined, 313

Redundancy
   defined, 162
   letter writing and, 166
Referral(s), 126
   card, 137f
   scheduling appointments for, 137
Registered Medical Assistant (RMA), 20, 328
   certification competency summary, 346–347
Registered nurses (RNs), 24
Reminder card, 133f, 138f
Reports
   case history and physical, 181f
   consulting physician's, 182f
   developing, 150–152
   formatting business, 183–186
   laboratory, 183f
Reproductive system, 11
Research
   centers, 6–7
   hospitals, 9
   online, 194–196
Residency, 4, 5
Respiratory system, 11
Resume, 317–319, 320f
Reversed charges, 104
Rheumatology, as subspecialty, 13f
RMA. *See* Registered Medical Assistant (RMA)
RNs. *See* Registered nurses (RNs)
Role Delineation Chart (RDC), 20, 23
Root Medical word, 4
Root words, 9

S
Sales representatives, scheduling appointment for,
     133–134
Scanner, defined, 145
Scheduling appointments, 127–128
School employment offices, job search process and, 315
Search engines, 195
Searching
   Internet, 194–195
   phrase, 195–196
Sentence structure, letter writing and, 165, 166f
Shipping services, 204
Skeletal system, 11
SOAP formula, 214, 225, 226f
Social policy, 42–43
Social security taxes, 250
Software, 145
   applications
     word processing, 173
   medical applications, 147–150
Solo-physician practices, types of, 5
SOMR. *See* Source-oriented medical record (SOMR)
Sorting mail, 208
Source-oriented medical record (SOMR), 214, 225
Specialized care centers, 8
Special mail services, 205–207

Special statement form, 265, 266f
Specialties/subspecialties
   dental, 12
   medical, 4, 12, 13–14f
Spell checking utilities, 186–187
Spreadsheet, 145, 148
Stored letter parts, defined, 162
Stream scheduling, 127
Subject filing, 234
Substance abuse, medical ethics and, 47–48
Suffixes, 9
Summons to court, 75, 76f
Supplies
   clinical, 152–153
   office, 153–154
   as responsibility of the manager, 330
Supply disposal, defined, 162
Surgery, scheduling appointments for, 136

T
Table of contents, business reports, 186
Tact, Medical Assistant and, 85, 87–88
Taxes
   federal and state withholding, 250
   social security, 250
Teaching hospitals, 9
Technicians, role of, 24–25
Telecommunications
   and confidentiality, 72–73
   medical, for diagnosis and treatment, 120
Telephone
   collections, 276–277
     dos and don'ts for, 277f
   turnoffs, 105–106
Telephone procedures
   answering services/machines, 119–120
   "hold" function etiquette, 105–106
   monthly telephone charges, 116–117
   screening incoming calls, 106–109
   taking messages, 110–111
     callback messages, 110
     emergency calls, 111
     for prescription refill requests, 110–111
     regarding an illness, 111
   telephone directory, 118–119
   telephone logs, 116, 117f
   telephone number file, 117–118, 118f
   time zones, 115
   types of calls
     collect calls, 114–115
     conference calls, 115
     credit card calls, 115
     direct distance dialing (DDD), 113–114
     local calls, 113
     long distance calls/alternative services, 113
     operator-assisted calls, 114
     station-to-station/person-to-person calls, 114
Terminology

abbreviations, 9–10
  medical, importance of, 172
  medical and nonmedical, 165f
  root words, prefixes, and suffixes, 9
Therapeutic radiological physics, as subspecialty, 14f
Therapeutic radiology, as subspecialty, 14f
Thesaurus, defined, 162
Third-party carriers, 271
Third-party payers, defined, 262
Third-party reimbursement, 4
Thoracic surgery, as subspecialty, 14f
Ticker file, 302–303
Time zones, 104, 115
Tone
  defined, 162
  letter writing and, 162–164
Tort law, 61
Touch, communication and, 91f
Traditional health coverage, 287–288
Training coworkers, 196–197
Train travel, 201
Transcription, 170, 172
  defined, 162
Transplantation, medical ethics and organ, 46
Travel arrangements, 198–201
  airline travel, 199
  automobile travel, 201
  international travel, 202
  itinerary preparation, 202
  lodging, 201
    ship travel, 199
    train, 201
    travel agencies, 198–199
Travel funds, 201–202, 203f
Triage, 126, 131
TRICARE, 294
Triple Option Plan (Cafeteria Plan), 8f, 290
Truth-in-lending letter, 277

U

Underlining mail, 208–209
Unnecessary/worthless services, medical ethics and, 48
Urinalysis, 222
Urinary system, 11

Urology, as specialty, 14f

V

Vaccinations, before traveling, 202
Vascular surgery, general, as subspecialty, 14f
Vendor, 162
Verbal communication, 89–90
Voice-activated dictation, 170
Voice mail, 120
Voice (tone of), and communication, 91f

W

Wave scheduling, 126, 127
Word choice, letter writing and, 164
Word processing, 145, 148, 167–191
  composing at the computer, 167, 168f
    input
      sources of, 169–172
  correspondence formatting, 173–182
    block/modified block formats, 174–177
    merged paragraphs, 178–179
    proofreading, 186–187
    spell checkers, 186–187
  input
    dictation and transcription, 170, 172
    rough draft, 169–170
  output, 173–187
    business report formatting
      job instructions, 183, 185f
    correspondence formatting
      second-page headings, 178
      stored letter parts, 178
    medical report formatting, 179–180
    memorandums, 179
  software, 173
    create/edit text, 173
Workers' compensation insurance, 286, 294, 295f

Y

Yellow pages, job search process and, 317
"You" viewpoint, 162, 163

Medical Assisting Administrative Skills CD-ROM

System Requirements

166 MHz Intel Pentium processor or greater

Microsoft® Windows® 95 or newer

32 MB of installed RAM

100 MB of available disk space

256-color monitor capable of 800 x 600 resolution

CD-ROM drive

Microsoft® Windows® compatible sound card

Set-Up Instructions

1. Insert disk into CD-ROM player. The *Medical Assisting Administrative Skills* CD-ROM should start up automatically. If it does not, go to step 2.

2. From My Computer, double click the icon for the CD drive.

3. Double click the *start.exe* file to start the program.

License Agreement for Delmar Learning, a division of Thomson Learning, Inc.

Educational Software/Data

You the customer, and Delmar Learning, a division of Thomson Learning, Inc. incur certain benefits, rights, and obligations to each other when you open this package and use the software/data it contains. BE SURE YOU READ THE LICENSE AGREEMENT CAREFULLY, SINCE BY USING THE SOFTWARE/DATA YOU INDICATE YOU HAVE READ, UNDERSTOOD, AND ACCEPTED THE TERMS OF THIS AGREEMENT.

Your rights:

1. You enjoy a non-exclusive license to use the software/data on a single microcomputer in consideration for payment of the required license fee, (which may be included in the purchase price of an accompanying print component), or receipt of this software/data, and your acceptance of the terms and conditions of this agreement.

2. You acknowledge that you do not own the aforesaid software/data. You also acknowledge that the software/data is furnished "as is," and contains copyrighted and/or proprietary and confidential information of Delmar Learning, a division of Thomson Learning, Inc. or its licensors.

There are limitations on your rights:

1. You may not copy or print the software/data for any reason whatsoever, except to install it on a hard drive on a single microcomputer and to make one archival copy, unless copying or printing is expressly permitted in writing or statements recorded on the diskette(s).

2. You may not revise, translate, convert, disassemble or otherwise reverse engineer the software/data except that you may add to or rearrange any data recorded on the media as part of the normal use of the software/data.

3. You may not sell, license, lease, rent, loan or otherwise distribute or network the software/data except that you may give the software/data to a student or and instructor for use at school or, temporarily at home.

Should you fail to abide by the Copyright Law of the United States as it applies to this software/data your license to use it will become invalid. You agree to erase or otherwise destroy the software/data immediately after receiving note of termination of this agreement for violation of its provisions from Delmar Learning.

Delmar Learning, a division of Thomson Learning, Inc gives you a LIMITED WARRANTY covering the enclosed software/data. The LIMITED WARRANTY follows this License.

This license is the entire agreement between you and Delmar Learning, a division of Thomson Learning, Inc. interpreted and enforced under New York law.

Limited Warranty

Delmar Learning, a division of Thomson Learning, Inc. warrants to the original licensee/purchaser of this copy of microcomputer software/data and the media on which it is recorded that the media will be free from defects in material and workmanship for ninety (90) days from the date of original purchase. All implied warranties are limited in duration to this ninety (90) day period. THEREAFTER, ANY IMPLIED WARRANTIES, INCLUDING IMPLIED WARRANTIES OF MERCHANTABILITY AND FITNESS FOR A PARTICULAR PURPOSE, ARE EXCLUDED. THIS WARRANTY IS IN LIEU OF ALL OTHER WARRANTIES, WHETHER ORAL OR WRITTEN, EXPRESS OR IMPLIED.

If you believe the media is defective please return it during the ninety day period to the address shown below. Defective media will be replaced without charge provided that it has not been subjected to misuse or damage.

This warranty does not extend to the software or information recorded on the media. The software and information are provided "AS IS." Any statements made about the utility of the software or information are not to be considered as express or implied warranties.

Limitation of liability: Our liability to you for any losses shall be limited to direct damages, and shall not exceed the amount you paid for the software. In no event will we be liable to you for any indirect, special, incidental, or consequential damages (including loss of profits) even if we have been advised of the possibility of such damages.

Some states do not allow the exclusion or limitation of incidental or consequential damages, or limitations on the duration of implied warranties, so the above limitation or exclusion may not apply to you. This warranty gives you specific legal rights, and you may also have other rights which vary from state to state. Address all correspondence to:

Delmar Learning, a division of Thomson Learning, Inc.
5 Maxwell Drive, P.O. Box 8007
Clifton Park, NY 12065-8007
Attention: Technology Department